Study Guide

Maternity & Women's Health Care

11th Edition

Deitra Leonard Lowdermilk, RNC-E, PhD, FAAN
Shannon E. Perry, RN, PhD, FAAN
Kitty Cashion, RN-BC, MSN
Kathryn Rhodes Alden, EdD, MSN, RN, IBCLC

Associate Editor
Ellen F. Olshansky, PhD, RN, WHNP-BC, NC-BC, FAAN

By
Karen A. Piotrowski, RNC, MSN
Associate Professor of Nursing
D'Youville College
Buffalo, New York

ELSEVIER

ELSEVIER

3251 Riverport Lane
St. Louis, Missouri 63043

STUDY GUIDE FOR
MATERNITY & WOMEN'S HEALTH CARE, 11th EDITION   ISBN: 978-0-323-26558-4

Previous editions copyrighted 2012, 2007, 2004, 2000.

Content Strategist: Sandra Clark
Content Development Manager: Laurie K. Gower
Senior Content Development Specialist: Heather Bays
Publishing Services Manager: Hemamalini Rajendrababu
Project Manager: Umarani Natarajan
Designer: Ashely Miner

Printed in the USA

Last digit is the print number: 9   8   7   6   5   4   3   2   1

Working together
to grow libraries in
developing countries

www.elsevier.com • www.bookaid.org

Introduction

This *Study Guide* is designed to help you effectively use the text *Maternity & Women's Health Care*, Eleventh Edition. In addition to reviewing content of the text, this *Study Guide* encourages you to think critically in applying your knowledge.

Chapter Review Activities focus on recall and application of critical concepts and essential terminology. These activities are specifically designed to help you to identify the important content of the chapter and to test your level of knowledge and understanding after reading the chapter. Completion of each of the activities will provide you with an excellent resource to use when you are reviewing important content before course examinations. The knowledge you attain by completing the activities will help you to develop the theoretical foundation that you will need to answer the Critical Thinking Exercises that follow, to successfully pass course examinations and the NCLEX-RN© Examination, and to manage the care of your clients in the clinical setting. Answers or answer guidelines for the activities are provided in the Answer Key located at the end of this *Study Guide*.

Critical Thinking Exercises focus primarily on the application of critical chapter content. Typical client care situations are presented and you are required to apply concepts found in the chapter to solve problems, to make decisions concerning care management, and to provide responses to a client's questions and concerns. These exercises may be completed by you on your own or with members of your study group. Completing the Critical Thinking Exercises will help you to prepare for clinical experiences, course examinations, and the NCLEX-RN© Examination, all of which focus on problem solving and application of nursing knowledge. Guidelines for completing the exercises and specific chapter sections, boxes, or tables where the content for the answer is found are provided in the Answer Key located at the end of the *Study Guide*.

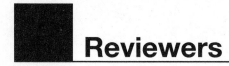

Reviewers

Diane Johnson, RNC, MSN
Nursing Program Director
University Department Chair
Keiser University
Jacksonville, Florida

Daryle Wane, PhD, ARNP-BC
Professor of Nursing
Pasco-Hernando Community College
New Port Richey, Florida

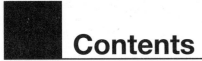

Contents

1 21st Century Maternity and Women's Health Nursing

I. LEARNING KEY TERMS

MATCHING: Match the definition in Column I with the appropriate descriptive term in Column II.

COLUMN I

1. _____ Number of live births in 1 year per 1000 population.

2. _____ Embryo or fetus that is removed or expelled from the uterus at 20 weeks of gestation or less, weighs 500 g or less, or measures 25 cm or less.

3. _____ Number of maternal deaths from births and complications of pregnancy, childbirth, and the puerperium (the first 42 days after termination of the pregnancy) per 100,000 live births.

4. _____ An infant who at birth demonstrates no signs of life, such as breathing, heartbeat, or voluntary muscle movements.

5. _____ Number of stillbirths and number of neonatal deaths per 1000 live births.

6. _____ Number of births per 1000 women between the ages of 15 and 44 years (inclusive), calculated on a yearly basis.

7. _____ Infant whose weight at birth is less than 2500 g (5 lb, 8 oz).

8. _____ Number of deaths of infants younger than 1 year of age per 1000 live births.

9. _____ Number of deaths of infants younger than 28 days of age per 1000 live births.

10. _____ Infant born before 38 weeks of gestation.

COLUMN II

A. Fertility rate
B. Infant mortality rate
C. Birth rate
D. Maternal mortality rate
E. Neonatal mortality rate
F. Perinatal mortality rate
G. Low-birth-weight infant
H. Abortus
I. Stillbirth
J. Preterm infant

FILL IN THE BLANKS: Insert the term that corresponds to each of the following definitions or descriptions.

11. _____ Specialty area of nursing practice that focuses on the care of childbearing women and their families through all stages of pregnancy and childbirth, as well as the first 4 weeks after birth.

12. _____ Health care that focuses on the physical, psychologic, and social needs of women throughout their lives.

13. _____ A set of science-based 10-year objectives that reflects the nation's agenda for improving health with the ultimate aims to increase the quality and years of healthy life and to eliminate health disparities.

14. _____ A set of eight goals to be achieved by 2015 that respond to the world's main development challenges and adopted by 189 nations under the auspices of the United Nations.

15. _____ Type of educational approach that involves faculty and students from two or more health professions who create and foster a learning environment that is collaborative and will facilitate improvement in patient care.

16. _____ An Act passed in 2010 that aims to make insurance affordable, contain costs, strengthen and improve Medicare and Medicaid, and reform the insurance market. Full implementation of this Act will occur over the next several years.

17. _____ Term used to refer to the forcing of individuals, mostly women and children, into hard labor, sex work, and even organ donation.

18. _____ Terms used to describe procedures in which part or all of the female external genitalia are removed for cultural or nontherapeutic reasons.

19. _____ Trained and experienced female labor attendants who provide a continual one-on-one caring presence throughout the labor and birth process.

20. _____ Term used to refer to a spectrum of abilities, ranging from reading an appointment slip to interpreting medication instructions.

21. _____ Comprehensive standardized language that describes interventions performed by generalist or specialist nurses.

22. _____ Health care that is based on information gained through research and clinical trials.

23. _____ Result of a collaboration that oversees up-to-date, systematic reviews of randomized controlled trials of health care and disseminates these reviews to provide the most reliable evidence about the effects of care. Care measures are ranked in six categories from beneficial forms of care to those that are ineffective and potentially harmful.

24. _____ Approach to care that measures effectiveness of care against benchmarks or standards. It is a measure of the value of nursing using quality indicators and answers the question: "Did the client benefit or not benefit from the care provided?"

25. _____ Guidelines for nursing practice that reflect current knowledge, represent levels of practice agreed on by leaders in the specialty, and can be used for clinical benchmarking.

26. _____ Term used to refer to the level of practice that a reasonably prudent nurse would provide in the same or similar circumstances.

27. _____ An evolving process that is used to identify risks, establish preventive practices, develop reporting mechanisms, and delineate procedures for managing lawsuits.

28. _____ Term used by The Joint Commission to describe an unexpected occurrence involving death or serious physical or psychologic injury or risk thereof.

29. _____ Failure to recognize or act on early signs of distress.

30. _____ Effort to provide nurses with the competencies to improve the quality and safety of the systems of health care in which they practice.

31. _____ Technique that gives a specific framework for communication among health care providers. It is an easy-to-remember, useful, concrete mechanism for communicating important information that requires a clinician's immediate attention.

32. _____ Approach developed by the Department of Defense's Patient Safety Program in collaboration with the Agency for Healthcare Research and Quality as a teamwork system for health professionals to provide higher quality, safer client care. It provides an evidence base to improve communication and teamwork skills.

II. REVIEWING KEY CONCEPTS

33. CITE four major maternal, infant, and child health objectives included in *Healthy People 2020*. IDENTIFY one strategy you would propose to facilitate achievement of each goal.

34. When assessing pregnant women, STATE what factors you would recognize as having the potential to contribute to the rate of infant mortality in the United States.

35. The health care system in the United States faces many problems. DESCRIBE how the nurse can effect change in each of the following areas to improve the quality and effectiveness of health care available to Americans:
    - Structure

    - Medical errors

    - Cost

    - Access

    - Health disparities

    - Health literacy

36. The number of high-risk pregnancies occurring in the United States is increasing. Briefly DISCUSS the factors that have been identified as contributing to this increase in the incidence of high-risk pregnancies.

37. IDENTIFY several factors and conditions that affect the health of women. For each factor and condition identified, DESCRIBE the effect it has had on women's health.

MULTIPLE CHOICE: Circle the correct option(s) and state the rationale for the option(s) chosen.

38. When caring for women, nurses should focus on helping their patients to decrease their risk for the leading cause of death for women, which is:
    A. Breast cancer
    B. Heart disease
    C. Cervical cancer
    D. Diabetes mellitus

39. A nurse manager of a prenatal clinic should recognize that the most significant barrier encountered by pregnant women in accessing health care is:
    A. Lack of transportation to the clinic
    B. Child care responsibilities
    C. Inability to pay
    D. Deficient knowledge related to the benefits of prenatal care

40. Both worldwide and in the United States, the leading cause of maternal mortality is:
    A. Hemorrhage
    B. Infection or sepsis
    C. Diabetes
    D. Cardiovascular disease, including hypertensive disorders

41. Knowledge of trends in fertility and birth rates and infant mortality rates can guide nurses in targeting health care resources to those areas and clients in most need of intervention. Which statements accurately reflect current trends in the United States? (Circle all that apply.)
    A. Women between ages 20 and 29 years have the highest birth rate.
    B. The incidence of LBW (low birth weight) is highest among non-Hispanic African-American women.
    C. The leading cause of neonatal death is premature birth.
    D. The infant mortality rate is a common indicator of the adequacy of prenatal care and the health of a nation as a whole.
    E. Hispanic women are twice as likely as non-Hispanic Caucasian women to die as a result of pregnancy.

42. After teaching a group of pregnant women about the hazards of cigarette smoking during pregnancy, a woman answers a question by listing the hazards. Which hazard, if included by the woman in her list, indicates the need for further teaching?
    A. Intrauterine growth restriction
    B. Congenital anomalies
    C. Low birth weight
    D. Premature labor and birth

43. Pregnant women who are obese are more likely to develop one or both of the two most frequently reported maternal risk factors. These factors are:
    A. Premature labor and infection
    B. Hemorrhage and hypertension associated with pregnancy
    C. Infection and diabetes
    D. Diabetes and hypertension associated with pregnancy

III. THINKING CRITICALLY

1. Imagine that you are the nursing director of an inner-city prenatal clinic that serves a large number of minority women, many of whom are younger than 20 years of age. DESCRIBE five nursing services you would provide for these women that would help to reduce the potential for maternal and infant morbidity and mortality and low birth weight. Use the statistical data and risk behaviors presented in Chapter 1 to support the types of services you propose.

2. SUPPORT the accuracy of the following statement: An emphasis on high-technology medical care and lifesaving techniques will not reduce the rate of preterm and low-birth-weight infants in the United States.

3. PROPOSE three changes in health care and its delivery that you believe would improve the health status and well-being of mothers and their infants and reduce the rate of infant and maternal mortality. SUPPORT your answer by using the content presented in Chapter 1 and your own experiences with the health care system.

4. Many barriers interfere with a woman's participation in early and ongoing prenatal care. DESCRIBE incentives and services that you would offer to pregnant women to encourage their participation in prenatal care. State the rationale for your proposals. Your answer should reflect an understanding of the barriers.

5. At the prenatal clinic where you work, a change in health care focus is being implemented that will involve pregnant women and their families more completely in their care and promote self-management. DESCRIBE the measures you would implement when caring for your clients that would support this change in focus.

6. Many clients who come to a prenatal clinic speak English as a second language and often have difficulty speaking fluently. EXPLAIN what measures nurses working in this clinic should use to ensure health literacy among their clients.

7. Medical errors are a leading cause of death in the United States. EXPLAIN the process that you will use as a student to prevent medical errors.

8. Imagine that you are the nurse manager of a postpartum unit that recently changed to a mother-baby form of care delivery. You now want to develop an evidence-based protocol that nurses on your unit will use to teach and guide breastfeeding women. Nurses on your unit are reluctant to participate in developing this protocol, stating, "The approach we use now when helping our breastfeeding moms works just fine—how can research make it better?" DESCRIBE the approach that you would use to convince these nurses that evidence-based practice enhances the quality and effectiveness of nursing care.

9. Explain how a nurse can use social media to improve the health care provided to pregnant women and their families. IDENTIFY the precautions that the nurse must take to ensure that patient confidentiality and privacy are protected.

10. DISCUSS two international concerns that have serious, detrimental effects on the health and safety of women and their children. EXPLAIN how nurses can address these concerns.

2 | Community Care: The Family and Culture

I. LEARNING KEY TERMS

MATCHING: Match the family described in Column I with the appropriate family category in Column II.

COLUMN I

1. _____ Miss M. lives with her 4-year-old adopted Korean daughter, Kim.

2. _____ Anne and Duane are married and live with their daughter, Susan, and Duane's mother, Ruth.

3. _____ Gloria and Andy are a married couple living with their new biologic baby girl, Annie, and their adopted son, Joseph.

4. _____ Tina and her brother Mark live with their grandmother, Irene, who is raising them.

5. _____ Carl and Allan are a gay couple living with Carl's daughter, Sally, and a son, Thomas, born through surrogacy whom they are raising together.

6. _____ The S. family consists of Jim; his second wife, Jane; and Jim's two daughters by a previous marriage.

7. _____ George and Denise, who are not married, live together with their daughter Rose.

COLUMN II

A. Cohabitating-parent family
B. Single-parent family
C. Homosexual family
D. Married-parent family
E. Extended family
F. Married blended family
G. No-parent family

MATCHING: Match the description in Column I with the appropriate cultural concept in Column II.

COLUMN I

8. _____ Mrs. M., a Mexican-American who just gave birth, tells the nurse not to include certain foods on her meal tray because her mother told her to avoid those foods while breastfeeding. The nurse tells her that she doesn't have to avoid any foods and should eat what is on the tray because it is good for her.

9. _____ Ms. P., an immigrant from Vietnam, has lived in the United States for 1 year. She tells you that although she enjoys the comfort of wearing blue jeans and sneakers for casual occasions, such as shopping, she still wears traditional or "conservative" clothing for family gatherings.

10. _____ A Cambodian family immigrated to the United States and has been living in Denver for more than 5 years. The parents express concern about their children ages 10, 13, and 16 years, stating, "The children act so differently now. They are less respectful to us, want to eat only American food, and go to rock concerts. It's hard to believe they are our children."

11. _____ The Amish represent an important ethnic community in Lancaster, Pennsylvania.

12. _____ A nurse who is caring for a Native-American couple following the birth of their daughter arranges for them to take the placenta home for a ceremonial burial.

COLUMN II

A. Cultural relativism
B. Ethnocentrism
C. Assimilation
D. Subculture
E. Acculturation

FILL IN THE BLANKS: Insert the cultural concept that corresponds to each of the following definitions.

13. _____ A unified set of values, attitudes, beliefs, and standards of behavior shared by a group of people and passed down from one generation to the next.

14. _____ A group existing within a larger cultural system that retains its own characteristics.

15. _____ Recognizing that people from different cultural backgrounds comprehend the same objects and situations differently and that a culture determines a person's viewpoint.

16. _____ Changes that occur within one group or among several groups when people from different cultures come into contact with one another and exchange and adopt each other's mannerisms, styles, and practices while retaining some of their own culture.

17. _____ Process in which one cultural group loses its cultural identity and becomes a part of the dominant culture.

18. _____ A belief that one's cultural way of doing things is the right way, supporting the notion that "My group is the best."

19. _____ Approach that involves acknowledging, respecting, and appreciating ethnic, cultural, and linguistic diversity.

20. _____ Type of time orientation that maintains a focus on achieving long-term goals; families or people who practice this time orientation are more likely to return for follow-up visits related to health care and to participate in primary prevention activities.

21. _____ Type of time orientation of families or people who are more likely to strive to maintain tradition or the status quo and have little motivation for formulating future goals.

22. _____ Type of time orientation of families or people who may have difficulty adhering to strict schedules and are often described as "living for the moment."

23. _____ Cultural concept that reflects dimensions of personal comfort zones. Actions such as touching, placing the woman in proximity to others, taking away personal possessions, and making decisions for the woman can decrease personal security and heighten anxiety.

24. _____ The primary unit of socialization and nurturing within a community that preserves and transmits culture.

25. _____ Family structure in which male and female partners and their children live as an independent unit, sharing roles, responsibilities, and economic resources.

26. _____ Family structure that includes the nuclear family and other people related by blood (kin), such as grandparents, aunts, uncles, and cousins.

27. _____ Family structure in which children live with two unmarried biologic or adoptive parents.

28. _____ Family category in which there is only one biologic or adoptive parent as head of the household who may or may not be living with other adults; it is becoming an increasingly recognized structure in our society.

29. _____ Family structure formed as a result of divorce and consisting of unrelated family members (stepparents, stepchildren, and stepsiblings) who join to create a new household.

30. _____ Family structure in which gay or lesbian couples may live together with or without children.

8

Chapter 2 Community Care: The Family and Culture

31. _____ Family structure in which children live independently in foster or kinship care, such as living with a grandparent.

32. _____ Family structure consisting of three or more generations of relatives (e.g., grandparents, children, and grandchildren).

33. _____ Family structure composed of biologic or adoptive married parents and their children.

34. _____ A family theory that views the family as a whole greater than the sum of its individual members and thus focuses on observing the interaction among family members rather than on studying family members individually.

35. _____ A family theory that focuses on the family as it moves through stages and relationships among family members as they progress through transitions.

36. _____ A family theory concerned with the way families react to stressful events; stress is studied within the internal and external contexts in which the family is living.

37. _____ A family theory that involves a strength-based approach in clinical practice with families as opposed to a deficit approach.

38. _____ A family theory with a focus on reducing cultural and environmental barriers that interfere with access to health care. Key elements include perceived susceptibility, perceived severity, perceived benefits, perceived barriers, cues to action, and confidence.

39. _____ A family theory based on the belief that behavior is a function of the interaction of traits and abilities with the environment. Major concepts include ecosystem, niches, adaptive range, and ontogenetic development.

40. _____ Term used for the family tree format of depicting relationships of family members over at least three generations; it provides valuable information about a family and its health.

41. _____ Term used for a graphic portrayal of social relationships of the woman and family, including school, work, religious affiliations, and club memberships.

42. _____ A community assessment technique that involves observing a community by traveling through it.

43. _____ Groups within the community that are more likely to experience health status problems and negative health outcomes as a result of a variety of sociocultural, economic, and environmental risk factors.

44. _____ Conditions that disproportionately affect certain racial, ethnic, or other groups.

45. _____ Level of preventive care that involves promoting healthy lifestyles to decrease the occurrence of illness and enhance general health and quality of life.

46. _____ Level of preventive care that involves early detection of a disease and prompt treatment with the goal of curing the disease or slowing its progression and preventing subsequent disability; populations at risk for certain diseases are targeted.

47. _____ Level of preventive care that focuses on rehabilitation of an individual who already has a disease back to as optimal a level of health as possible.

48. DISCUSS why the nurse should take each of the following "products of culture" into consideration when providing care within a cultural context:

    A. Communication

    B. Personal space

    C. Time orientation

    D. Family roles

49. IDENTIFY the key components of culturally competent care. DISCUSS how you have tried to include these components as you plan care for and provide care to your patients.

50. STATE the rationale for the increasing emphasis on home- and community-based health care. How has this trend changed the demands placed on the community-based nurse?

51. Community health promotion requires the collaborative efforts of many individuals and groups within a community. CITE several programs that could be established to promote the health of a community's childbearing families.

52. EXPLAIN why each of the groups listed below has been identified as a vulnerable population of women:
    - Adolescent girls and older women
    - Racial and ethnic minorities
    - Incarcerated women
    - Immigrant, refugee, and migrant women
    - Rural women
    - Homeless women

53. DESCRIBE the ways in which nurses can provide care to perinatal clients using the telephone.

MULTIPLE CHOICE: Circle the correct option(s) and state the rationale for the option(s) chosen.

54. A family with open boundaries:
    A. Uses available support systems to meet its needs
    B. Is more prone to crisis, related to increased exposure to stressors
    C. Discourages family members from setting up channels
    D. Strives to maintain family stability by avoiding outside influences

55. Which nursing action is most likely to reduce a woman's anxiety and enhance her personal security as it relates to the concept of personal space needs?
    A. Touching the woman before and during procedures
    B. Providing explanations when performing tasks
    C. Making eye contact as much as possible
    D. Reducing the need for the woman to make decisions

56. A Native-American woman gave birth to a girl 12 hours ago. The nurse notes that the woman keeps her baby in the bassinet except for feeding and states that she will wait until she returns home to begin breastfeeding. The nurse recognizes that this behavior is most likely a reflection of:
    A. Embarrassment
    B. Delayed attachment
    C. Disappointment that the baby is a girl
    D. Cultural beliefs regarding the best way to care for newborns

57. When caring for a pregnant woman who is Hispanic, the nurse should recognize that the woman may be guided by which of the following cultural beliefs and practices during her pregnancy? (Circle all that apply.)
    A. Cool air currents can be dangerous during pregnancy.
    B. Prenatal care should begin very early in pregnancy.
    C. Milk should be avoided because it results in big babies and difficult births.
    D. Drinking chamomile tea should be avoided because it can cause preterm labor.
    E. The advice of both mothers and mothers-in-law should be followed during pregnancy.
    F. Pelvic examinations should not be performed by a male health care provider.

58. Regarding pregnancy and childbirth, European-American women are likely to believe that: (Circle all that apply.)
    A. The father of the baby should be actively involved in the labor and birth
    B. Pregnancy requires medical attention, so prenatal care should begin early in pregnancy
    C. Birthing at home should be valued
    D. Pregnant women should participate in childbirth education
    E. The doctor is the head of the obstetric care team
    F. Mothers should not begin to breastfeed until milk comes in

59. A student nurse is planning to communicate with her postpartum client using an interpreter. Her instructor should provide further guidance if the student:
    A. Arranges for a female from the woman's country of origin to act as interpreter
    B. Stops periodically during the interaction to ask the interpreter how things are going
    C. Asks the woman questions while looking at the interpreter
    D. Gathers culturally appropriate learning aids and reading materials to use during the interaction

60. Which health services represent the primary level of preventive care? (Circle all that apply.)
    A. Breast self-examination and testicular self-examination education programs
    B. Providing flu immunizations in pharmacies
    C. A safer-sex informational pamphlet provided to adolescents during a health education class
    D. Blood pressure and cholesterol screening at a health fair
    E. Instituting a wheelchair, cane, and walker exchange program for persons whose health insurance does not cover these items
    F. A car-seat fitting fair at local automobile dealerships

61. A student nurses' association is planning a health fair that will emphasize secondary-level prevention activities. Which activity would the faculty adviser tell them to eliminate because it does not fit into their stated focus?
   A. Teaching participants how to check their radial pulse for rate and regularity
   B. Blood glucose monitoring
   C. Demonstration of relaxation measures to manage stress
   D. Breast models that participants can use to learn breast palpation techniques

62. When making a home visit, it is essential that the nurse use appropriate infection control measures. Of the measures listed below, which one is the most important?
   A. Including personal protective equipment in the home care bag
   B. Designating a dirty area with a trash bag to collect soiled equipment and supplies
   C. Wearing clean vinyl gloves for procedures that involve touching the client
   D. Performing hand hygiene using either soap and running water or a self-drying antiseptic solution

III. THINKING CRITICALLY

1. Nurses must avoid making stereotypical assumptions when caring for pregnant women from specific sociocultural or religious groups. EXPLAIN the process you would follow when providing culturally competent care that is reflective of a pregnant woman's unique values, beliefs, and behavioral patterns.

2. Imagine that you are a nurse working in a clinic that provides prenatal services to a multicultural community predominated by Hispanic-American, African-American, and Asian-American families. DESCRIBE how you would adapt care measures to reflect the cultural beliefs and practices of pregnant women and their families from each of the following cultural groups.
   A. Hispanic-American

   B. African-American

   C. Asian-American

3. Pamela is a 20-year-old Native American. She is 3 months pregnant and has come to the prenatal clinic on the reservation where she lives for her first visit to obtain prenatal vitamins, which her friends at work told her are important.
   A. STATE the questions the nurse should ask to determine Pamela's cultural expectations about childbearing.

   B. DESCRIBE the communication approach you would consider when interviewing Pamela.

C. IDENTIFY the Native-American beliefs and practices regarding childbearing that may influence Pamela's approach to her pregnancy and birth.

4. A nurse has been providing care to a Hispanic family. This family recently experienced the birth of twin girls at 38 weeks of gestation. It is the first birth experience for both parents and the first grandchildren for the extended family. Both newborns are healthy and living at home. DESCRIBE the cultural beliefs and practices that the family, as Hispanic, might use as guidelines to provide care to their newborn twin girls.

5. The nurse-midwife at a prenatal clinic has been assigned to care for a Sunni refugee couple from Iraq who recently immigrated to the United States. The woman has just been diagnosed as 2 months pregnant. Neither she nor her husband speaks English. OUTLINE the process that this nurse should use when working with a translator to facilitate communication with this couple to enhance care management.

6. Imagine that you are a nurse who has just been hired to provide home health care. Before you begin seeing your clients, you realize that it would be helpful for you to become familiar with the neighborhood and resources in the community where your clients live.
   A. You decide to conduct a community walkthrough (walking survey) of your client's community. DESCRIBE how you would go about conducting this survey and gathering data.

   B. LIST the data you would consider essential to gather.

   C. DISCUSS how you would use the findings from your walking survey when providing health care to the clients you will be visiting.

7. Marie is a single parent of two young children, ages 4 years and 1 year. She and her children have been homeless for 3 months since her husband abandoned her and she lost her job because she had no one to help her care for her children.

   A. IDENTIFY the types of health problems to which Marie and her children are most vulnerable, and discuss the rationale for their increased risk for these health problems.

   B. Women who are homeless can become pregnant. What factors related to being homeless could increase Marie's risk for becoming pregnant? If she did become pregnant, EXPLAIN why it would be considered a high-risk pregnancy.

   C. EXPLAIN how you, as a nurse, would provide health care services to Marie and her children.

8. Consuelo is the wife of a migrant laborer. She and her husband, along with their two children, have been working on a California farm for 2 weeks. She has arrived at a health center established for migrant laborers. Consuelo states that she is 4 months pregnant. As the woman's health nurse practitioner assigned to care for Consuelo, DESCRIBE what approaches you would use to ensure that she obtains quality health care that addresses her unique health risks as a migrant worker.

9. WRITE a series of questions that you would ask when making a postpartum follow-up call to a woman who gave birth 3 days ago.

10. Eileen gave birth to a son 36 hours ago. A home care nurse has been assigned to visit Eileen and her husband in their home to assess the progress of her recovery after birth, the health status of her newborn son, and the adaptation of family processes to the responsibilities of newborn care.

    A. OUTLINE the approach the nurse should take in preparing for this visit.

    B. DESCRIBE the nurse's actions during the visit using the care management (nursing) process as a format.

C. DISCUSS how the nurse should end the visit.

D. IDENTIFY interventions the nurse should implement at the conclusion of the visit with Eileen and her husband.

E. SPECIFY how the nurse should protect her personal safety both outside and inside Eileen's home.

F. CITE the infection control measures the nurse should use when conducting the visit and providing care in Eileen's home.

11. Angela has recently been diagnosed with hyperemesis gravidarum and has been hospitalized to stabilize her fluid and electrolyte balance. The hospital-based nurse must evaluate Angela for referral to home care.
    A. STATE the criteria that this nurse should follow to determine Angela's readiness for discharge from hospital to home care.

    B. Angela has been discharged and will be receiving parenteral nutrition in her home. DISCUSS the additional information required related to high-technology home care.

    C. IDENTIFY specific home environment criteria that must be met to ensure the safety and effectiveness of Angela's treatment.

12. A nurse is seeking funding to start a home care agency designed to provide home visits to postpartum women and their families within 1 week of birth and follow-up visits as indicated. STATE the points the nurse should emphasize as a rationale for the importance of this health care service and the cost effectiveness of funding such a service.

3 Nursing and Genomics

I. LEARNING KEY TERMS

MATCHING: Match the description in Column I with the appropriate genetic concept in Column II.

COLUMN I

1. _____ An individual's observable expression of his or her genetic makeup.

2. _____ Condition in which there is a mixture of cells, some with a normal number of chromosomes and others either missing a chromosome or containing an extra chromosome.

3. _____ Failure of chromosomes to separate.

4. _____ Basic physical units of inheritance that are passed from parents to offspring and contain the coded information (DNA) needed to determine an individual's unique characteristics.

5. _____ An abnormality in chromosome number in which the numeric deviation is not the exact multiple of the haploid set.

6. _____ An individual's collection of genes or entire genetic makeup.

7. _____ Union of a normal gamete and a gamete containing an extra chromosome, resulting in a cell with 47 chromosomes.

8. _____ A portion of the chromosome is rearranged in reverse order.

9. _____ X, Y.

10. _____ A cell with the correct or normal number of chromosomes within it.

11. _____ Entire set of genetic instructions found in the nucleus of each human cell.

12. _____ Having two copies of the same allele for the same trait.

13. _____ Genes at corresponding loci on homologous chromosomes that code for different forms or variations of the same trait.

14. _____ Chromosomal material is exchanged between two chromosomes.

15. _____ Matched chromosomes, each having the same number and arrangement of genes.

16. _____ Loss of chromosomal material and partial monosomy for the chromosome involved.

17. _____ There are 22 pairs of these on each chromosome, one from each parent; they control most traits in the body.

18. _____ Threadlike strands of genes and other DNA in a cell nucleus.

19. _____ Union of a normal gamete and a gamete missing a chromosome, resulting in a cell with 45 chromosomes.

20. _____ A spontaneous and permanent change in normal gene structure.

21. _____ Pictorial analysis of the number, form, and size of an individual's chromosomes.

22. _____ Having two different alleles for a given trait.

COLUMN II

A. Genome
B. Chromosome
C. Homozygous
D. Gene
E. Sex chromosomes
F. Karyotype
G. Aneuploidy
H. Autosomes
I. Trisomy
J. Nondisjunction
K. Monosomy
L. Translocation
M. Mutation
N. Heterozygous
O. Alleles
P. Deletion
Q. Mosaicism
R. Euploid
S. Phenotype
T. Inversion
U. Genotype
V. Homologous

FILL IN THE BLANKS: Insert the term that corresponds to each of the following descriptions related to the study of genes and chromosomes.

23. _____ The study of individual genes.

24. _____ The study of all genes in the human genome together, including their interactions with each other and the environment and the influence of other psychosocial and cultural factors.

25. _____ Testing that involves the analysis of human DNA, RNA, chromosomes, or proteins to detect abnormalities related to an inherited condition.

26. _____ Tests used to directly examine the DNA and RNA that make up a gene.

27. _____ Tests that look at markers coinherited with a gene that causes a genetic condition.

28. _____ Tests that examine the protein products of genes.

29. _____ Tests that examine chromosomes.

30. _____ Tests used to identify individuals who have a gene mutation for a genetic condition but do not show symptoms of the condition because it is an autosomal recessive condition.

31. _____ Tests used to clarify the genetic status of asymptomatic family members. There are two specific types of these tests, namely, _____ tests (gene mutation is present and symptoms are certain to appear if the individual lives long enough) and _____ tests (gene mutation is present but this positive result does not indicate that there is a 100% risk of developing the condition).

32. _____ The use of genetic information to individualize drug therapy. Primary benefits are the potential to reduce adverse drug reactions and to develop target therapies.

33. _____ Therapeutic approach that is based on the use of genetic information to correct inherited diseases.

FILL IN THE BLANKS: Insert the term that corresponds to each of the following descriptions related to patterns of genetic transmission.

34. _____ Phenotypic characteristics resulting from two or more genes on different chromosomes acting together; it involves a combination of genetic and environmental factors.

35. _____ Phenotypic characteristics controlled by a single gene; it is also known as single-gene inheritance.

36. _____ Inherited disorder in which only one copy of a variant gene is needed for phenotypic expression.

37. _____ Inherited disorder in which both genes of a pair are forms associated with the disorder to be expressed.

38. _____ Disorder that follows the autosomal recessive pattern of inheritance; it occurs when a gene mutation reduces the efficiency of encoded enzymes to a level at which normal metabolism cannot occur.

39. _____ Form of inheritance that mimics autosomal dominant inheritance, except that male-to-male transmission cannot occur unless the father has Klinefelter syndrome due to XY disomy.

40. _____ Form of inheritance in which the abnormal gene is carried on the female chromosome; if the male receives the abnormal gene, the disorder will be expressed; a common example of this type of disorder is hemophilia.

41. IDENTIFY five genetics-related activities that reflect the minimal amount of genetic and genomic competency expected of all nurses.

42. Couples referred for genetic counseling receive an estimation of risk for the genetic disorder of concern. EXPLAIN the difference between an estimate of occurrence risk and an estimation of recurrence risk.

43. Many nurses specialize in the area of genetic counseling. DISCUSS the major ethical, legal, and social implications (ELSI) associated with genetic testing that should guide the practice of these nurses.

MULTIPLE CHOICE: Circle the correct option(s) and state the rationale for the option(s) chosen.

44. Based on genetic testing of a newborn, a diagnosis of neurofibromatosis is made. The parents ask the nurse if this could happen to future children. Because this is an example of autosomal dominant inheritance, the nurse tells the parents:
    A. "For each pregnancy, there is a 50/50 chance the child will be affected by neurofibromatosis."
    B. "This will not happen again because the neurofibromatosis was caused by the harmful genetic effects of the infection you had during pregnancy."
    C. "For each pregnancy there is a 25% chance the child will be a carrier of the defective gene but unaffected by the disorder."
    D. "Because you already have had an affected child, there is a decreased chance of this happening in future pregnancies."

45. A female carries the gene for hemophilia on one of her X chromosomes. Her father does not have hemophilia. Now that she is pregnant she asks the nurse how this might affect her baby. The nurse should tell her:
    A. A female baby has a 50% chance of also being a carrier.
    B. A male baby can be a carrier or have hemophilia.
    C. Female babies are never affected by this disorder.
    D. Hemophilia is always expressed if a male inherits the defective gene.

46. A pregnant woman carries a single gene for cystic fibrosis, an inborn error of metabolism. The father of her baby does not carry this gene. Which of the following is true regarding the genetic pattern of the inborn error of metabolism as it applies to this family?
    A. The pregnant woman has cystic fibrosis herself.
    B. There is a 50% chance her baby will have the disorder.
    C. There is a 25% chance her baby will be a carrier.
    D. There is no chance her baby will be affected by this disorder.

47. A woman has been diagnosed with factor V Leiden (FVL). The nurse caring for this woman would be alert for which of the following problems?
    A. Breast cancer
    B. Postpartum hemorrhage
    C. Deep vein thrombosis (DVT)
    D. Placenta previa

1. A nurse is providing genetic counseling to a pregnant woman and her partner. They are unsure about whether they should undergo genetic testing to determine if they are carriers of a genetic disorder. IDENTIFY the factors this nurse should keep in mind that can influence her clients' decision to have genetic testing or to refuse it.

2. SUPPORT this statement: All nurses must possess a basic understanding of and expertise in genetics to provide holistic family-centered care.

3. Angela has come for her first prenatal visit. IDENTIFY the questions the nurse should ask during the health history interview to determine if factors are present that would place Angela at risk for giving birth to a baby with an inheritable disorder.

4. Rachel and Joshua, who are Jewish, are newly married and planning for pregnancy. They express to the nurse their concern that Rachel has a history of Tay-Sachs disease in her family. Joshua has never investigated his family history.
   A. DESCRIBE the nurse's role in the process of assisting the couple to determine their genetic risk.

   B. Both Rachel and Joshua are found to be carriers of the disorder. DISCUSS the estimation of risk and interpretation of risk as it applies to the couple in terms of giving birth to a child who is normal, is a carrier, or is affected by the disorder.

   C. OUTLINE the nurse's role in the education and emotional support of the couple now that a diagnosis and estimation of risk have been made.

Assessment and Health Promotion

I. LEARNING KEY TERMS

FILL IN THE BLANKS: Insert the term that corresponds to each of the following descriptions related to the female reproductive system and breasts. Use the anatomic drawings (Figs. 4-1, 4-2, 4-4, and 4-6) in your text to visualize each of the structures as you insert the terms.

1. _____ Fatty pad that lies over the anterior surface of the symphysis pubis.

2. _____ Two rounded folds of fatty tissue covered with skin that extend downward and backward from the mons pubis; their purpose is to protect the inner vulvar structures.

3. _____ Two flat reddish folds composed of connective tissue and smooth muscle, which are supplied with extremely sensitive nerve endings.

4. _____ Hoodlike covering of the clitoris.

5. _____ Fold of tissue under the clitoris.

6. _____ Thin, flat tissue formed by the joining of the labia minora; it is underneath the vaginal opening at the midline.

7. _____ Small structure underneath the prepuce composed of erectile tissue with numerous sensory nerve endings; it increases in size during sexual arousal.

8. _____ Almond-shaped area enclosed by the labia minora that contains openings to the urethra, Skene glands, vagina, and Bartholin glands.

9. _____ Bladder opening found between the clitoris and the vagina.

10. _____ Skin-covered muscular area between the fourchette and the anus that covers the pelvic structures.

11. _____ Fibromuscular collapsible tubular structure that extends from the vulva to the uterus and lies between the bladder and rectum. Its mucosal lining is arranged in transverse folds called

_____. _____ and _____ glands secrete mucus that lubricates the vagina.

12. _____ Anterior, posterior, and lateral pockets that surround the cervix.

13. _____ Muscular pelvic organ located between the bladder and the rectum and just above the vagina. The _____ is a deep pouch, or recess, posterior to the cervix formed by the posterior ligament.

14. _____ Upper triangular portion of the uterus.

15. _____ Also known as the lower uterine segment, it is the short constricted portion that separates the corpus of the uterus from the cervix.

16. _____ Dome-shaped top of the uterus.

17. _____ Highly vascular lining of the uterus.

18. _____ Layer of the uterus composed of smooth muscles that extend in three different directions.

19. _____ Lower cylindric portion of the uterus composed of fibrous connective tissue and elastic tissue.

20. _____ Passage that connects the uterine cavity to the vagina. The opening between the uterus and this passage is the _____. The opening between this passage and the vagina is the _____.

21. _____ Location in the cervix where the squamous and columnar epithelia meet (the transformation zone); it is the most common site for neoplastic changes; cells from this site are scraped for the _____ test.

22. _____ Passageways between the ovaries and the uterus; they are attached at each side of the dome-shaped uterine fundus.

23. _____ Almond-shaped organs located on each side of the uterus. Their two functions are _____ and the production of the hormones _____, _____, and _____.

24. _____ Structure that protects the bladder, uterus, and rectum; accommodates the growing fetus during pregnancy; and anchors support structures.

25. _____ The paired mammary glands.

26. _____ Segment of mammary tissue that extends into the axilla.

27. _____ Mammary papilla.

28. _____ Pigmented section of wrinkled skin that surrounds the nipple.

29. _____ Sebaceous glands that cause the areola to appear rough.

30. _____ Breast structures that are lined with epithelial cells that secrete colostrum and milk.

31. _____ Layer of breast tissue below the epithelium that contracts to expel milk from the acini forward toward the nipple.

MATCHING: Match the descriptions related to the menstrual cycle in Column I with the appropriate term in Column II.

COLUMN I

32. _____ The first menstruation.

33. _____ Transitional stage between childhood and sexual maturity.

34. _____ Transitional phase during which ovarian function and hormone production decline.

35. _____ The last menstrual period dated with certainty once 1 year has passed after menstruation ceases.

36. _____ Period preceding the last menstrual period that lasts about 4 years; during this time ovarian function declines, ova diminish, more menstrual cycles become anovulatory, and irregular bleeding occurs.

37. _____ Periodic uterine bleeding that begins approximately 14 days after ovulation and lasts an average of 5 days.

38. _____ The cycle that involves cyclic changes in the lining of the uterus.

39. _____ Phase of the menstrual cycle during which the uterine lining grows rapidly and thickens from about the fifth day to the time of ovulation.

40. _____ Phase of the menstrual cycle during which the uterine lining becomes luxuriant with blood and glandular secretions suitable to protect and nurture a fertilized ovum.

41. _____ Phase during which the blood supply to the functional uterine lining is blocked and necrosis develops; the functional layer separates from the basal layer and menstrual bleeding begins.

42. _____ Cycle that involves secretion of hormones required to stimulate ovulation.

43. _____ Cycle that involves the changes in the ovary, leading to ovulation. It consists of two phases, namely, follicular and luteal.

44. _____ Structure that encloses the developing ovum; it ruptures at the time of ovulation, releasing the ovum.

45. _____ Hormone secreted by the hypothalamus when ovarian hormones are reduced to a low level. It stimulates the pituitary gland to secrete two critical hormones.

46. _____ Pituitary hormone that stimulates the development of follicles in the ovary.

47. _____ Pituitary hormone that stimulates the expulsion of the ovum from the graafian follicle and formation of the corpus luteum.

48. _____ Ovarian hormone that stimulates the thickening of the endometrium that occurs after menstruation and prior to ovulation; it is also responsible for changes in the cervix and cervical mucus.

49. _____ Stretchable quality of the cervical mucus at the time of ovulation.

50. _____ Ovarian hormone that is responsible for the changes in the endometrium that occur after ovulation to facilitate implantation should fertilization occur; it is also responsible for the rise in temperature that occurs after ovulation.

51. _____ Oxygenated fatty acids classified as hormones. They are thought to play an essential role in ovulation, transport of sperm, regression of the corpus luteum, and menstruation. By increasing the myometrial response to oxytocin, they also play a role in labor and dysmenorrhea.

COLUMN II

A. Menstruation
B. Hypothalamic-pituitary cycle
C. Gonadotropin-releasing hormone (GnRH)
D. Prostaglandins
E. Menarche
F. Luteinizing hormone
G. Graafian follicle
H. Spinnbarkeit
I. Secretory phase
J. Progesterone
K. Puberty
L. Ovarian cycle
M. Proliferative phase
N. Climacteric
O. Follicle-stimulating hormone
P. Perimenopause
Q. Estrogen
R. Ischemic phase
S. Menopause
T. Endometrial cycle

52. It is essential that guidelines for laboratory and diagnostic procedures be followed exactly to ensure the accuracy of the results obtained. OUTLINE the guidelines that should be followed when performing a Pap test in terms of each of the following:

    A. Client preparation

    B. Timing during examination when the specimen is obtained

    C. Sites for specimen collection

    D. Handling of specimens

    E. Frequency of performance

53. During a clinical examination of a woman's breasts the nurse identifies a lump in one of the breasts. CITE the characteristics that the nurse should document regarding the palpated lump.

MULTIPLE CHOICE: Circle the correct option(s) and state the rationale for the option(s) chosen.

54. A 20-year-old woman tells the nurse that she performs breast self-examination (BSE) on a regular basis. The nurse evaluates the woman's understanding of BSE and ability to perform the technique correctly. Which actions by the woman indicate that she needs further instruction regarding BSE? (Circle all that apply.)

    A. Performs BSE every month on the first day of her menstrual cycle.
    B. Observes the size of her breasts, direction of her nipples, and appearance of her skin, including the presence of dimpling, when looking at her breasts in the mirror.
    C. Lies down on a bed and puts a pillow under the shoulder of the breast she is going to palpate. Then she places the arm on that side under her head.
    D. Uses the tips of two fingers to palpate her breast.
    E. Palpates her breast, using an overlapping circular pattern around her entire breast.
    F. Palpates her breasts again, including up into her axillae, while taking a shower.

55. When palpating the small breasts of a young, slender woman the nurse should:
    A. Wear clean gloves
    B. Lift the hands when moving from one segment of the breast to another
    C. Use both hands
    D. Follow a systematic, overlapping pattern

56. A nurse instructed a female client regarding vulvar self-examination (VSE). Which statement made by the client indicates that further instruction is needed?
    A. "I will perform this examination at least once a month, especially if I change sexual partners or am sexually active."
    B. "I will become familiar with how my genitalia look and feel so that I will be able to detect changes."
    C. "I will use the examination to determine when I should get medications at the pharmacy for infections."
    D. "I will wash my hands thoroughly before and after I examine myself."

57. A women's health nurse practitioner is going to perform a pelvic examination on a female client. Which nursing action would be least effective in enhancing the client's comfort and relaxation during the examination?
    A. Encourage the client to ask questions and express feelings and concerns before and after the examination.
    B. Ask the client questions as the examination is performed.
    C. Allow the client to keep her shoes and socks on when placing her feet in the stirrups.
    D. Instruct the client to place her hands over her diaphragm and take deep, slow breaths.

58. When assessing women it is important for a nurse to keep in mind the possibility that they are victims of violence. The nurse should:
    A. Use an abuse assessment screen during the assessment of every woman
    B. Recognize that abuse rarely occurs during pregnancy
    C. Assess a woman's legs and back as the most commonly injured areas
    D. Notify the woman's partner immediately if abuse is suspected

59. A 52-year-old woman asks the nurse practitioner about how often she should be assessed for the common health problems that women of her age could experience. The nurse recommends:
    A. An endometrial biopsy every 3 to 4 years
    B. A fecal occult blood test annually
    C. A mammogram every other year
    D. Bone mineral density testing annually

60. Which statement is most accurate regarding persons who should participate in preconception counseling?
    A. All women and their partners as they make decisions about their reproductive future, including becoming parents
    B. Women older than 40 years of age who wish to become pregnant
    C. Sexually active women who do not use birth control
    D. Women with chronic illnesses such as diabetes who are planning to get pregnant

61. To enhance the accuracy of the Pap test, the nurse should instruct the woman to:
    A. Schedule the test just prior to the onset of menses
    B. Stop taking birth control pills for 2 days before the test
    C. Avoid intercourse for 24 to 48 hours before the test
    D. Douche with a specially prepared antiseptic solution on the night before the test

III. THINKING CRITICALLY

1. A nurse is teaching a group of young adult women about health promotion activities. As part of the discussion the nurse identifies preconception care as an important health promotion activity. One woman in the class asks, "I know you need to go for checkups once you are pregnant, but why would you need to see a doctor before you get pregnant? Isn't that a big waste of time and money?" EXPLAIN how the nurse should respond to this woman's question.

2. A group of nurse practitioners and midwives is establishing a women's health clinic in a large metropolitan area of New York. They will be serving a multiethnic population that consists of women ranging from adolescence to old age.
   A. Using your awareness that women most often initially seek health care for reproductive concerns, IDENTIFY the services that the nurses at this new clinic should plan to offer.

   B. CITE the factors (barriers) that could interfere with the women in this community seeking health care at the clinic. Based on these barriers, DESCRIBE strategies these nurses could use to reduce the barriers to care and to encourage the women to participate in the services offered at the clinic.

   C. Major goals of the nurses at this clinic are to promote the health of women in the community and prevent illness. DISCUSS the types of services that the nurses should place a high priority on offering to achieve their goals. Include a rationale for each service proposed.

3. An inner-city women's health clinic serves a diverse population in terms of age, ethnic background, and health problems. DESCRIBE how the women's health nurse practitioner should adjust the approach for the following women with special needs. Each of the factors should influence a women's health nurse practitioner's approach when assessing the health of the women who come to the clinic for care.
   A. Adolescents

   B. Midlife and older women

   C. Women with disabilities

   D. Abused women

4. During a routine checkup for her annual Pap test, Julie, who is 26 years old, asks the nurse for advice regarding nutrition and exercise. Her body mass index (BMI) is 32 and she wants to "lose weight sensibly and keep it off." DISCUSS the advice the nurse should give to Julie.

5. Alice, a 30-year-old client, comes to the women's health clinic complaining of fatigue, insomnia, and feeling anxious. She works as a stockbroker for a major Wall Street brokerage firm. Alice states that although she enjoys the challenge of her job, she never can seem to find time for herself or to socialize with her friends. Alice tells the nurse practitioner that she has been drinking more and has started smoking again to help her to relax. She is glad that she has lost some weight, attributing this to her diminished appetite.
   A. STATE the physical and emotional signs of stress that the nurse should take note of when assessing Alice.

   B. DISCUSS how the nurse can help Alice to cope with stress and its consequences in a healthy manner.

   C. Alice expresses interest in attempting to stop smoking. "I felt so much better when I stopped the first time. That was more than 2 years ago and now here I am back at it again." DESCRIBE an approach the nurse could use to help Alice achieve a desired change in health behavior that is long-lasting.

6. During a routine women's health checkup, a woman expresses concern to the nurse practitioner about the increase in violence against women. She states: "One of my friends was raped and a colleague at work was beaten by her boyfriend." DISCUSS how the nurse practitioner should respond to this woman's concern, including measures she could use to protect herself from violence and injury.

7. IMAGINE that you are a nurse working at a clinic that provides health care to women. DESCRIBE how you would respond to each of the following concerns or questions of women who have come to the clinic for care.
   A. Serena, 17 years old, has just been scheduled for her first women's health checkup, which will include a pelvic examination and Pap test. She nervously asks if there is anything she needs to do to prepare for the examination.

   B. Andrea is trying to get pregnant. She wonders if there are signs she could observe in her body that would indicate that she is ovulating and therefore able to conceive a baby with her partner.

C. While you are teaching a group of women of various ages about BSE, they ask you to describe the normal characteristics of the female breast and how these characteristics change as a woman gets older.

D. Anne, 24 years old, asks the nurse about a recommended douche to use a couple of times a week to stay "nice and clean down there."

8. Julie, a 21-year-old client, has come to the women's health clinic for a women's health checkup. During the health history interview she becomes very anxious and states: "I have to tell you this is my first examination. I am very scared. My friends told me that it hurts a lot to have this examination." DESCRIBE how the nurse should respond in an effort to reduce Julie's anxiety.

9. As a nurse working in a women's health clinic, you have been assigned to interview Angie, a 25-year-old new client, to obtain her health history.
   A. LIST the components that should be emphasized in gathering Angie's history.

   B. WRITE a series of questions that you would ask to obtain data related to Angie's reproductive and sexual health and practices.

   C. DISCUSS the therapeutic techniques that you would use to facilitate communication. GIVE an example of each technique.

10. Self-examination of the breasts and vulva (genitalia) are important assessment techniques to teach a woman. OUTLINE the procedure you would use to teach each technique to one of your clients. INCLUDE the teaching methodologies you would use to enhance learning.
   Breast self-examination

   Vulvar (genital) self-examination

11. Lu Chen is a 25-year-old exchange student from China who has been living in the United States for 3 months. This is the first time that she has been away from home. She comes to the university women's health clinic for a checkup and to obtain birth control. DESCRIBE how the nurse assigned to Lu Chen would approach and communicate with her in a culturally sensitive manner.

12. Nurses working in women's health care must be aware of the growing problem of violence against women. All women should be screened when being assessed during health care for the possibility of abuse.
    A. DESCRIBE how you as a nurse would adjust the environment where the health history interview and physical examination will take place to elicit a woman's confidence and trust.

    B. IDENTIFY indicators of possible abuse that you would look for before the appointment and then during the health history interview and physical examination.

    C. STATE the questions you would ask to screen for abuse.

    D. DISCUSS the approach you would take if abuse is confirmed during the assessment.

13. When teaching a group of preadolescent girls about menstruation, one student asks the nurse, "What will happen to me when all of this stuff starts?" DESCRIBE what the nurse should tell the girls about the changes they can expect and what will happen to their bodies during each of the following components of the menstrual cycle:
    Hypothalamic-pituitary cycle

    Ovarian cycle

    Endometrial cycle

14. As a student you may be assigned to assist a health care provider during the performance of a pelvic examination for one of your clients.
   A. DESCRIBE how you would:
   Prepare your client for the examination

   Support your client during the examination

   Assist your client after the examination

   B. DESCRIBE how you would assist the health care provider who is performing the examination.

15. Lara, 16 years old, has come to the women's health clinic where you are a women's health nurse practitioner. This is her first visit and she is accompanied by her mother. During the history Lara asks her mother to leave so she can have privacy. She expresses to you that her major concerns are that she still has not had her first menstrual period and her breasts are not developing. You note that she is very thin. When you weigh her you discover that her BMI is 16. Despite this, Lara is concerned that she has gained half a pound since her last weighing at home. She checks her weight several times a week.
   A. DESCRIBE how you would address the nutritional problem that Lara is exhibiting.

   B. COMPARE and CONTRAST each of the following eating disorders:
   Anorexia nervosa

   Bulimia nervosa

   Binge-eating disorder

5 Violence Against Women

I. LEARNING KEY TERMS

FILL IN THE BLANKS: Insert the term that corresponds to the description related to violence against women.

1. _____ The most common form of violence against women. It refers to the actual or threatened physical, sexual, psychologic, or emotional abuse by a spouse, ex-spouse, boyfriend, girlfriend, ex-boyfriend, ex-girlfriend, date, or cohabitating partner.

2. _____ View of violence based on three phases in an intimate partner violence (IPV) relationship. The first phase is a period of _____, leading to the second phase involving acute _____, followed by the third phase of calm and remorse called the _____ phase.

3. _____ A contemporary view of violence with the primary theme of male dominance and coercive control.

4. _____ View of violence based on the dynamic relationship between the individual and the environment. The _____ is the center of the model and includes her intimate partner and their relationship as part of her immediate environment. At the next level or _____ are her children, family, friends, and the people and activities in her day-to-day life that are important to her. The _____ represents the community resources such as women's groups, violence prevention programs, and local resources. The _____ refers to organizations and formal agencies, health care systems, and providers such as nurses, the police, and the legal system. Finally, all of these are influenced by the _____, which includes the larger sociocultural beliefs, myths, and media. The _____ represents the influence of events over time.

5. _____ Broad term that encompasses a wide range of sexual victimization.

6. _____ Unwelcome, degrading sexual remarks, jokes, contact, or behavior such as exhibitionism that makes the work or other environment uncomfortable or difficult.

7. _____ Intentional, unwanted, completed or attempted touching of the victim's genitals, anus, groin, or breasts, directly or through clothing as well as by voyeurism. It also includes exhibitionism, exposing someone to pornography, or images taken of the victim in a private context.

8. _____ Forced sexual intercourse or penetration of the mouth, anus, or vagina by a body part or object without consent; it may or may not include the use of a weapon.

9. _____ Penetration by a person who is 18 years or older of a person under the age of consent; specifics vary from state to state.

10. _____ Noncoital sexual activity between a child and adolescent or adult.

11. _____ Cluster of characteristic symptoms and related behaviors experienced by women in the weeks and months after they have been sexually assaulted. The three phases are _____

_____, _____, and _____.

12. _____ A nurse educated in the specialty of forensic nursing and who is prepared to examine women who have been raped.

II. REVIEWING KEY CONCEPTS

13. Nurses caring for women should be alert for the presence of sociologic factors that have been associated with violence. IDENTIFY several of these factors that should be included as part of the assessment of women.

14. STATE how cultural beliefs and values can affect violence against women: its occurrence, how it is viewed, and the help sought by and provided to women who are abused. CITE examples from specific cultures.

15. Nurses working in women's health care should be aware of the characteristics typical of women who are abused and the persons who abuse them.
    A. CONTRAST the characteristics of women who are most likely to be in abusive relationships with the characteristics of women who are most likely to be in nonviolent relationships.

    B. CITE the characteristics of women who are most likely to seek assistance when they are abused.

    C. EXPLAIN why some women may not seek help when they are in an abusive relationship.

    D. CREATE a profile of persons most likely to become abusive partners.

16. A nurse is presenting a class related to IPV to a group of female college students. An expected outcome of this class is: *Women will describe the many forms that abuse can take.* DESCRIBE the information this nurse should present to the class to ensure that the outcome is achieved.

17. Clarise is a victim of IPV by her male partner. DESCRIBE how the nurse caring for Clarise could use the ABCDEs tool to provide Clarise with the support she needs.

18. Nurses play an essential role in preventing the cycle of violence against women in our society. DESCRIBE several strategies that school nurses can use to accomplish this goal.

19. Nurses working with victims of rape must realize that women are often reluctant to report the rape. INDICATE the factors that can deter women from reporting that they have been raped.

MULTIPLE CHOICE: Circle the correct option(s) and state the rationale for the option(s) chosen.

20. Men who are likely to abuse their female partners often exhibit which of the following characteristics? (Circle all that apply.)
    A. Low self-esteem
    B. Assertiveness
    C. Ability to express feelings verbally
    D. Intense interest in spending all of his time doing things with his partner
    E. Tolerance for frustration

21. A characteristic of women in abusive relationships is which of the following?
    A. Masochism
    B. Willingness to take a stand no matter what the cost
    C. Absence of typical feminine characteristics such as nurturing and compassion
    D. Tendency to isolate themselves from social relationships

22. A nurse caring for pregnant women needs to be aware that physical abuse during pregnancy can result in which of the following outcomes? (Circle all that apply.)
    A. Excessive weight gain
    B. Use of alcohol or tobacco as a means of coping
    C. Increased risk for giving birth to a low-birth-weight (LBW) baby
    D. Postterm pregnancy
    E. Sexually transmitted infections (STIs)

23. Which of the following women is most likely to seek assistance when battered?
    A. A woman with a career
    B. A woman who has been battered for the first time
    C. A woman who, as a child, saw her mother being abused by her father
    D. A woman who was abused as a child

24. A woman suspects that she has been raped by her date and that he put a "roofie" (flunitrazepam [Rohypnol]) in the wine she was drinking. What signs would she describe to the sexual assault nurse examiner (SANE) to help confirm that her suspicions are correct? (Circle all that apply.)
    A. Remembering what happened clearly
    B. Severe headache in the morning
    C. Feeling as if sex has occurred
    D. Feeling more intoxicated than usual with a similar amount of alcohol
    E. Feeling fuzzy or woozy on awakening

1. SUPPLY the facts to disprove each of the following myths concerning violence against women.
   A. IPV is primarily a problem of families who are at a low socioeconomic level and poorly educated.

   B. Violence affects only a small percentage of women in this country.

   C. Victims and perpetrators of IPV cannot change.

   D. Battered women usually provoke their attack because they have a need to be beaten.

   E. Being pregnant protects a woman from IPV.

2. OUTLINE an assessment format based on the ecological framework for IPV.

3. As a nurse working in a women's health clinic, you must be alert to cues indicative of physical abuse.
   A. IDENTIFY the cues you would look for.

   B. Carol, a 24-year-old married client, comes to the clinic to confirm her belief that she is pregnant. During the assessment phase of the visit, you note cues that lead you to suspect that Carol is being abused by her husband. DISCUSS the approach you would take to confirm your suspicion that Carol is being abused.

   C. Carol admits that her husband beats her sometimes and that "it has been increasing." Now she is afraid it will get worse because she "was not supposed to get pregnant." DISCUSS the nursing actions you could take to help Carol.

D. LIST the possible reasons that Carol, now that she is pregnant, is experiencing an escalation of battering and abuse from her husband.

E. SPECIFY what you should avoid as you work with Carol.

F. EXPLAIN how you would determine the degree of danger Carol faces.

G. DISCUSS how Carol's pregnancy could be adversely affected by the violence she is experiencing.

H. DESCRIBE the behaviors Carol most likely would exhibit as an indication of her readiness to leave the abusive relationship.

I. IDENTIFY your legal responsibilities regarding confirmation that Carol is being abused and reporting the abuse to authorities who can help Carol.

4. Marie has been raped. She is admitted to the emergency department for examination.
    A. EXPLAIN the advantage of having a SANE nurse care for Marie.

    B. DESCRIBE the nurse's responsibility in assessing Marie and in collecting and preserving the physical evidence of her rape.

C. DISCUSS the nursing actions that should be used to meet the emotional needs of Marie at this time.

D. OUTLINE how Marie's emotions and behaviors will be expressed and will change as she progresses through the phases of the rape-trauma syndrome. IDENTIFY how a rape-trauma counselor should assess Marie during each phase.

E. SPECIFY the interventions required prior to discharging Marie.

6 Reproductive System Concerns

I. LEARNING KEY TERMS

FILL IN THE BLANKS: Insert the term that corresponds to each of the following descriptions related to menstrual disorders and experiences.

1. _____ Absence of menstrual flow. It is a clinical symptom of a variety of disorders but most commonly a result of pregnancy and is a classic sign of anorexia nervosa.

2. _____ Absence of menstrual flow related to a problem of the central hypothalamic-pituitary axis.

3. _____ Interrelatedness of disordered eating, amenorrhea, and altered bone mineral density.

4. _____ Collective term used to describe pain and discomfort associated with the menstrual cycle. The three main conditions included are _____, _____, and _____.

5. _____ Pain that occurs during or shortly before menstruation; it is one of the most common gynecologic problems in women of all ages.

6. _____ Painful menstruation that occurs as a result of increased uterine activity due to myometrial contractions induced by excessive release of prostaglandins in the second half of the menstrual cycle; it is associated with ovulatory cycles.

7. _____ Acquired menstrual pain that typically develops after age 25 years and is associated with pelvic pathology.

8. _____ A cluster of physical and psychologic symptoms beginning in the luteal phase of the menstrual cycle and followed by a symptom-free period.

9. _____ A more severe variant of premenstrual syndrome (PMS) with an emphasis on symptoms associated with mood disturbances, such as marked irritability, dysphoria, mood lability, anxiety, fatigue, appetite changes, and a sense of feeling overwhelmed.

10. _____ Menstrual disorder characterized by the presence and growth of endometrial glands and stroma outside the uterus.

11. _____ Infrequent menstrual periods characterized by intervals of 40 to 45 days or longer.

12. _____ Scanty bleeding at normal intervals.

13. _____ or _____ Any episode of bleeding (e.g., spotting, menses, hemorrhage) that occurs at a time other than the normal menses.

14. _____ Small amount of bleeding or spotting that occurs at the time of ovulation (14 days before onset of the next menses); it is considered to be normal.

15. _____ Bleeding that occurs when the contraceptive pill does not maintain a sufficiently hypoplastic endometrium, resulting in shedding of the endometrium in small amounts at a time.

16. _____ or _____ Excessive menstrual bleeding, either in duration or amount.

17. _____ Any form of uterine bleeding that is irregular in amount, duration, or timing and not related to regular menstrual bleeding.

18. _____ Excessive uterine bleeding with no demonstrable organic cause, genital or extragenital; it is most frequently associated with anovulation.

19. _____ First menstrual period.

20. _____ Complete cessation of menses, said to have occurred when menstrual flow or spotting has ceased for 1 year.

21. _____ or _____ Period that encompasses the transition from normal ovulatory cycles to cessation of menses; it is marked by irregular menstrual cycles.

22. _____ Cessation of the menstrual cycle that occurs as a result of hysterectomy and bilateral oophorectomy.

23. _____ The period of time after menopause occurs.

24. _____ Painful intercourse.

25. _____ Visible red flush of the skin with perspiration.

26. _____ Sudden warm sensation in the neck, head, and chest.

27. _____ Profuse perspiration and heat radiating from the body that disrupts sleep.

28. _____ Generalized metabolic disease characterized by decreased bone mass and increased incidence of bone fractures.

29. _____ or _____ Substances found in certain plant foods (e.g., red clover, wild yams, dandelion greens, cherries, alfalfa sprouts, black beans, soybeans) that are capable of interacting with estrogen receptors in the body.

II. REVIEWING KEY CONCEPTS

30. When caring for perimenopausal women it is important not only to recognize the expected changes associated with this period of transition but also to be able to explain to these women why these changes occur. IDENTIFY the manifestations and physiologic basis for each of the following expected changes:
    ■ Bleeding

    ■ Genital changes

- Vasomotor instability

- Mood and behavioral responses

MULTIPLE CHOICE: Circle the correct option(s) and state the rationale for the option(s) chosen.

31. Which woman is at greatest risk for developing hypogonadotropic amenorrhea?
    A. A 48-year-old woman in Weight Watchers who lost 20 pounds over 6 months
    B. A 14-year-old figure skater
    C. An 18-year-old softball player
    D. A 30-year-old (G3 P3003) breastfeeding woman

32. Pharmacologic preparations can be used to treat primary dysmenorrhea. Choose the preparation that is least effective in relieving the symptoms of primary dysmenorrhea.
    A. Combined oral contraceptive pill (OCP)
    B. Naproxen sodium (Anaprox)
    C. Acetaminophen (Tylenol)
    D. Ibuprofen (Motrin)

33. Women experiencing primary dysmenorrhea should be advised to avoid:
    A. Pretzels and potato chips
    B. Valerian
    C. Cranberry juice
    D. Whole-grain cereals

34. The nurse counseling a 30-year-old woman regarding effective measures to use to relieve symptoms associated with PMS could suggest that she: (Circle all that apply.)
    A. Decrease intake of fruits, especially peaches and watermelon
    B. Take a bugleweed or evening primrose oil supplement
    C. Limit alcohol intake to less than 1 oz per day
    D. Reduce exercise during the luteal phase of the menstrual cycle when symptoms are at their peak
    E. Eat small, more frequent meals and snacks

35. A 28-year-old woman has been diagnosed with endometriosis. She has been placed on a course of treatment with danazol (Danocrine). The woman exhibits understanding of this treatment when she states: (Circle all that apply.)
    A. "Because this medication stops ovulation, I do not need to use birth control."
    B. "I will experience more frequent and heavier menstrual periods when I take this medication."
    C. "I should follow a low-fat diet because this medication can increase the level of cholesterol in my blood."
    D. "I can experience a decrease in my breast size, oily skin, and hair growth on my face as a result of taking this medication."
    E. "I will need to spray this medication into my nose twice a day."
    F. "I may need to use a lubricant during intercourse to reduce discomfort."

36. A female client, age 26 years, describes scant bleeding between her menstrual periods. The nurse records this finding as:
    A. Metrorrhagia
    B. Oligomenorrhea
    C. Menorrhagia
    D. Hypomenorrhea

39

37. Dysfunctional uterine bleeding (DUB) is most likely to occur when women:
    A. Experience ovulatory cycles
    B. Weigh less than their expected body weight
    C. Experience signs of the onset of perimenopause
    D. Secrete high levels of prostaglandin

38. A 55-year-old woman tells the nurse that she has started to experience pain when she and her husband have intercourse. The nurse would record that this woman is experiencing:
    A. Dyspareunia
    B. Dysmenorrhea
    C. Dysuria
    D. Dyspnea

39. A 65-year-old woman is beginning treatment with alendronate sodium (Fosamax). Which statement by this woman indicates the need for further instructions?
    A. "I will take this medication first thing in the morning."
    B. "I will sit in a chair and read a book for about 30 minutes after I take this medication."
    C. "I will take this medication with a full glass of water."
    D. "I will eat my breakfast just before I take the medication."

40. Herbal preparations can be used as part of the treatment for a variety of menstrual disorders. Which herb is beneficial for a woman experiencing menorrhagia?
    A. Ginger
    B. Shepherd's purse
    C. Black cohosh root
    D. Black haw

III. THINKING CRITICALLY

1. Maria is a 16-year-old gymnast who has been training vigorously for a placement on the U.S. Olympic team. She has been experiencing amenorrhea, and the development of her secondary sexual characteristics has been limited. Maria expresses concern because her nonathletic friends have all been menstruating for at least 1 year and have well-developed breasts. After a health assessment, Maria is diagnosed with hypogonadotropic amenorrhea.
   A. STATE the risk factors for this disorder that Maria most likely exhibited during the assessment process.

   B. STATE one nursing diagnosis reflective of Maria's concern.

   C. WRITE two expected outcomes for a plan of care for Maria.

   D. OUTLINE a typical care management plan for Maria that addresses the issues associated with hypogonadotropic amenorrhea.

E. At Maria's all-female high school there is a large athletic department that emphasizes participation and excellence in a variety of sports. As the school nurse, you are concerned that there are other students like Maria who may be exhibiting signs of the female athlete triad. You have decided to institute an education program aimed at prevention and early detection of the triad.

    1. STATE which sports you should emphasize in your program.

    2. STATE what measures you should include in your program as a means of prevention and early detection of the female athlete triad.

2. Mary, a 17-year-old who experienced menarche at age 16, comes to the women's health clinic for a routine checkup. She complains to the nurse that her past few periods have been very painful. "I have missed a few days of school because of it. What can I do to reduce the pain that I feel during my periods?" Physical examination and testing reveal normal structure and function of Mary's reproductive system. A medical diagnosis of primary dysmenorrhea is made.

    A. WRITE several questions that the nurse should ask Mary to obtain a full description of her pain.

    B. STATE the priority nursing diagnosis appropriate for Mary.

    C. DESCRIBE what a nurse should tell Mary about the physiologic basis for her pain.

    D. IDENTIFY several relief measures, including alternative therapies, for primary dysmenorrhea that a nurse could suggest to Mary.

3. Susan experiences physical and psychologic signs and symptoms associated with premenstrual syndrome (PMS) during every ovulatory menstrual cycle.

    A. LIST the signs and symptoms most likely described by Susan that led to the diagnosis of PMS.

    B. IDENTIFY one nursing diagnosis that may be appropriate for Susan when she is experiencing the signs and symptoms of PMS.

C. DESCRIBE the approach a nurse would use in helping Susan to deal with this menstrual disorder.

D. STATE the symptoms that Susan would describe that could indicate she is also experiencing premenstrual dysphoric disorder (PMDD).

4. Lisa is 26 years old and has been diagnosed recently with endometriosis.
   A. LIST the signs and symptoms Lisa most likely exhibited that led to this medical diagnosis.

   B. Lisa asks, "What is happening to my body as a result of this disease?" DESCRIBE the nurse's response.

   C. Lisa asks about her treatment options. "Are there medications I can take to make me feel better?" DESCRIBE the action, effect, and potential side effects for each of the following pharmacologic approaches to treatment.
   Oral contraceptive pills

   Gonadotropin-releasing hormone agonists

   Androgen derivatives

   D. IDENTIFY support measures that a nurse can suggest to assist Lisa in coping with the effects of endometriosis.

5. Jane, a 46-year-old slender, Caucasian secretary, is at the beginning of the perimenopausal period. Her health history reveals a high intake of fast foods, coffee, and diet soft drinks, especially Pepsi, along with a smoking habit of one pack per day. Jane states that her favorite leisure activities are reading, needlework, and playing Bingo two evenings a week. She expresses concern about the development of osteoporosis because her mother experienced the stress fractures and dowager's hump characteristic of this disorder. Jane requests information concerning what she can do to prevent this from happening to her.

   A. IDENTIFY the risk factors for osteoporosis present in this situation.

   B. DISCUSS the information you should give Jane regarding prevention measures that would reduce her risk for developing osteoporosis and its sequelae.

   C. LIST the signs Jane would exhibit if she begins to develop osteoporosis.

6. Heidi is a 50-year-old client who is experiencing the changes typical of perimenopause. Her body mass index (BMI) is 30. During a routine gynecologic checkup at the women's health clinic she tells her nurse practitioner that she is having a hard time coping with hot flashes, stress incontinence, and insomnia. Heidi also expresses concern about the vaginal dryness she is experiencing, because it has resulted in discomfort and even pain when she and her husband have intercourse. She is also worried that her bones will get thin just like her mother's and grandmother's did. Heidi asks the nurse if there is anything she could suggest to reduce the discomfort associated with all of these problems. She tells the nurse that several of her friends have been taking hormones and seem to be doing better, stating, "They told me that hormones cure everything from hot flashes to bad bones."

   A. DESCRIBE the relief measures the nurse practitioner should suggest to Heidi regarding:
      Hot flashes and flushes

      Insomnia

      Urogenital symptoms (e.g., vaginal dryness, stress incontinence, dyspareunia)

   B. DISCUSS the approach the nurse practitioner should use to help Heidi decide about menopausal hormonal therapy (MHT).

C. Heidi decides to try MHT using a combined estrogen-progestin transdermal patch (CombiPatch). SPECIFY the instructions that Heidi should be given regarding this treatment to ensure its safety and effectiveness.

D. Heidi tells her nurse practitioner that she is very concerned about her potential for heart disease as a result of what is happening to her body with menopause. She asks the nurse why these changes occur and what she can do to promote her cardiac health. DISCUSS how the nurse should respond.

E. Heidi is a computer expert and enjoys using the Internet to research a variety of topics and "chat" with persons who share her interests in quilting and mystery novels. DESCRIBE how the nurse could use Heidi's interest in and expertise with computers to direct her to appropriate websites that would provide her with reliable information and support during the perimenopausal period.

7 Sexually Transmitted and Other Infections

I. LEARNING KEY TERMS

FILL IN THE BLANKS: Insert the term that corresponds to each of the following descriptions related to infections.

1. _____ Infections or infectious disease syndromes primarily transmitted by close intimate contact. The most common infections of this type in women are , _____,

   _____, _____, _____,

   _____ and _____.

2. _____ Precautions used during sexual activity to prevent the transmission of pathogens.

3. _____ The physical barrier promoted for the prevention of sexual transmission of human immunodeficiency virus (HIV) and other sexually transmitted infections (STIs).

4. _____ Bacterial infection that is the most commonly reported STI in American women. This infection is often silent and is highly destructive to the female reproductive tract.

5. _____ The oldest communicable disease in the United States and second most common in terms of reported cases. Because it is a reportable communicable disease, health care providers are legally responsible for reporting all cases to health authorities.

6. _____ One of the earliest described STIs. It is caused by *Treponema pallidum*, a motile spirochete. _____ Primary lesion that appears 5 to 90 days after infection.

   _____ Broad, painless, pink-gray wartlike infectious lesion that may develop on the vulva, the perineum, or the anus.

7. _____ Infectious process that most commonly involves the uterine (fallopian) tubes, uterus, and more rarely ovaries and peritoneal surfaces.

8. _____ Infection that is the most common viral STI seen in ambulatory health care settings; also called genital warts. _____ The visible lesions caused by infection with certain strains of this virus. _____ and _____ Vaccines currently available to protect against some of the most common strains of this infection.

9. _____ Viral infection that is transmitted sexually and is widespread in the United States. It is characterized by painful, recurrent genital ulcers.

10. _____ Viral infection acquired primarily through a fecal-oral route by ingestion of contaminated food—particularly milk, shellfish, or polluted water—or person-to-person contact.

11. _____ Viral infection involving the liver that is transmitted parenterally, perinatally, and through intimate contact. A vaccine is available to protect infants, children, and adults.

12. _____ Viral infection of the liver that is a major bloodborne infection in the United States. It is transmitted parenterally and through intimate contact. There is no vaccine available to provide protection against this infection.

13. _____ A retrovirus that is transmitted primarily through exchange of body fluids. Severe depression of the _____ system is associated with this infection and characterizes _____.

14. _____ A normal vaginal flora found in nonpregnant women. It is present in 25% of healthy pregnant women. It has been associated with poor pregnancy outcomes and neonatal morbidity and mortality resulting from vertical transmission from the birth canal of the infected mother to the infant during birth.

15. _____ Vaginal infection formerly called nonspecific vaginitis, *Haemophilus vaginitis*, or *Gardnerella*. It is the most common type of vaginal infection and is characterized by discharge that is usually profuse, thin, and white, gray, or milky in appearance with a characteristic "fishy" odor.

16. _____ A yeast infection that is the second most common type of vaginal infection in the United States. It is characterized by itching and a thick, white, lumpy discharge with a cottage cheese–like consistency. A yeasty or musty odor may be present.

17. _____ A vaginal infection caused by an anaerobic one-celled protozoan with characteristic flagella. It is characterized by a copious yellowish green, frothy, mucopurulent, malodorous discharge.

18. _____ A group of infections that can affect a pregnant woman and her fetus. The infecting organisms are capable of crossing the placenta and adversely affecting the development of the fetus.

19. _____ A protozoal infection associated with the consumption of raw or undercooked meat or exposure to litter used by infected cats.

20. _____ German or 3-day measles; the virus is transmitted by droplets.

21. _____ Viral infection that may be asymptomatic or present with mild influenza-like symptoms. It is transmitted by transfusion of infected blood, sexual contact, or contact with contaminated saliva or urine. It can lead to profound neurologic and sensory disorders if transmitted to the fetus.

22. _____ Infection control measures that must be followed by health care providers when caring for all clients.

II. REVIEWING KEY CONCEPTS

23. When assessing sexually active adults, the nurse must be alert for client behaviors that increase the risk for acquiring STIs. IDENTIFY two STI risk behaviors for each of the following categories:
Partners

Practices (sexual and drug use)

24. Nurses who work on childbirth and postpartum units and in newborn nurseries must be guided by infection control principles when caring for their clients. DESCRIBE one implementation measure for each Standard Precautions category:
- Hand hygiene
- Use of personal protective equipment (PPE)
- Respiratory hygiene and cough etiquette
- Safe injection practices

25. OUTLINE the clinical manifestations and management guidelines for each common reproductive tract infection.
    - Chlamydia
    - Gonorrhea
    - Syphilis
    - Human papillomavirus
    - Genital herpes simplex virus
    - Bacterial vaginosis
    - Candidiasis
    - Trichomoniasis

26. STATE the infections represented by the group of infections known collectively as TORCH.

MULTIPLE CHOICE: Circle the correct option(s) and state the rationale for the option(s) chosen.

27. Infections of the female midreproductive tract such as chlamydia are dangerous primarily because they:
    A. Are asymptomatic or silent
    B. Cause infertility
    C. Lead to pelvic inflammatory disease (PID)
    D. Are difficult to treat effectively

28. A finding associated with human papillomavirus (HPV) infection includes:
    A. White, curdlike adherent discharge
    B. Soft papillary swellings occurring singly or in clusters
    C. Vesicles progressing to pustules and then to ulcers
    D. Yellow to green frothy, malodorous discharge

29. A recommended medication effective in the treatment of vulvovaginal candidiasis is:
    A. Metronidazole
    B. Clotrimazole
    C. Benzathine penicillin G
    D. Acyclovir

30. A woman is determined to be group B streptococci (GBS) positive at the onset of her labor. The nurse should prepare this woman for:
    A. Cesarean birth
    B. Isolation of her newborn after birth
    C. Intravenous antibiotic prophylaxis (IAP) using penicillin G during labor
    D. Application of acyclovir to her labial lesions

31. When providing a woman who is recovering from primary herpes with information regarding the recurrence of herpes infection of the genital tract, the nurse tells her that: (Circle all that apply.)
    A. Fever and flulike symptoms occur only with primary infection
    B. Little can be done to control the recurrence of infection
    C. Transmission of the virus is possible only when lesions are open and draining
    D. Itching and tingling often occur as prodromal symptoms prior to the appearance of vesicles
    E. Cleaning lesions twice a day with saline will help to prevent secondary infections
    F. Acyclovir therapy will cure herpes

32. A nurse is teaching a 20-year-old woman about risk-reduction measures. Which measure should the nurse emphasize as the most important?
    A. Using a female condom
    B. Knowing her partner
    C. Reducing the number of partners
    D. Getting the HPV vaccination

33. Cervical neoplasia has been linked to which of the following sexually transmitted infections?
   A. Herpes simplex virus (HSV)
   B. Human papillomavirus (HPV)
   C. Human immunodeficiency virus (HIV)
   D. Chlamydia

34. A nurse has just taught a group of parents at a grade school PTA meeting regarding the vaccine Gardisil. Which statement by one of the parents would indicate a need for further instructions?
   A. "I should make sure that my child receives this vaccine before becoming sexually active."
   B. "This vaccine will prevent my child from being infected by some of the most common strains of HPV that can cause cervical cancer."
   C. "My child will need to receive the vaccine in two doses every 6 months for 1 year."
   D. "Both my daughter and my son should receive the vaccine around the age of 11 to 12 years."

III. THINKING CRITICALLY

1. Terry, 20 years old, comes to a women's health clinic for her first visit.
   A. During the health history interview it is imperative that the nurse practitioner determine Terry's risk for contracting an STI, including HIV. DESCRIBE the approach you would take to determine this woman's risk for STIs.

   B. Terry asks the nurse about measures she can use to protect herself from STIs. CITE the major points that the nurse practitioner should emphasize when teaching Terry about prevention measures.

   C. Terry tells the nurse that she does not know if she could ever tell a partner that he must wear a condom. DESCRIBE the approach the nurse can take to enhance Terry's assertiveness and communication skills.

   D. Terry asks the nurse if it is too late for her to get the immunization for HPV. She states that she heard it prevents cervical cancer and therefore she would not need to bother getting a Pap test every year. DISCUSS what the nurse should tell Terry.

2. Martha is 4 weeks pregnant. As part of her prenatal assessment it is discovered that she is HIV positive.
   A. STATE the modes of HIV transmission that could relate to Martha.

   B. LIST the clinical manifestations she most likely exhibited during her seroconversion to HIV positivity.

C. OUTLINE the care management approach that nurses should use when caring for Martha during her pregnancy and after she gives birth.

D. IDENTIFY the measures that can be used to reduce the risk of transmission of HIV from Martha to her baby.

3. Suzanne, a 20-year-old client, is admitted for suspected severe, acute PID.
   A. IDENTIFY the risk factors for PID that the nurse should be looking for in Suzanne's health history.

   B. A complete physical examination is performed to determine if the criteria for PID are met. SPECIFY the criteria that Suzanne's health care provider should be alert for during the examination.

   C. Suzanne is hospitalized when the diagnosis of PID secondary to chlamydial infection is confirmed. Intravenous (IV) antibiotics will be used as the primary medical treatment followed by oral antibiotics at the time of discharge. STATE three priority nursing diagnoses that are likely to be present during the acute stage of Suzanne's infection and treatment.

   D. OUTLINE a nursing management plan for Suzanne.

   E. LIST the recommendations for Suzanne's self-management during the recovery phase.

   F. IDENTIFY the reproductive health risks that Suzanne may face as a result of the pelvic infection she experienced.

4. Laura has come to the women's health clinic on her campus because she has been informed that her boyfriend has been diagnosed with gonorrhea.
   A. STATE the essential areas of assessment the nurse should keep in mind when interviewing Laura during the health history and performing a physical examination.

   B. Diagnostic testing confirms that Laura has gonorrhea. Laura is very upset by the diagnosis, stating, "This is just awful—what kind of sex life can I have now?" CITE a nursing diagnosis that reflects Laura's concern.

   C. OUTLINE a therapeutic plan that will assist Laura to take control of her self-management and prevent future infections.

5. Cheryl, 27 years old, is being treated for HPV. A primary diagnosis identified for Cheryl is acute pain related to lesions on the vulva and around the anus secondary to HPV infection. STATE the measures the nurse could suggest to Cheryl to reduce the pain from the condylomata and enhance their healing.

6. Mary, 20 years old, has just been diagnosed with a primary genital herpes simplex infection. In addition to the typical systemic symptoms, Mary exhibits multiple, painful genital lesions.
   A. Relief of pain and healing without the development of a secondary infection are two expected outcomes for care. IDENTIFY several measures that the nurse can suggest to Mary to help her achieve the expected outcomes of care.

   B. Mary asks the nurse if there is anything she can do so that this infection does not return and to prevent transmission of the infection to her new partner. DISCUSS what the nurse should tell Mary about the recurrence of herpes infection and the influence of self-care measures.

7. Gloria tested positive for hepatitis B. DESCRIBE the measures that the nurse should teach Gloria in an effort to decrease the risk for transmission of the virus to other people in Gloria's life.

8. Sonya is concerned that she has been exposed to HIV and has come to the women's health clinic for testing.

A. During the health history the nurse questions Sonya about behaviors that could have placed her at risk for HIV transmission. CITE the behaviors that the nurse would be looking for.

B. EXPLAIN the testing procedure that most likely will be followed to determine Sonya's HIV status.

C. OUTLINE the counseling protocol that should guide the nurse when caring for Sonya before and after the test.

D. Sonya's test result is negative. DISCUSS the instructions the nurse should give Sonya regarding guidelines she should follow to reduce her risk for the transmission of HIV with future sexual partners.

8 Contraception and Abortion

I. LEARNING KEY TERMS

FILL IN THE BLANKS: Insert the term that corresponds to each of the following descriptions regarding methods to prevent or plan pregnancy.

1. _____ The intentional prevention of pregnancy during sexual intercourse.

2. _____ The device and/or practice used to decrease the risk of conceiving, or bearing, offspring.

3. _____ The conscious decision about when to conceive or to avoid pregnancy, throughout the reproductive years.

4. _____ Percentage of contraceptive users expected to have an unplanned pregnancy during the first year, even when they use a method consistently and correctly.

5. _____ Method that requires the male partner to withdraw his penis from the woman's vagina before he ejaculates.

6. _____ Methods that depend on identifying the beginning and end of the fertile period of the menstrual cycle; they provide contraception by relying on avoidance of intercourse during fertile periods.

7. _____ Method based on the number of days in each cycle, counting from the first day of menses. The fertile period is determined after accurately recording the lengths of menstrual cycles for at least 6 months.

8. _____ Method based on monitoring and recording cervical secretions; each day the woman asks herself: (1) "Did I note secretions today?" and (2) "Did I note secretions yesterday?" If the answer to either question is yes, she should avoid coitus or use a backup method of birth control. If the answer to both questions is no, her probability of getting pregnant is very low.

9. _____ Method that requires the woman to recognize and interpret cyclic changes in the amount and consistency of cervical mucus that characterize her own unique pattern of changes at the time of ovulation.

10. _____ Term used to refer to the stretchiness of cervical mucus.

11. _____ Method based on variations in a healthy woman's lowest body temperature taken immediately after waking and before getting out of bed.

12. _____ Term used to refer to the decrease and subsequent increase in temperature associated with ovulation.

13. _____ Method that combines the basal body temperature (BBT) and cervical mucus methods with awareness of secondary phase-related symptoms of the menstrual cycle.

14. _____ Methods based on detecting the sudden surge of luteinizing hormone (LH) that occurs approximately 12 to 24 hours before ovulation.

15. _____ Chemical that reduces the mobility of sperm and attacks the sperm flagella and body. When inserted into the vagina it acts as a chemical barrier to sperm.

53

16. _____ Thin, stretchable sheath that covers the penis or is inserted into the vagina.

17. _____ Shallow, dome-shaped latex or silicone device with a flexible rim that covers the cervix, resulting in a mechanical barrier to sperm.

18. _____ A silicone device that fits snugly around the base of the cervix close to the junction of the cervix and vaginal fornices.

19. _____ A small round polyurethane device that contains spermicide. It fits over the cervix and has a woven polyester loop to facilitate its removal.

20. _____ Form of oral contraceptive pill that provides a fixed dosage of estrogen and progesterone.

21. _____ Form of oral contraceptive pill that alters the amount of progestin and sometimes the amount of estrogen within each cycle.

22. _____ Bleeding that occurs from 1 to 4 days after the last combined oral contraceptive is taken.

23. _____ Contraceptive form that delivers continuous levels of norelgestromin and ethinyl estradiol; a patch is applied to intact skin of the upper outer arm, the upper torso, the lower abdomen, or the buttocks on the same day once a week for 3 weeks followed by a week without the patch.

24. _____ Flexible device worn in the vagina to deliver continuous levels of etonogestrel and ethinyl estradiol; the device is worn for 3 weeks, followed by a week without the device.

25. _____ Progestin-only contraceptive pill.

26. _____ Progestin-only intramuscular (IM) injection providing contraception for approximately 3 months.

27. _____ Form of hormonal contraception in which a single flexible rod containing progestin is implanted subdermally, usually into the inner aspect of the upper arm. _____ Implantable progestin using two rods.

28. _____ Small T-shaped device inserted into the uterine cavity. It is loaded with copper or levonorgestrel.

29. _____ Surgical procedures intended to render the person infertile. For the female, the _____ are occluded. For the male, the _____ are occluded during a _____.

30. _____ Procedure used to restore tubal continuity (reanastomosis).

31. _____ Temporary method of birth control based on the surge of prolactin that occurs with breastfeeding. An elevated prolactin level inhibits estrogen production and suppresses ovulation and the return of menses.

32. _____ Purposeful interruption of a pregnancy before 20 weeks of gestation. If it is performed at the woman's request, it is termed an _____. If it is performed for reasons of maternal or fetal health or disease, it is termed a _____.

33. _____ Surgical method of performing an early induced abortion (8 to 12 weeks of gestation); it is the most common abortion procedure used in the first trimester.

34. _____ Induced early abortion method using one of three drugs, namely,

_____, _____, or _____.

35. _____ Surgical method used for a second-trimester abortion. It accounts for almost all procedures performed in the United States and results in more complications and greater costs than first-trimester abortions.

II. REVIEWING KEY CONCEPTS

36. A nurse is working with a couple to help them choose a method of contraception that is right for them.
    A. LIST the factors that can influence the effectiveness of the contraceptive method they choose.

    B. Informed consent is a vital component when helping this couple to choose a contraceptive. STATE the elements of informed consent that need to be met and documented as part of the decision-making process.

37. A woman is a little uncomfortable about checking her cervical mucus and asks the nurse what she could possibly discover by doing this assessment. STATE the useful purpose of self-evaluation of cervical mucus.

38. June's religious and cultural beliefs prohibit her from using any artificial method of birth control. She is interested in learning about fertility awareness methods (natural family planning) for contraception. FILL IN THE BLANKS in each of the following statements concerning this method.
    A. The two principal problems with fertility awareness methods are difficulty in determining the exact time of

    _____ and difficulty in _____ for several days before

    and after ovulation. Women with _____ have the greatest risk for failure.

    B. Using the calendar method, June and her husband would abstain from day _____

    to day _____ of her menstrual cycle because her shortest cycle was 23 days and her longest cycle was 33 days.

    C. Basal body temperature (BBT) will _____ about _____

    degrees Celsius at about the time of ovulation. After ovulation, because of increasing levels of _____

    _____, the BBT will _____ about _____

    degrees Celsius. This change in BBT will last until _____ days before menstruation.

    D. The ovulation method would require June to recognize and interpret the cyclic changes in the characteristics

    of her _____, such as _____ and _____

    _____.

    E. The symptothermal method combines _____ with _____

    _____ methods in addition to awareness of secondary phase-related symptoms of the menstrual cycle.

    F. The home predictor test for ovulation detects the sudden surge of _____ in the

    urine that occurs approximately _____ hours before ovulation.

39. Alice and Bob use nonprescription chemical and mechanical contraceptive barriers. LABEL each of the following actions with "C" if correct or "I" if incorrect. INDICATE how the action should be changed for those actions labeled "I."

A. _____ When using a vaginal foam, Alice applies it just inside her vagina.

B. _____ Alice avoids using a spermicide with nonoxynol-9 as a lubricant if she and her husband plan to have anal intercourse.

C. _____ Alice reapplies the spermicide before each act of intercourse.

D. _____ Alice uses a female condom when her husband uses a condom during her fertile period because they want to have the added protection against getting pregnant.

E. _____ Bob applies a condom over his erect penis, leaving an empty space at the tip.

F. _____ Bob often lubricates the outside of a latex condom with Vaseline, a petroleum-based lubricant.

G. _____ Alice and Bob will reuse the female condom if they have intercourse more than once because it is more expensive than the male condom.

MULTIPLE CHOICE: Circle the correct option(s) and state the rationale for the option(s) chosen.

40. A single young-adult woman received instructions from the nurse regarding the use of an oral contraceptive. The woman demonstrates a need for further instruction if she:
    A. Stops asking her sexual partners to use condoms with spermicide
    B. States that her menstrual periods should be shorter with less blood loss
    C. Takes a pill every morning
    D. Uses a barrier method of birth control if she misses two or more pills

41. Oral contraception in the form of a combination of low-dose estrogen and progesterone:
    A. Reduces the pH of cervical mucus, thereby destroying sperm
    B. Protects against iron deficiency anemia by reducing menstrual blood loss
    C. Prevents the transmission of sexually transmitted infections
    D. Is 90% effective in preventing pregnancy when used correctly

42. For some women the most distressing side effect of progestin-only contraception is:
    A. Irregular vaginal bleeding
    B. Headache
    C. Nervousness
    D. Nausea

43. A 36-year-old woman has chosen depot medroxyprogesterone acetate (DMPA, Depo-Provera) as the method of contraception most suitable for her lifestyle. Which statement made by the woman indicates a lack of understanding and a need for further instruction by the nurse?
    A. "I will need to receive another injection every 4 weeks."
    B. "I am going to watch my diet and exercise, because weight gain is common."
    C. "If I plan to continue with the Depo-Provera, I should have my bone density assessed."
    D. "This method will result in a smaller amount of thicker cervical mucus."

44. A woman with an IUD should confirm its placement by checking the IUD's string:
    A. After menses ceases
    B. After intercourse
    C. Two days after ovulation
    D. During menstrual bleeding

45. When teaching women about the effective use of chemical barriers, the nurse should tell them to:
    A. Insert at least 2 hours prior to intercourse
    B. Use nonoxynol-9 (N-9) to inhibit the transmission of HIV
    C. Douche immediately after the last act of intercourse
    D. Reapply before each act of coitus

46. When using a cervical cap (FemCap), the woman should be taught to:
   A. Apply spermicide only to the outside of the cap and around the rim
   B. Leave it in place for a minimum of 6 hours after the last act of coitus
   C. Continue to use the cap during menstrual periods
   D. Check the position of the cap and insert additional spermicide before each act of coitus

47. Joyce has chosen the diaphragm as her method of contraception. Which actions indicate that Joyce is using the diaphragm effectively? (Circle all that apply.)
   A. Joyce came to be refitted after healing was complete following the term vaginal birth of her son.
   B. Joyce applies a spermicide only to the rim of the diaphragm just before insertion.
   C. Joyce empties her bladder before inserting the diaphragm and after intercourse.
   D. Joyce applies more spermicide for each act of intercourse.
   E. Joyce removes the diaphragm within 1 hour of intercourse.
   F. Joyce always uses the diaphragm during her menstrual periods.

48. A woman must assess herself for signs that ovulation is occurring. Which signs are associated with ovulation? (Circle all that apply.)
   A. Increase in the level of LH in her urine 12 to 24 hours before ovulation
   B. Spinnbarkeit
   C. Drop in BBT during the luteal phase of her menstrual cycle
   D. Softened moist cervix, which opens and rises in the vagina
   E. Decreased libido

49. A woman has had a ParaGard T380A IUD inserted. The nurse should recognize that the woman needs further teaching if she says: (Circle all that apply.)
   A. "This IUD remains effective for 10 years."
   B. "It is normal to experience an increase in bleeding and cramping within the first year after it has been inserted."
   C. "My IUD works by releasing progesterone."
   D. "I should avoid using NSAIDs such as Motrin if I have cramping."
   E. "I must use risk prevention measures, including condoms, to prevent infections in my uterus."

50. A 40-year-old male has elected to have a vasectomy because he no longer wants to worry that a sexual partner will become pregnant. The nurse describes the procedure along with care requirements before and after the procedure. Which statements by the client indicate the need for further instruction? (Circle all that apply.)
   A. "I am glad I will not need to use a condom. I hate them!"
   B. "I will use ice packs for a few hours after I get home to reduce swelling and discomfort."
   C. "I will wear a scrotal support for a few days to reduce discomfort."
   D. "I will need to wait about 3 weeks before resuming sexual intercourse."
   E. "I should not expect to see a decrease in the amount of semen I ejaculate."

III. THINKING CRITICALLY

1. A nurse working in a women's health clinic should be aware that toxic shock syndrome (TSS) is a possible complication for women who use a diaphragm or cervical cap as their method of contraception.
   A. CITE the prevention measures that the nurse should teach women to use to reduce their risk for TSS.

   B. IDENTIFY the clinical manifestations of TSS that the nurse should be alert for when assessing women who use diaphragms or cervical caps.

2. Kathy, an 18-year-old client, has come to Planned Parenthood for information on birth control methods and assistance with making her choice. She tells the nurse that she is planning to become sexually active with her boyfriend of 6 months and is worried about getting pregnant. She says, "I know I should know more about all of this but I just don't."

   A. STATE the nursing diagnosis that reflects Kathy's concern.

   B. OUTLINE the approach the nurse should use to help Kathy make an informed decision in choosing contraception that is right for her.

3. June plans to use combined oral contraceptive (COC) pills.

   A. DESCRIBE the mode of action for this type of contraception.

   B. LIST the advantages of using COC pills.

   C. IDENTIFY the factors that, if present in June's health history, would constitute absolute or relative contraindications to the use of oral contraception with estrogen and progesterone.

   D. When caring for June, the nurse must be alert for signs that she is experiencing adverse reactions related to the changing levels of estrogen and progesterone. SPECIFY the estrogen and progesterone reactions the nurse should discuss with June.

   E. Using the acronym ACHES, IDENTIFY the signs and symptoms that would require June to stop taking the pill and notify her health care provider.

   A

   C

H

E

S

F. SPECIFY the instructions the nurse should give June about taking the pill to ensure maximum effectiveness.

4. Beth has decided to try the cervical cap (FemCap) as her method of contraception.
   A. IDENTIFY factors that, if present in Beth's health history, would make her a poor candidate for this contraceptive method.

   B. Following assessment, Beth is determined to be a good candidate for using the cervical cap. DESCRIBE the principles that the nurse should teach Beth to guide her in the safe and effective use of this method.

5. Anita has just had a ParaGard T380A copper IUD inserted. SPECIFY the instructions that the nurse should give Anita before she leaves the women's health clinic after the insertion.

6. Judy (6-4-0-2-4) and Allen, both age 36 years, are contemplating sterilization now that their family is complete. They are seeking counseling regarding this decision.
   A. DESCRIBE the approach a nurse should use in helping Judy and Allen to make the right decision.

   B. The couple decides that Allen will have a vasectomy. DISCUSS the preoperative and postoperative care and instructions required for Allen.

7. Edna is 20 years old and unmarried. She is 8 weeks pregnant and unsure about what to do. She comes to the women's health clinic and asks for the nurse's help in making her decision, stating, "I just cannot support a baby right now. I am alone and trying to finish my education. What can I do?"

A. CITE the nursing diagnosis reflective of Edna's current dilemma.

B. DESCRIBE the approach the nurse should take in helping Edna to make a decision that is right for her.

C. Edna elects to have an abortion. A vacuum aspiration will be performed in the morning. Edna asks what will happen to her as part of the abortion procedure. DESCRIBE how the nurse should respond to Edna's question.

D. IDENTIFY three nursing diagnoses related to Edna's decision and the procedure she is facing.

E. DESCRIBE the nursing measures related to the physical care and emotional support that Edna will require as part of this procedure.

F. OUTLINE the discharge instructions that Edna should receive.

8. A woman is 7 weeks pregnant and seeking an elective abortion. At this stage of gestation she would be a candidate for a medical abortion. CITE the three drugs that are used for this purpose in the United States, and DESCRIBE how each drug works.

9. Marlee comes to the women's health clinic to report that she had unprotected intercourse on the previous night. She is worried about getting pregnant because she is at midcycle and has already noticed signs of ovulation. Marlee tells the nurse that she hardly knows her partner and that her emotions just got the best of her. She is very anxious and asks the nurse what her options are.

A. DESCRIBE the approach this nurse should use to assist Marlee with her concerns.

B. After considering her options, Marlee elects to use Plan B. EXPLAIN what the nurse should tell Marlee about each of the following:
   - What Plan B entails

   - Timing of administration

   - Measures to decrease nausea and vomiting

C. Prior to leaving, Marlee tells the nurse that she is so glad that the Plan B regimen will mean that she will not have to worry about pregnancy. STATE how the nurse should respond.

9 Infertility

I. LEARNING KEY TERMS

MATCHING: Match the description in Column I with the appropriate term in Column II.

COLUMN I

1. _____ Basic test for male infertility.

2. _____ Test that uses fluid infused into the uterus via the cervix to help define the uterine cavity and the depth of the uterine lining via vaginal ultrasound.

3. _____ Examination of the lining of the uterus to assess its response to progesterone and to detect secretory changes and receptivity to implantation. It is not done if pregnancy is possible.

4. _____ Use of a flexible scope threaded through the cervix to view the uterine cavity directly.

5. _____ Examination of the uterine cavity and tubes using radiopaque contrast material instilled through the cervix. It is often used to determine tubal patency and to release a blockage if present.

6. _____ Test used to visualize pelvic tissues and structures for a variety of reasons; it may be accomplished via a transabdominal or transvaginal approach.

7. _____ Visualization of pelvic structures intraperitoneally outside the uterus by inserting a small endoscope through an incision in the anterior abdominal wall.

COLUMN II

A. Laparoscopy
B. Ultrasonography
C. Endometrial biopsy
D. Hysterosalpingography
E. Semen analysis
F. Sonohysterography
G. Hysteroscopy

FILL IN THE BLANKS: Insert the term that corresponds to each of the following descriptions related to alterations in fertility.

8. _____ Term that refers to subfertility, a prolonged time to conceive.

9. _____ Term that refers to an inability to conceive.

10. _____ Collective term used to designate a variety of alternative measures to help infertile couples achieve the goal of a successful pregnancy and live birth; it involves fertility treatments in which both eggs and sperm are handled.

11. _____ A woman's eggs are collected from her ovaries, fertilized in the laboratory with sperm, and transferred to her uterus once normal embryo development has occurred.

12. _____ Selection of one sperm cell that is injected directly into the egg to achieve fertilization.

13. _____ Oocytes are retrieved from the ovary, placed into a catheter with sperm, and immediately transferred into the fimbriated end of the uterine tube; fertilization takes place in the uterine tube.

14. _____ After in vitro fertilization the ova are placed in one uterine tube during the zygote stage.

15. _____ Sperm from a person other than the male partner are used to inseminate the female partner.

16. _____ Embryo(s) from one couple are transferred to the uterus of another woman who has contracted with the couple to carry the baby to term. This woman has no genetic investment in the child.

17. _____ Process by which a woman is inseminated with the semen from the infertile woman's partner and then carries the fetus until birth.

18. _____ The zona pellucida is penetrated chemically or manually to create an opening for the dividing embryo to hatch and to implant into the uterine wall.

19. _____ A donated embryo is transferred to the uterus of an infertile woman at the appropriate time (normal or induced) of the menstrual cycle.

20. _____ Form of early testing designed to eliminate embryos with serious genetic defects before implantation through one of the ARTs and to avoid future termination of pregnancy for genetic reasons.

21. _____ Procedure used to freeze embryos, sperm, ovarian tissue, or oocytes for later implantation.

22. _____ Prepared sperm is placed in the uterus at ovulation.

II. REVIEWING KEY CONCEPTS

23. STATE the type of infertility problem that each of the following medications is designed to treat, and explain the mechanism of action. (Note: You may want to consult the *Physicians' Desk Reference* (PDR) or a nurse's drug manual for more in-depth information on each of these medications.)
clomiphene citrate

follitropins (purified FSH)

Gonadotropin-releasing hormone (GnRh) antagonists (ganirelix acetate)

progesterone

menotropins (human menopausal gonadotropin)

human chorionic gonadotropin (hCG)

metformin

MULTIPLE CHOICE: Circle the correct option(s) and state the rationale for the option(s) chosen.

24. A woman must assess herself for signs that ovulation is occurring. Which of the following is a sign associated with ovulation?
    A. Reduction in level of luteinizing hormone (LH) in the urine 12 to 24 hours prior to ovulation
    B. Spinnbarkeit
    C. Drop in basal body temperature (BBT) following ovulation
    D. Increased thickness of cervical mucus

25. Lifestyle and sexual practices can affect fertility. Which of the following practices could enhance a couple's ability to conceive?
    A. Use balanced nutrition and exercise to achieve a normal body mass index (BMI).
    B. Abstain from alcohol.
    C. Avoid the use of lubricants during intercourse.
    D. Relax in a hot tub every day before going to bed.

26. A woman taking human menopausal gonadotropins for infertility should understand which of the following regarding this medication?
    A. She should take the medication orally, once a day after breakfast.
    B. The medication stimulates the pituitary gland to produce the follicle-stimulating hormone (FSH) and the luteinizing hormone (LH).
    C. She must report for ultrasound testing as scheduled to monitor follicular development.
    D. Progesterone should be administered after seven doses of the gonadotropins have been taken.

27. An infertile woman is given clomiphene citrate (Clomid) to achieve which of the following therapeutic outcomes?
    A. Stimulate the pituitary gland to secrete FSH and LH
    B. Enhance the development of a secretory endometrium
    C. Induce the formation of the corpus luteum
    D. Increase the secretion of favorable cervical mucus to enhance sperm viability

28. When caring for a woman who is scheduled for a hysterosalpingogram, the nurse should do which of the following?
    A. Ensure that the woman is in the secretory phase of her menstrual cycle.
    B. Explain to the woman that the procedure will allow her to conceive.
    C. Report any uterine cramping immediately because it may indicate that the woman's uterus was perforated during the procedure.
    D. Change the woman's position if she complains of shoulder pain following the procedure.

III. THINKING CRITICALLY

1. Mary and Jim have come for their first visit at the fertility clinic. The nurse needs to instruct them about the interrelated structures, functions, and processes essential for conception, emphasizing that they are a biologic unit of reproduction.
    A. PREPARE a lesson plan that explains each component required for normal fertility. INCORPORATE anatomic illustrations to clarify descriptions.

B. SUPPORT the following statement: Assessment of infertility must involve both partners.

2. Mark and his wife, Mary, are undergoing testing for impaired fertility.
   A. DESCRIBE the nursing support measures that should be used when working with this couple.

   B. LIST the components of the assessment for both Mary and Mark.
      Assessment for the woman

      Assessment for the man

   C. Mark must provide a specimen of semen for analysis. DESCRIBE the procedure he should follow to ensure accuracy of the test.

   D. During the assessment process Mark, whose BMI is 31, admits that he smokes a pack of cigarettes every 1 or 2 days and drinks at least two beers each weekday and a few more on the weekend. He tells the nurse that he does this as a way of relieving the stress associated with his job, along with using the hot tub that he and his wife recently installed every evening before bed. DISCUSS how the nurse should respond to these lifestyle patterns.

3. ARTs are being developed and perfected, creating a variety of ethical, legal, financial, and psychosocial concerns. DISCUSS the issues and concerns engendered by these alternative technologies.

4. Suzanne has been scheduled for a diagnostic laparoscopy to determine the basis of her infertility.
   A. INDICATE when during the menstrual cycle this test should be performed.

B. SPECIFY the measures required to prepare Suzanne for this procedure.

C. Suzanne asks the nurse why the test is needed and what will be done during the test. DESCRIBE the nurse's response.

D. SPECIFY the postprocedural care measures required, including the discharge instructions that Suzanne should receive.

5. Sara and Ben have been trying to conceive for 3 years. They have come to an infertility clinic to find out what is wrong. They are distraught because they have been trying for so long to get pregnant. They tell the nurse that they just cannot believe what is happening to them. "None of our friends and no one in our family is having a problem. What's wrong with us?" A diagnosis of infertility is made, necessitating that Sara and Ben make decisions about treatments, use of alternative birth technologies, and adoption.
   A. IDENTIFY the responses that Sara and Ben might exhibit related to the diagnosis of infertility. DESCRIBE one nursing action for each of the responses you have identified.

   B. DISCUSS how the nurse should guide this couple through the decision-making process that is required to determine a course of action that is right for both of them.

   C. The nurse is aware that Sara and Ben, as a devout Jewish couple, may be influenced by cultural and religious beliefs and practices as they make decisions regarding assessment and treatment for infertility. EXPLAIN the approach the nurse should take to identify and then incorporate these beliefs and practices in planning care with the couple.

10 Problems of the Breast

I. LEARNING KEY TERMS

MATCHING: Match the description in Column I with the appropriate benign breast disorder in Column II.

COLUMN I

1. _____ Most common benign breast problem characterized by lumpiness, with or without tenderness, in both breasts.

2. _____ Breast pain.

3. _____ Breast hyperplasia characterized by very large, heavy, pendulous breasts.

4. _____ Discrete, usually solitary lump less than 3 cm in diameter; it is unresponsive to dietary changes or hormone therapy and is the most common solid mass of the breast.

5. _____ Spontaneous, bilateral milky sticky breast discharge unrelated to malignancy.

6. _____ Underdevelopment of breast tissue.

7. _____ Most common benign reactive inflammatory lesion of the breasts, most frequently occurring in middle-aged women. Pain, redness of the skin, nipple inversion, dilated ducts, and greenish nipple discharge are hallmark findings of this disorder.

8. _____ Small, nonpalpable benign lesions in the terminal nipple ducts most often occurring in women 30 to 50 years of age; it is characterized by a serous, serosanguineous, or bloody nipple discharge.

COLUMN II

A. Fibroadenoma
B. Fibrocystic changes
C. Intraductal papilloma
D. Mammary duct ectasia (periductal mastitis)
E. Mastalgia
F. Galactorrhea
G. Macromastia
H. Micromastia

II. REVIEWING KEY CONCEPTS

9. DEFINE each of the following treatment approaches used in the care of women with breast cancer and briefly describe the rationale for their selection.
   A. Chemoprevention

   B. Lumpectomy

   C. Mastectomy (segmental, modified radical, total [simple], preventive/prophylactic)

D. Breast reconstruction (simultaneous or delayed, implant, flap procedure)

E. Radiation (accelerated, brachytherapy, partial)

F. Adjuvant systemic therapy (adjuvant chemotherapy, hormonal therapy, chemotherapy)

MULTIPLE CHOICE: Circle the correct option(s) and state the rationale for the option(s) chosen.

10. When teaching a group of women about breast cancer, the nurse should emphasize: (Circle all that apply.)
    A. The incidence of breast cancer is highest among African-American women.
    B. One in eight American women will develop breast cancer in their lifetime.
    C. The mortality rate from breast cancer has been declining since 1990.
    D. Breast cancer is most prevalent among women in their 30s and 40s.
    E. Most women diagnosed with breast cancer have a family history of the disease.

11. The physician of a 46-year-old premenopausal woman with breast cancer has prescribed tamoxifen (Nolvadex) beginning in the postoperative period following a lumpectomy. What should the nurse teach this woman regarding tamoxifen?
    A. It will help to relieve postoperative discomfort.
    B. She will take 100 mg of tamoxifen four times a day.
    C. Tamoxifen works by blocking the action of progesterone on breast tissue.
    D. She may experience hot flashes and menstrual irregularities when taking tamoxifen.

12. When providing discharge instructions to a woman who had a modified right radical mastectomy, the nurse should emphasize the importance of:
    A. Reporting any tingling or numbness in her incisional site or right arm immediately
    B. Telling health care providers to take a blood pressure or draw blood from her left arm
    C. Learning how to use her left arm to write and accomplish the activities of daily living, such as brushing her hair
    D. Avoiding the use of any deodorant in her right axillary area

13. A 26-year-old woman has just been diagnosed with fibrocystic changes in her breasts. Which nursing diagnosis is appropriate for this woman?
    A. Acute pain related to cyclic enlargement of breast cysts
    B. Risk for infection related to altered integrity of the areola associated with accumulation of a thick sticky discharge from both nipples
    C. Anxiety related to anticipated surgery to remove the cysts in her breasts
    D. Fear related to high risk for breast cancer

14. When assessing a woman with a diagnosis of fibroadenoma, the nurse would expect to find:
    A. Bilateral tender lumps behind the nipple
    B. Milky discharge from one or both nipples
    C. Soft and nonmovable lumps
    D. Firm, well-delineated, movable lump in one breast

70

15. The doctor has prescribed raloxifene hydrochloride for a 58-year-old postmenopausal woman. Which statements indicate that the woman understands the nurse's instructions regarding this medication? (Circle all that apply.)
    A. "I should stop taking my calcium supplement when I am taking this medication."
    B. "This drug can reduce my risk for breast cancer."
    C. "I must take this medication in the morning 1 hour before breakfast."
    D. "I will report to my doctor if I notice swelling in my hands and feet."
    E. "I may start experiencing hot flashes again when taking this medication."

III. THINKING CRITICALLY

1. Breast cancer is a major health problem facing women in the United States. Imagine that you are a nurse who has been invited to discuss the issue of breast cancer with a group of women.
    A. OUTLINE the information that you would give these women about the risk factors associated with breast cancer.

    B. The ages of the women in your class range from 26 to 65 years. SPECIFY the breast screening examinations you would recommend for women across the life span. INDICATE the frequency with which each examination should be performed, according to the American Cancer Society.

    C. DISCUSS several factors that could inhibit these women from participating in the breast screening examinations you identified. SUGGEST several strategies that can be used to overcome these inhibiting factors.

    D. One of the women asks you to discuss the signs associated with breast cancer. DISCUSS the clinical manifestations that are strongly suggestive of breast cancer.

    E. Another woman asks you what would happen if she finds a lump in her breast. SPECIFY the diagnostic tests she could anticipate.

    F. Finally, a woman asks whether breast cancer is hereditary, as she had heard. She further states that she must not have the gene for breast cancer because no one in her family that she knows of has or has had breast cancer. STATE how the nurse should respond.

2. Jane's mother died from breast cancer at the age of 36. Now, at 30 years of age, Jane is concerned about her chances of developing breast cancer herself. She asks you about tests available to detect the gene for breast cancer and wonders if she should have a test performed. She doesn't want to take it if it's not necessary because it is so expensive. Further, she is worried that if her test is positive she will lose her health insurance coverage. DISCUSS your response to Jane's concerns.

3. Mary Anne, a 24-year-old, comes to the women's health clinic complaining that her breasts feel lumpy.
   A. OUTLINE the assessment process that should be used to determine the basis for Mary Anne's complaint.

   B. A diagnosis of fibrocystic breast changes is made. DESCRIBE the clinical manifestations Mary Anne most likely exhibited to support this diagnosis.

   C. STATE one nursing diagnosis that the nurse would identify as a priority when preparing a plan of care for Mary Anne.

   D. IDENTIFY measures the nurse could suggest to Mary Anne for lessening the symptoms she experiences related to fibrocystic changes.

   E. Mary Anne expresses fear that she is now at very high risk for breast cancer. DESCRIBE how the nurse should respond to Mary Anne's expressed fear.

4. Molly, 50 years old, found a lump in her left breast during a breast self-examination (BSE). She comes to the women's health clinic for help.
   A. DESCRIBE the diagnostic protocol that should be followed to determine the basis for the lump Molly found in her breast.

   B. Molly's lump is diagnosed as cancerous. DESCRIBE the emotional effect that this diagnosis and the related treatment is likely to have on Molly and her family.

C. Molly elects to have a modified radical mastectomy based on the information provided by her oncologist regarding her cancer and in consultation with her husband. IDENTIFY two priority nursing diagnoses and OUTLINE the nursing care management for each of the following phases of Molly's treatment.
Preoperative phase

Immediate postoperative phase

D. Molly will be discharged within 48 hours after her surgery. DESCRIBE the instructions that the nurse should give Molly to prepare her for self-care at home.

E. DISCUSS support measures the nurse should use to address the concerns that Molly and her husband will most likely experience and express.

5. Susan has been diagnosed with breast cancer. Her initial treatment included a lumpectomy. In addition, Susan's physician has prescribed adjuvant hormonal therapy using tamoxifen. EXPLAIN to Susan and her family what this medication is and how it works. USE a drug manual to obtain information regarding administration, dosage, and side effects that you will incorporate in a teaching plan to ensure that Susan takes the medication effectively and safely.

6. Annie is a 36-year-old client about to begin chemotherapy for treatment of breast cancer.
A. OUTLINE a teaching plan the nurse would use to prepare Annie and her family for what to expect regarding this treatment method.

B. IDENTIFY two priority nursing diagnoses the nurse should address when developing a plan of care for Annie during her treatment. DESCRIBE two nursing interventions for each nursing diagnosis identified, including the use of alternative therapies.

I. LEARNING KEY TERMS

MATCHING: Match the description in Column I with the appropriate disorder in Column II.

COLUMN I

1. _____ The most common malignancy of the female reproductive system, usually seen in women between the ages of 50 and 65 years.

2. _____ Herniation of the anterior rectal wall through the relaxed or ruptured vaginal fascia and rectovaginal septum.

3. _____ Development of multiple follicular cysts that occurs when an endocrine imbalance results in high levels of estrogen, testosterone, and luteinizing hormone and decreased secretion of follicle-stimulating hormone.

4. _____ Spectrum of disorders arising from the placental trophoblast; it includes hydatidiform mole, invasive mole, and choriocarcinoma.

5. _____ Tumors that are on pedicles, usually originating from the mucosa of the cervix or endometrium.

6. _____ Perforations between genital tract organs, with most occurring between the bladder and the vagina.

7. _____ Germ cell tumors, usually occurring in childhood; they contain substances such as hair, teeth, sebaceous secretions, and bones.

8. _____ Protrusion of the bladder downward into the vagina that develops when supporting structures in the vesicovaginal septum are injured.

9. _____ Slow-growing benign tumors arising in uterine muscle tissue; their growth is influenced by ovarian hormones.

10. _____ Spread of cancer from its original site.

11. _____ Vulvar pain syndrome or vulvovestibulitis; chronic pain disorder of the vulvar area.

12. _____ The most common benign lesion of the vulva.

13. _____ Form of cancer that is strongly linked to the human papillomavirus (types 16 and 18); it is the third most common reproductive cancer.

14. _____ Reproductive cancer with a high mortality rate as a result of being frequently diagnosed in an advanced stage; it is the second most frequently occurring reproductive cancer.

15. _____ Downward displacement of the uterus as a result of diminished pelvic support.

COLUMN II

A. Cystocele
B. Leiomyomas (fibroid tumors)
C. Endometrial cancer
D. Cervical cancer
E. Ovarian cancer
F. Rectocele
G. Polyps
H. Genital fistulas
I. Bartholin cyst
J. Gestational trophoblastic disease (GTD)
K. Uterine prolapse
L. Polycystic ovary syndrome (PCOS)
M. Dermoid cysts
N. Vulvodynia
O. Metastasis

FILL IN THE BLANKS: Insert the treatment that corresponds to each of the following descriptions.

16. _____ Device used to support pelvic organs such as the uterus and hold them in the correct position.

17. _____ Surgery used to repair a cystocele.

18. _____ Surgery used to repair a rectocele.

19. _____ Surgical removal of a leiomyoma (fibroid).

20. _____ Injection of polyvinyl alcohol (PVA) pellets into selected blood vessels to block the blood supply to a leiomyoma (fibroid) in order to cause shrinkage and resolution of symptoms.

21. _____ Use of electrocauterization to destroy small fibroids through a laparoscopic (abdominal) or hysteroscopic (vaginal) approach.

22. _____ Vaporization of tissue inside the uterus.

23. _____ Surgical removal of the entire uterus.

24. _____ Surgical removal of both ovaries and both uterine tubes.

25. _____ Examination of the cervix using a stereoscopic binocular microscope that magnifies the view of the cervix.

26. _____ Removal of a wedge of tissue from the exocervix and endocervix to establish a diagnosis or effect a cure.

27. _____ Treatment that involves destroying abnormal cells by freezing them. Cells slough off and are replaced with the regeneration of normal tissue.

28. _____ Treatment for cervical intraepithelial neoplasia that involves use of a wire loop electrode that can excise and cauterize with minimal tissue damage.

29. _____ Surgical procedure involving the removal of the uterus, tubes, ovaries, and upper third of the vagina along with certain pelvic ligaments and lymph nodes and a portion of the parametrium while preserving the bladder, rectum, and ureters.

30. _____ Surgical removal of the perineum, pelvic floor, levator muscles, all reproductive organs, pelvic lymph nodes, rectum, sigmoid colon, urinary bladder, and distal ureters. A colostomy and ileal conduit are constructed.

31. _____ Surgical removal of all of the vulva (mons pubis, labia majora and minora, and possibly the clitoris).

32. _____ Surgical removal of entire vulva, deep tissues, and the clitoris.

II. REVIEWING KEY CONCEPTS

33. EXPLAIN why ovarian cancer is called the silent disease.

MULTIPLE CHOICE: Circle the correct option(s) and state the rationale for the option(s) chosen.

34. A 60-year-old woman has been diagnosed with a mild prolapse of her uterus. The nurse practitioner could suggest that this woman: (Circle all that apply.)
    A. Assume a knee-chest position for a few minutes several times a day
    B. Use a specially fitted pessary to support her uterus and hold it in the correct position
    C. Begin progestin-only hormone replacement therapy
    D. See a surgeon to discuss the possibility of having an anterior repair (colporrhaphy) performed
    E. Perform Kegel exercises several times each day

Chapter **11** **Structural Disorders and Neoplasms of the Reproductive System**

35. A 35-year-old woman has recently been diagnosed with two leiomyomas in the body of her uterus. This woman can expect to experience which clinical manifestations? (Circle all that apply.)
    A. Shrinkage of tumors if she becomes pregnant
    B. Diarrhea
    C. Dysmenorrhea
    D. Acute abdominal pain
    E. Abnormal uterine bleeding

36. Which measure is the *least* effective in relieving the stress urinary incontinence experienced by a 60-year-old woman with pelvic relaxation?
    A. Performing Kegel exercises
    B. Reducing her intake of oral fluids to 1 L or less per day
    C. Emptying her bladder on a regular basis every 2 hours
    D. Participating in a smoking cessation program to relieve her smoker's cough

37. A 38-year-old premenopausal woman has had a total abdominal hysterectomy (TAH) performed as a result of fibroid tumors that have been increasing in size and causing menorrhagia. Postoperative care for this woman would include instructions regarding:
    A. Taking hormone replacement therapy (HRT), which will begin prior to discharge
    B. Avoiding vigorous exercise and heavy lifting for at least 6 weeks
    C. Performing a Betadine douche daily for the first week postoperatively
    D. Turning, coughing, and deep breathing every 4 hours for the first 24 hours

38. A woman has been diagnosed with carcinoma in situ (CIS) of the cervix. The nurse should prepare this woman for which treatment measure?
    A. Uterine artery embolization (UAE)
    B. Radical hysterectomy
    C. Cervical conization with follow-up Pap tests and colposcopy
    D. Intracavitary and external radiation therapy

III. THINKING CRITICALLY

1. When caring for women across the life span, it is critical that the nurse be alert for risk factors associated with the three most common types of reproductive system cancers.
    A. IDENTIFY the risk factors that increase a woman's vulnerability to the following:
    Endometrial cancer

    Ovarian cancer

    Cervical cancer

    B. DESCRIBE how you as a nurse would use this information when providing health care to women.

Chapter **11** Structural Disorders and Neoplasms of the Reproductive System

2. Denise (6-5-0-1-5), a 60-year-old postmenopausal client, has been diagnosed with a moderate uterine prolapse along with cystocele and rectocele.
   A. DESCRIBE the clinical manifestations Denise most likely exhibited to lead to this diagnosis.

   B. IDENTIFY two priority nursing diagnoses related to the signs and symptoms Denise is most likely experiencing. WRITE one expected outcome for each of the nursing diagnoses identified.

   C. OUTLINE the care management approach recommended for Denise's health problem.

   D. Denise will use a pessary during the day until a surgical repair can be accomplished.
      1. IDENTIFY one nursing diagnosis associated with pessary use.

      2. SPECIFY the instructions the nurse should give to Denise regarding the use and care of a pessary.

   E. Denise has a vaginal hysterectomy and an anterior and posterior colporrhaphy. OUTLINE the postoperative care Denise will require in order to heal without complications.

3. Marie, age 40 years, has been diagnosed with two leiomyomas (fibroid tumors).
   A. DESCRIBE the clinical manifestations most likely exhibited by Marie.

   B. COMPARE the commonly used therapeutic approaches for fibroid tumors. INCLUDE in your answer the criteria that Marie's gynecologist will consider when making a recommendation for treatment.

   C. After consultation with her gynecologist, Marie chooses uterine artery embolization as her treatment. OUTLINE a plan of care for Marie during her preoperative and postoperative periods.

4. Louise, age 60 years, has been diagnosed with endometrial cancer. Because of the early stage of the carcinoma, a total abdominal hysterectomy and bilateral salpingo-oophorectomy is the form of treatment chosen.

   A. IDENTIFY one nursing diagnosis relevant for the preoperative period and one nursing diagnosis relevant for the postoperative period. STATE an expected outcome for each nursing diagnosis identified.

   B. OUTLINE the nursing care and support required for each of the following stages in Louise's treatment.
     Preoperative stage

     Postoperative stage

   C. SPECIFY the instructions that Louise should receive about caring for herself once at home in preparation for discharge.

   D. DISCUSS how Louise's cultural beliefs could affect her responses to her diagnosis of cancer and the need to have her reproductive organs removed.

   E. IDENTIFY one nursing diagnosis associated with Louise's likely emotional response to her diagnosis and treatment.

   F. DISCUSS the support measures the nurse could use to meet Louise's emotional and psychosocial needs as she recovers.

5. Laura has been diagnosed with invasive carcinoma of the cervix and is about to begin a course of radiation therapy.

   A. IDENTIFY two priority nursing diagnoses associated with the course of treatment that Laura is about to undergo. WRITE one expected outcome for each nursing diagnosis identified.

Chapter **11** **Structural Disorders and Neoplasms of the Reproductive System**

B. USE the following outline to summarize the care and support Laura will require at each stage of her treatment regimen.

External radiation
- Pretreatment care

- Care during treatment

- Posttreatment care and instructions

Internal radiation
- Pretreatment care

- Care during treatment

- Posttreatment care and instructions

C. DESCRIBE the self-protection measures the nurse should use when caring for a woman receiving internal radiation therapy.

6. Pat is recovering from a radical vulvectomy that was performed to treat invasive vulvar cancer.
   A. IDENTIFY three nursing measures related to the expected outcome: Pat will heal without the development of infection.

Chapter **11** **Structural Disorders and Neoplasms of the Reproductive System**

B. IDENTIFY three nursing measures related to the expected outcome: Pat will maintain appropriate sexual functioning.

C. DISCUSS the discharge instructions Pat should receive.

7. DISCUSS the issues and emotions that can confront a pregnant woman, her family, and her health care providers when the woman is diagnosed with cancer.

8. Angela has been diagnosed with advanced ovarian cancer. Metastasis has occurred and as a result she will be starting another course of chemotherapy.
   A. OUTLINE the measures you would recommend to relieve the following anticipated problems associated with chemotherapy.
   Altered taste and anorexia

   Nausea and vomiting

   Stomatitis

   Constipation

   Diarrhea

   B. DESCRIBE the approach you would use to support Angela and her family as they cope with the effects of the chemotherapy and the diagnosis of advanced cancer.

12 Conception and Fetal Development

I. LEARNING KEY TERMS

FILL IN THE BLANKS: Insert the term that corresponds to each of the following descriptions related to conception and fetal development.

1. _____ Union of a single egg and sperm. It marks the beginning of a pregnancy.

2. _____ Male and female germ cell. The male germ cell is a _____ _____ and the female germ cell is an _____.

3. _____ The process by which body (somatic) cells replicate to yield two cells, each with the same genetic makeup as the parent cell.

4. _____ The process by which germ cells divide and decrease their chromosome number by half.

5. _____ A cell with 23 single chromosomes.

6. _____ A cell with 46 chromosomes or 23 pairs.

7. _____ Process whereby gametes are formed and mature. For the male the process is called _____ and for the female the process is called _____.

8. _____ Process of successful penetration of the membrane surrounding the ovum by a sperm.

9. _____ The first cell of the new individual.

10. _____ The 16-cell solid ball of cells that develops within 3 days of fertilization.

11. _____ Term used to refer to the solid cell ball when a cavity becomes recognizable within it. The outer layer of cells surrounding this cavity is called the _____.

12. _____ Attachment process whereby the blastocyst burrows into the endometrium at 6 to 10 days after conception.

13. _____ Fingerlike projections develop from the trophoblast and extend into the blood-filled spaces of the endometrium.

14. _____ Term used to refer to the endometrium after implantation.

15. _____ The term used to refer to the developing baby from day 15 until about 8 weeks after conception.

Chapter **12** Conception and Fetal Development

16. _____ The term used to refer to the developing baby from 9 weeks of gestation to the end of pregnancy.

17. _____ Membranes that surround the developing baby and the fluid. The _____ is the outer cell layer of these membranes and the _____ is the inner cell layer.

18. _____ Fluid that surrounds the developing baby in utero. _____ refers to a decreased amount of the fluid (<300 mL). _____ refers to an excessive amount of the fluid (>2 L).

19. _____ Structure that connects the developing baby to the placenta. It contains three vessels, namely, two _____ and one _____. _____ is the connective tissue that prevents compression of the blood vessels to ensure continued nourishment of the developing baby. When it is wrapped around the fetal neck, it is called a _____.

20. _____ Structure composed of 15 to 20 lobes called cotyledons; it serves as a means of metabolic exchange and produces several hormones, including _____, which is the hormone that is the basis of pregnancy tests.

21. _____ Capability of fetus to survive outside the uterus.

22. _____ Special circulatory pathway that allows fetal blood to bypass the lungs.

23. _____ Shunt that allows most fetal blood to bypass the liver and pass into the inferior vena cava.

24. _____ Opening between the atria of the fetal heart.

25. _____ Formation of blood.

26. _____ Surface-active phospholipids that must be present in fetal and newborn lungs to facilitate breathing after birth. The _____ ratio can be performed using amniotic fluid to determine fetal lung maturity.

27. _____ Maternal perception of fetal movement that occurs sometime between 16 and 20 weeks of gestation.

28. _____ Dark green to black tarry substance that contains fetal waste products and accumulates in the fetal intestines.

29. _____ Twins that are formed from two zygotes. They are also called _____ twins.

30. _____ Twins that are formed from one fertilized ovum that then divides. They are also called _____ twins. _____ Term used to describe twins when there is an incomplete embryonic division.

31. _____ Disorders that are present at birth as a result of genetic inheritance, environmental factors, or inadequate maternal nutrition.

32. _____ Environmental substances or exposures that cause abnormal fetal development.

33. Each of the following structures plays a critical role in fetal growth and development. DESCRIBE the functions of these structures.
    - Yolk sac

    - Amniotic fluid and membranes

    - Umbilical cord

    - Placenta

34. NAME the three primary germ layers and identify the tissues or organs that develop from each layer.

MULTIPLE CHOICE: Circle the correct option(s) and state the rationale for the option(s) chosen.

35. When teaching a class of pregnant women about fetal development, the nurse would include which statements? (Circle all that apply.)
    A. "The sex of your baby is determined by the 9th week of pregnancy."
    B. "Your baby will be able to suck and hiccup while in your uterus."
    C. "The baby's heart begins to pump blood during the 10th week of pregnancy."
    D. "The baby's heartbeat will be audible using a special ultrasound stethoscope beginning at the 18th week of pregnancy."
    E. "You should be able to feel your baby move by week 16 to 20 of pregnancy."
    F. "By the 24th week of your pregnancy you will notice your baby responding to sounds in the environment, including music and your voice."

36. The results of an amniocentesis show that the pregnant woman's lecithin-sphingomyelin (L/S) ratio is 2:1. This result indicates that:
    A. The woman is in her second trimester of pregnancy
    B. The newborn should be able to maintain effective respiration after birth
    C. The fetus most likely has developed a renal problem
    D. An open neural tube defect is present

37. If a pregnant woman's intake of iron is sufficient, her newborn will have enough iron stored in its liver to last approximately how many months after birth?
   A. 1 month
   B. 3 months
   C. 5 months
   D. 9 months

38. When caring for pregnant women, the nurse would recognize that a woman with which disorder has the greatest risk for giving birth to a macrosomic newborn?
   A. Diabetes
   B. Anemia
   C. Hyperthyroidism
   D. Hypertension

III. THINKING CRITICALLY

1. IMAGINE that you are a nurse-midwife working in partnership with an obstetrician. FORMULATE a response to each of the following concerns or questions directed to you from some of your prenatal clients.
   A. June (2 months pregnant), Mary (5 months pregnant), and Alice (7 months pregnant) each ask for a description of their fetus at the present time.
   June

   Mary

   Alice

   B. Jessica states that a friend told her that babies born after about 35 weeks have a better chance of survival because they can breathe more easily. She asks if this is true.

   C. Beth, who is 1 month pregnant, states that she heard that women who are pregnant experience quickening. She wants to know what that means and if it hurts.

   D. Susan, who is 6 months pregnant, states that she read in a magazine that a fetus can actually hear and see. She feels that this is totally unbelievable!

E. Alexa is 2 months pregnant. She asks how the sex of her baby is determined and if a sonogram can tell whether she is having a boy or a girl.

F. Karen is pregnant for the first time. She reveals that she has a history of twins in her family. She wants to know what causes twin pregnancies to occur and what the difference is between identical and fraternal twins.

G. Louise is beginning her second trimester. She tells the nurse that a friend who just had a baby told her that her position and activity can affect how her baby grows and develops. Louise asks if this is true.

13 Anatomy and Physiology of Pregnancy

I. LEARNING KEY TERMS

MATCHING: Match the assessment finding in Column I with the appropriate descriptive term in Column II.

COLUMN I

1. _____ Menstrual bleeding no longer occurs.
2. _____ Fundal height decreased and fetal head descended into the pelvis.
3. _____ Cervix and vagina are violet-bluish in color.
4. _____ Swelling of ankles and feet at the end of the day.
5. _____ Cervical tip softened.
6. _____ Lower uterine segment is soft and compressible.
7. _____ Fetal head rebounds with gentle, upward tapping through the vagina.
8. _____ White or slightly gray mucoid vaginal discharge with faint, musty odor.
9. _____ Enlarged sebaceous glands in areola on both breasts.
10. _____ Plug of mucus fills endocervical canal.
11. _____ Pink stretch marks or depressed streaks on breasts and abdomen.
12. _____ Creamy white to yellowish to orange premilk fluid expressed from nipples.
13. _____ Cheeks, nose, and forehead blotchy; brownish hyperpigmentation.
14. _____ Pigmented line extending up abdominal midline.
15. _____ Red raised nodule on gums; bleeds after brushing teeth.
16. _____ Heartburn experienced after supper.
17. _____ Lumbosacral curve accentuated.
18. _____ Paresthesia and pain in right hand radiating to elbow.
19. _____ Spotting following cervical palpation or intercourse.
20. _____ Hematocrit decreased to 36% and hemoglobin to 11 g/dL.
21. _____ Vascular spiders on neck and thorax.
22. _____ Palms pinkish red and mottled.
23. _____ Abdominal wall muscles separated.
24. _____ Varicosities around the anus.

COLUMN II

A. Colostrum
B. Operculum
C. Amenorrhea
D. Angiomas
E. Pyrosis
F. Friability
G. Striae gravidarum
H. Physiologic anemia
I. Linea nigra
J. Ballottement
K. Chadwick sign
L. Diastasis recti abdominis
M. Lordosis
N. Leukorrhea
O. Chloasma (mask of pregnancy; facial melasma)
P. Lightening
Q. Hemorrhoids
R. Palmar erythema
S. Goodell sign
T. Physiologic/dependent edema
U. Hegar sign
V. Montgomery tubercles/glands
W. Carpal tunnel syndrome
X. Epulis (gingival granuloma gravidarum)

FILL IN THE BLANKS: Insert the term that corresponds to each of the following descriptions related to pregnancy.

25. _____ Pregnancy.

26. _____ The number of pregnancies in which the fetus or fetuses have reached 20 weeks of gestation, not the number of fetuses (e.g., twins) born. The numeric designation is not affected by whether the fetus is born alive or is stillborn (i.e., showing no signs of life at birth).

27. _____ A woman who is pregnant.

28. _____ A woman who has never been pregnant and is not currently pregnant.

29. _____ A woman who has not completed a pregnancy with a fetus or fetuses beyond 20 weeks of gestation.

30. _____ A woman who is pregnant for the first time.

31. _____ A woman who has completed one pregnancy with a fetus or fetuses who have reached 20 weeks of gestation.

32. _____ A woman who has had two or more pregnancies.

33. _____ A woman who has completed two or more pregnancies to 20 weeks of gestation.

34. _____ Capacity to live outside the uterus at about 22 to 25 weeks of gestation.

35. _____ Designation given to a pregnancy that has reached 20 weeks of gestation but ends before completion of 37 weeks of gestation.

36. _____ Designation given to a pregnancy from the beginning of week 38 of gestation to the end of week 42 of gestation.

37. _____ Designation given to a pregnancy that goes beyond 42 weeks of gestation.

38. _____ Presence of this biochemical marker in maternal urine or serum results in a positive pregnancy test result.

39. _____ Pregnancy-related changes felt by the woman.

40. _____ Pregnancy-related changes that can be observed by an examiner.

41. _____ Signs that can be attributed only to the presence of a fetus.

42. _____ Uterine contractions that can be felt through the abdominal wall soon after the fourth month of pregnancy.

43. _____ A rushing or blowing sound of maternal blood flow through the uterine arteries to the placenta that is synchronous with the maternal pulse.

44. _____ Sound of fetal blood coursing through the umbilical cord; it is synchronous with the fetal heart rate.

45. _____ Fetal movements first felt by the pregnant woman from 14 to 18 weeks of gestation.

46. _____ Change in blood pressure as a result of compression of abdominal blood vessels and decrease in cardiac output when a pregnant woman lies on her back.

47. _____ Itching of the skin that occurs during pregnancy; _____ a common dermatosis that can occur during pregnancy.

48. _____ Nonfood cravings for substances such as ice, clay, and laundry starch.

49. _____ Excessive salivation.

50. DESCRIBE the obstetric history for each of the following women, using both the 2-digit and the 5-digit systems.

    A. Nancy is pregnant. Her first pregnancy resulted in a stillbirth at 36 weeks of gestation, and her second pregnancy resulted in the birth of her daughter at 42 weeks of gestation.

    B. Marsha is 6 weeks pregnant. Her previous pregnancies resulted in the live birth of a daughter at 40 weeks of gestation, the live birth of a son at 38 weeks of gestation, and a spontaneous abortion at 10 weeks of gestation.

    C. Linda is experiencing her fourth pregnancy. Her first pregnancy ended in a spontaneous abortion at 12 weeks of gestation, the second resulted in the live birth of twin boys at 32 weeks of gestation, and the third resulted in the live birth of a daughter at 39 weeks of gestation.

51. When assessing a pregnant woman a nurse should keep in mind that baseline vital sign values will change as she progresses through her pregnancy. DESCRIBE how each of the following changes as pregnancy progresses.

    ■ Blood pressure

    ■ Heart rate and patterns

    ■ Respiratory rate and patterns

    ■ Body temperature

52. CALCULATE the mean arterial pressure (MAP) for each of the following blood pressure (BP) readings.

    ■ 120/76 mm Hg

Chapter **13 Anatomy and Physiology of Pregnancy**

- 114/64 mm Hg

- 110/80 mm Hg

- 150/90 mm Hg

53. SPECIFY the value changes that occur in the following laboratory tests. STATE the rationale for these changes in terms of the expected physiologic adaptations to pregnancy.
    - Complete blood count (CBC): hematocrit, hemoglobin, white blood cell count, platelets

    - Clotting activity

    - Acid-base balance

    - Urinalysis

54. DISCUSS how and why the levels of each of the following substances change during pregnancy.
    - Parathyroid hormone

    - Insulin

- Estrogen

- Progesterone

- Thyroid hormones

- Human chorionic gonadotropin (hCG)

MULTIPLE CHOICE: Circle the correct option(s) and state the rationale for the option(s) chosen.

55. When assessing pregnant women during routine prenatal checkups, which findings would be categorized as probable signs of pregnancy? (Circle all that apply.)
    A. Human chorionic gonadotropin in the urine
    B. Breast tenderness
    C. Morning sickness
    D. Fetal heart sounds
    E. Ballottement
    F. Hegar sign

56. A pregnant woman with four children reports the following obstetric history: a stillbirth at 32 weeks of gestation, triplets (two sons and a daughter) born via cesarean section at 30 weeks of gestation, a spontaneous abortion at 8 weeks of gestation, and a daughter born vaginally at 39 weeks of gestation. What accurately expresses this woman's current obstetric history, using the 5-digit system?
    A. 5-1-4-1-4
    B. 4-1-3-1-4
    C. 5-2-2-0-3
    D. 5-1-2-1-4

57. An essential component of prenatal health assessment of pregnant women is the determination of vital signs. An expected change in vital sign findings as a result of pregnancy is:
    A. Increase in systolic BP by 30 mm Hg or more after assuming a supine position
    B. Increase in diastolic BP by 5 to 10 mm Hg beginning in the first trimester
    C. Increased awareness of the need to breathe as pregnancy progresses
    D. Gradual decrease in baseline pulse rate of approximately 20 beats/minute

58. A woman exhibits understanding of the instructions for performing a home pregnancy test to maximize accuracy if she:
    A. Uses urine collected at the end of the day, just before going to bed
    B. Avoids using Tylenol or aspirin for a headache for about 1 week prior to performing the test
    C. Performs the test on the day she expects her menstrual period to occur
    D. Records the day of her last menstrual period and her usual cycle length

59. During an examination of a pregnant woman, the nurse notes that the woman's cervix is soft on its tip. The nurse documents this finding as:
   A. Friability
   B. Goodell sign
   C. Chadwick sign
   D. Hegar sign

III. THINKING CRITICALLY

1. DESCRIBE how a nurse should respond to each of the following client concerns and questions.
   A. Tina is 16 weeks pregnant. She calls the prenatal clinic to report that she noticed slight painless spotting this morning. She reveals that she did have intercourse with her partner the night before.

   B. Lisa suspects that she is pregnant because her menstrual period is already 3 weeks late. She asks her friend, who is a nurse, how to use the pregnancy test that she just bought so that she can obtain the best results.

   C. Joan is 3 months pregnant. She tells the nurse that she is worried because a friend told her that vaginal and bladder infections are more common during pregnancy. She wants to know if this could be true and, if so, why.

   D. Tammy, who is 20 weeks pregnant, tells the nurse that she has noted some "problems" with her breasts. There are "little pimples" near her nipples and her breasts feel "lumpy and bumpy" and "leak a little" when she performs a breast self-examination (BSE).

   E. Tamara is concerned because she read in a book about pregnancy that a pregnant woman's position could affect her circulation, especially to the baby. She asks what positions are good for her circulation now that she is pregnant.

   F. Beth, a pregnant client, calls to tell the nurse that she had a nosebleed this morning and has noticed occasional feelings of fullness in her ears. She asks if these occurrences are anything to worry about.

   G. Karen is 7 months pregnant and works as a secretary full time. She asks the nurse if she should take a "water pill" that a friend gave her, because she has noticed that her ankles "swell up" at the end of the day.

H. Jan is in her third trimester of pregnancy. She tells the nurse that her posture seems to have changed and that she occasionally experiences low back pain.

I. Monica, who is 36 weeks pregnant with her first baby, calls the clinic stating that she knows the baby is coming because she felt some uterine contractions before getting out of bed in the morning. Monica confirms that they seem to have decreased in intensity and frequency since she has gotten out of bed and walked around.

J. Nina is a primigravida who is at 32 weeks of gestation. When she comes for a prenatal visit she reports that she has been experiencing occasional periods of shortness of breath during the day and sometimes has to use an extra pillow to sleep comfortably. Nina expresses concern that she is developing a breathing problem.

K. Shade, a primigravida, is at 26 weeks of gestation. She has recently begun to experience difficulty moving her bowels. Shade reports that she has a bowel movement every 2 days or so now instead of daily and that her stool is firmer and a little harder to pass.

2. Accurate BP readings are critical if significant changes in the cardiovascular system are to be detected as a woman adapts to pregnancy during the prenatal period. WRITE a protocol for BP assessment that can be used by nurses working in a prenatal clinic to ensure accuracy of the results obtained during BP assessment.

14 Nursing Care of the Family During Pregnancy

I. LEARNING KEY TERMS

FILL IN THE BLANKS: Insert the term that corresponds to each of the following descriptions.

1. _____ Indicators of pregnancy that can be caused by conditions other than gestation and are not reliable for diagnosis; they include subjective symptoms and objective signs.

2. _____ Indicators of pregnancy that are detected by an examiner and are related mainly to physical changes in the uterus; they strongly suggest pregnancy but are not conclusive.

3. _____ Indicators of pregnancy that are attributed directly to the fetus.

4. _____ Method used to determine the expected date of birth (EDB) by subtracting

_____ and adding _____ and _____

(if appropriate) to the first day of the last normal menstrual period (LNMP). Alternatively, _____

_____ can be added to the first day of the LNMP and counting forward _____.

5. _____ One of three periods of pregnancy, each of which is approximately 3 months in length.

6. _____ Change in blood pressure that can occur when a pregnant woman lies on her

back and the _____ and the _____ are compressed by abdominal contents, including the uterus.

7. _____ Uterine measurement that is performed beginning in the second trimester as one indicator of the progress of fetal growth.

8. _____ Test used to determine whether the nipple is everted or inverted, achieved by placing thumb and forefinger on the areola and gently pressing inward.

9. _____, _____, _____,

_____, and _____ Developmental tasks that are accomplished by parents as they adapt to the changes of pregnancy and impending parenthood.

10. _____ Rapid unpredictable changes in mood related to profound hormonal changes and concerns about finances and changed lifestyle.

11. _____ Emotional state of having conflicting feelings about a pregnancy simultaneously; it is considered a normal response to pregnancy.

12. As a pregnant woman establishes a relationship with her fetus and emotional attachment begins, she progresses through three phases. In phase one she accepts the _____ and needs to be able to state _____. In phase two the woman accepts the _____. She can now say _____. Finally, in phase three the woman prepares realistically for the _____ and _____. She expresses the thought _____ _____.

13. _____ Phenomenon of an expectant father experiencing pregnancy-like symptoms such as nausea, weight gain, and other physical symptoms.

14. _____ The first period of paternal adaptation, during which the father accepts the _____. During the second or _____ phase, the father adjusts to the reality of the pregnancy. The developmental task is to _____. The father becomes actively involved in the pregnancy and the relationship with his child during the third or _____ phase. The developmental task is to negotiate with his partner the role he is to play in _____ and to prepare for _____.

15. _____ Cultural practices that tell a woman what to do during pregnancy.

16. _____ Cultural practices that tell a woman what not to do during pregnancy; they establish _____.

17. _____ Multiple marker screen involving two blood tests and one ultrasound offered to women who start prenatal care before 14 weeks of gestation; it is used to identify such conditions as Down syndrome, neural tube defects, and abdominal wall abnormalities.

18. _____ Genetic testing technology used to identify fetuses at risk for trisomies 21, 18, and 13 and sex chromosome abnormalities.

19. _____ Woman professionally trained to provide physical, emotional, and informational support to women and their partners during labor and birth.

20. _____ Tool that can be used by parents to explore their childbirth options and choose those that are most important to them; it serves as a tentative guide because the realities of what is feasible may change as the actual labor and birth progress.

II. REVIEWING KEY CONCEPTS

21. CALCULATE the expected date of birth (EDB) for each of the following pregnant women using Nägele's rule.
    A. Diane's last normal menses began on May 5, 2014, and ended on May 10, 2014.

    B. Sara had intercourse on February 21, 2014. She has not had a menstrual period since the one that began on January 14, 2014, and ended 5 days later.

C. Beth's last normal menstrual period began on September 4, 2014, and ended on September 10, 2014. Beth noted that her basal body temperature (BBT) rose on the morning of September 28, 2014.

22. Cultural beliefs and practices are important influencing factors during the prenatal period.
    A. DESCRIBE how cultural beliefs can affect a woman's participation in prenatal care as it is defined by Western medicine's view of pregnancy and its problems.

    B. IDENTIFY one prescription and one proscription for each of the following areas. EXPLAIN how these beliefs can affect prenatal health care and practices.
       ■ Emotional response

       ■ Clothing

       ■ Physical activity and rest

       ■ Sexual activity

       ■ Diet

23. OUTLINE the assessment measures that should be used and the data that should be collected during each component of the initial prenatal visit and the follow-up prenatal visits.

INITIAL PRENATAL VISIT
Health History Interview

Physical Examination

Laboratory and Diagnostic Testing

FOLLOW-UP PRENATAL VISITS
Updating History Interview

Physical Examination

Fetal Assessment

Laboratory and Diagnostic Testing

24. Marie asks the nurse what can be done during a prenatal visit to ensure that her baby is healthy and doing well. IDENTIFY and DESCRIBE what the nurse could tell Marie about the components of fetal assessment that will determine her baby's health status.

25. Nurses responsible for the care management of pregnant women must be alert for warning signs of complications that women could develop as pregnancy progresses from trimester to trimester.
    A. LIST the signs of potential complications (warning signs) for each trimester of pregnancy. INDICATE possible cause(s) for each sign listed.

    B. DESCRIBE the approach a nurse should take when discussing potential complications with a pregnant woman and her family.

26. Nurses working in a prenatal clinic become concerned that the fundal height measurement technique they used was inconsistent and resulted in variations in findings. They decide to create a protocol for fundal measurement that will facilitate accuracy. DISCUSS what they should include in the protocol that they create.

27. IDENTIFY four factors that a nurse should use to estimate the gestational age of a fetus.

28. Prevention of injury is an important goal for nurses as they teach pregnant women about how to care for themselves during pregnancy.
    A. DESCRIBE three principles of body mechanics that a pregnant woman should be taught to prevent injury.

    B. IDENTIFY five safety guidelines that the nurse should include in a pamphlet titled "Safety During Pregnancy" that will be distributed to pregnant women during prenatal visits.

29. During the third trimester, parents often make a decision concerning the method they will use to feed their newborn. LIST reasons cited for choosing to bottle-feed rather than breastfeed. As a nurse, how might you address these reasons to help the parents to consider the possibility of breastfeeding?

MULTIPLE CHOICE: Circle the correct option(s) and state the rationale for the option(s) chosen.

30. A nurse is assessing a pregnant woman during a prenatal visit. Several presumptive indicators of pregnancy are documented. Presumptive indicators include: (Circle all that apply.)
    A. Nausea and vomiting
    B. Quickening
    C. Hegar sign
    D. Palpation of fetal movement by the nurse
    E. Amenorrhea
    F. Positive pregnancy test

31. A woman's last normal menstrual period (LNMP) began on November 9, 2014, and ended on November 14, 2014. Using Nägele's rule, the estimated date of birth is:
    A. July 2, 2015
    B. July 7, 2015
    C. August 16, 2015
    D. August 21, 2015

32. A woman at 30 weeks of gestation assumes a supine position for a fundal measurement and Leopold maneuvers. She begins to complain about feeling dizzy and nauseated. Her skin feels damp and cool. The nurse's first action is to:
    A. Assess the woman's blood pressure and pulse
    B. Provide the woman with an emesis basin
    C. Elevate the woman's legs 20 degrees from her hips
    D. Turn the woman onto her left side

33. During an early-bird prenatal class, a nurse teaches a group of newly diagnosed pregnant women about their emotional reactions during pregnancy. What topics should the nurse discuss with the women? (Circle all that apply.)
    A. Sexual desire (libido) usually increases during the second trimester of pregnancy.
    B. A referral for counseling should be sought if a woman experiences conflicting feelings about her pregnancy in the first trimester.
    C. Rapid, unpredictable mood swings reflect gestational bipolar disorder.
    D. A quiet period of introspection is often experienced around the time a woman feels her baby move for the first time.
    E. A woman's own mother is usually her greatest source of emotional support during pregnancy.
    F. Attachment to her baby begins late in the third trimester, when she begins attending childbirth preparation classes and realizes that the baby will arrive soon.

34. The nurse evaluates a pregnant woman's knowledge about prevention of urinary tract infections (UTIs) at the prenatal visit following a class on infection prevention that the woman attended. The nurse recognizes that the woman needs further instruction when she tells the nurse about which measures that she now uses to prevent urinary tract infections. (Circle all that apply.)
    A. "I drink about one quart of fluid a day."
    B. "I have stopped using bubble baths and bath oils."
    C. "I have started wearing panty hose and underpants with a cotton crotch."
    D. "I have intercourse with my husband only once a week now because it could lead to bladder infections."
    E. "If I drink cranberry juice at least twice a day, I will not get an infection."

35. Doulas are becoming important members of a laboring woman's health care team. Which activity should be expected as part of the doula's responsibilities?
    A. Monitoring hydration of the laboring woman, including adjusting intravenous (IV) flow rates
    B. Interpreting electronic fetal monitoring tracings to determine the well-being of the maternal-fetal unit
    C. Eliminating the need for the husband or partner to be present during labor and birth
    D. Providing continuous support throughout labor and birth, including explanations of labor progress

III. THINKING CRITICALLY

1. A health history interview of the pregnant woman by the nurse is included as part of the initial prenatal visit.
    A. STATE the purpose of the health history interview.

    B. WRITE two questions for each component that is included in the initial health history interview. Questions should be clear, concise, and understandable. Most of the questions should be open-ended to elicit the most complete response from the client.

    C. WRITE four questions that should be included when doing an updating health history interview during follow-up visits.

102

2. IMAGINE that you are a nurse working in a prenatal clinic. You have been assigned to be the primary nurse for Martha, an 18-year-old, who has come to the clinic for confirmation of pregnancy. She tells you that she knows she is pregnant because she has already missed three periods and a home pregnancy test that she did last week was positive. Martha states that she has had very little contact with the health care system and the only reason she came today is because her boyfriend insisted that she "make sure" she is really pregnant. DESCRIBE the approach that you would take regarding data collection and the nursing intervention that is appropriate for this woman.

3. Terry is a primigravida in her first trimester of pregnancy. She is accompanied by her husband, Tim, to her second prenatal visit. ANSWER each of the following questions asked by Terry and Tim.
   A. "At the last visit I was told that my baby's estimated date of birth is December 25, 2014! Can I really count on my baby being born on Christmas Day?"

   B. "Before I became pregnant, my friend told me I should be doing Kegel exercises. I was too embarrassed to ask her about them. What are they and is it safe for me to do them while I am pregnant?"

   C. "What effect will pregnancy have on our sex life? We are willing to abstain during pregnancy if we must to keep our baby safe."

   D. "This morning sickness I am experiencing is driving me crazy. I become nauseated in the morning and again late in the afternoon. Occasionally I vomit or have the dry heaves. Will this last for my entire pregnancy? Is there anything I can do to feel better?"

4. Tara is 2 months pregnant. She tells the nurse at the prenatal clinic that she is used to being active and that she exercises every day. Now that she is pregnant she wonders if she should shorten or stop her exercise routine. DISCUSS the nurse's response to Tara.

5. WRITE one nursing diagnosis for each of the following situations. STATE one expected outcome and LIST appropriate nursing measures for the nursing diagnosis you identified.
   A. Beth is 6 weeks pregnant. During the health history interview she tells you that she has limited her intake of fluids and tries to hold her urine for as long as she can because "I just hate having to go to the bathroom so frequently."

Nursing Diagnosis	Expected Outcome	Nursing Measures

   B. Doris, who is 23 weeks pregnant, tells you that she is beginning to experience more frequent lower back pain. You note that when she walked into the examining room, her posture exhibited a moderate degree of lordosis and neck flexion. She was wearing shoes with 2-inch-high narrow heels.

Nursing Diagnosis	Expected Outcome	Nursing Measures

   C. Lisa, a primigravida at 32 weeks of gestation, comes for a prenatal visit accompanied by her partner, the father of the baby. They both express anxiety about the impending birth of the baby and how they will handle the experience of labor. Lisa is especially concerned about how she will survive the pain, and her partner is primarily concerned about how he will help Lisa to cope with labor and ensure that she and the baby are safe.

Nursing Diagnosis	Expected Outcome	Nursing Measures

6. Jane is a primigravida in her second trimester of pregnancy. ANSWER each of the following questions asked by Jane during a prenatal visit.
   A. "Why do you measure my abdomen every time I come in for a checkup?"

B. "How can you tell if my baby is doing okay?"

C. "I am going to start changing the way that I dress now that I am beginning to show. Do you have any suggestions I could follow, especially because I have a limited amount of money to spend?"

D. "What can I do about gas and constipation? I never had much of a problem before I was pregnant."

E. "Since yesterday I have started to feel itchy all over. Do you think I am coming down with some sort of infection?"

F. "I will be flying to Chicago to visit my father in 1 month. Is airline travel safe for me when I am 5 months pregnant?"

7. While a nurse is measuring a pregnant woman's fundus, the woman becomes pale and diaphoretic. The woman, who is at 23 weeks of gestation, states that she feels dizzy and lightheaded.
A. STATE the most likely explanation for the assessment findings exhibited by this woman.

B. DESCRIBE the nurse's immediate action.

8. Kelly is a primigravida in her third trimester of pregnancy. ANSWER each of the following questions asked by Kelly during a prenatal visit.
A. "My husband and I have decided to breastfeed our baby but friends told me it is very difficult if my nipples do not come out. Is there any way I can tell now if my nipples are okay for breastfeeding?"

B. "My ankles are swollen by the time I get home from work late in the afternoon (Kelly teaches second grade). I have been trying to drink about 3 liters of fluid every day. Should I reduce the amount of liquid I am drinking or ask my doctor for a water pill?"

C. "I woke up last night with a terrible cramp in my leg. It finally went away but my husband and I just did not know what to do. What if this happens again tonight?"

9. Tanisha, a pregnant woman at 26 weeks of gestation, and her husband, George, tell the nurse at a prenatal visit that their friends who live in another state had a baby 2 months ago and employed a doula to help them during childbirth. Their friends recommended that they do the same because the doula was wonderful. Tanisha and George are unsure whether they should spend the extra money, asking the nurse exactly what doulas do and where they could find one.
   A. DESCRIBE what the nurse should tell this couple about the role of the doula during labor and birth, including how it could be of benefit to them.

   B. STATE what the nurse should tell this couple about how to find a doula and the importance of interviewing her before they make a commitment to ensure that she is a good "fit" for them.

10. Carol is 4 months pregnant and is beginning to "show." She asks the nurse what she should expect as a reaction from her 13-year-old daughter and 3-year-old son. DESCRIBE the response the nurse would make.

11. Your neighbor, Jane Smith, is in her second month of pregnancy. Knowing that you are a nurse, her husband, Tom, confides in you that he just "cannot figure Jane out. One minute she is happy and the next minute she is crying for no reason at all! I do not know how I will be able to cope with this for 7 more months."
    A. WRITE a nursing diagnosis and expected outcome that reflects Tom's concern.

    B. DISCUSS how you would respond to his concern.

12. Jim's partner, Mary, is 5 months pregnant. He tells you that sometimes he feels "left out" of Mary's pregnancy and asks you if he is important to Mary as her partner and the father of the baby. SPECIFY how you would answer his question.

13. Jennifer (2-1-0-0-1) and her husband, Dan, are beginning their third trimester of a low-risk pregnancy. As you work with them on their birth plan, they tell you that they are having trouble making a decision about their choice of a birth setting. They experienced a delivery room birth with their first child. Jennifer states, "My first pregnancy was perfectly normal just like this one but the birth was disappointing, so medically focused with monitors, IVs, and staying in bed." They ask you for your advice about the different birth settings they have heard and read about, namely, labor, delivery, recovery, and postpartum (LDRP) rooms at their local hospital, the birthing center a few miles from their home, and even their own home. DESCRIBE the approach you would take to guide Jennifer and Dan in their decision making regarding a birth setting.

14. Tony and Andrea are considering the possibility of giving birth to their second baby at home. They have been receiving prenatal care from a certified nurse-midwife who has experience with home birth. Their 5-year-old son and both sets of grandparents want to be present for the birth.
   A. DISCUSS the decision-making process that Tony and Andrea should follow to ensure that they make an informed decision that is right for them and their family.

   B. Tony and Andrea decide that home birth is an ideal choice for them. OUTLINE the preparation measures you would recommend to them to ensure a safe and positive experience for everyone.

Chapter **14** **Nursing Care of the Family During Pregnancy**

15 Maternal and Fetal Nutrition

FILL IN THE BLANKS: Insert the term that corresponds to each of the following descriptions.

1. _____ Birth weight of 2500 g or less.

2. _____ The best way to ensure that adequate nutrients are available for the developing fetus.

3. _____ Nutrient, the adequate intake of which is important for decreasing risk for _____ or failures in the closure of the neural tube. An intake of _____ _____ daily is recommended for all women capable of becoming pregnant.

4. _____ Recommendations for daily nutritional intakes that meet the needs of almost all healthy members of the population.

5. _____ Method used to evaluate the appropriateness of weight for height. If the calculated value is less than 18.5, the person is considered to be _____. If the calculated value is between 18.5 and 24.9, the person is considered to be _____. If the calculated value is between 25 and 29.9 the person is considered to be _____, and if the calculated value is 30 or greater, the person is considered to be _____.

6. _____ Presence of ketones in the urine as a result of catabolism of fat stores; it is associated with the occurrence of _____.

7. _____ Normal adaptation that occurs during pregnancy when the plasma volume increases more rapidly than red blood cell (RBC) mass.

8. _____ Inability to digest milk sugar because of the absence of the lactase enzyme in the small intestine.

9. _____ The practice of consuming nonfood substances such as _____ _____, _____, and _____ or excessive amounts of foodstuffs that are low in nutritional value, such as _____, _____ _____, _____, and _____.

10. _____ Urge to consume specific types of foods, such as ice cream, pickles, and pizza, during pregnancy.

11. _____ Infection that can occur as a result of consuming certain foods such as unpasteurized milk or products made with unpasteurized milk, raw fish or seafood, raw dough or batter, and unpasteurized juice; it increases the risk for miscarriage, premature birth, and stillbirth.

12. _____ Body measurements such as height and weight.

13. _____ Guide that can be used to make daily food choices during pregnancy and lactation, just as during other stages of the life cycle.

14. _____ A discomfort most commonly experienced in the first trimester of pregnancy; it usually causes only mild to moderate nutritional problems but may be a source of substantial discomfort.

15. _____ Severe and persistent vomiting during pregnancy causing weight loss, dehydration, and electrolyte abnormalities.

16. _____ Discomfort of pregnancy characterized by infrequent and difficult passage of hard, dry stool.

17. _____ Discomfort of pregnancy that is usually caused by reflux of gastric contents into the esophagus.

II. REVIEWING KEY CONCEPTS

18. INDICATE the importance of each of the following nutrients for healthy maternal adaptation to pregnancy and optimum fetal growth and development. INDICATE three food or fluid sources for each of the nutrients.

NUTRIENT	IMPORTANCE FOR PREGNANCY	MAJOR FOOD SOURCES
PROTEIN		
IRON		
CALCIUM		
SODIUM		
FAT-SOLUBLE VITAMINS		
WATER-SOLUBLE VITAMINS		

19. When assessing pregnant women, it is critical that nurses be alert for factors that could place women at nutritional risk so that early intervention can be implemented. NAME five such indicators or risk factors of which the nurse should be aware. CITE three strategies a nurse could use in an attempt to reduce nutritional risk for pregnant women based on the risks named.

20. CITE the pregnancy-related risks associated with the following nutritional problems.
    A. Underweight women

B. Inappropriate weight gain during pregnancy (inadequate or excessive)

C. Obese women

21. At her first prenatal visit, Marie, a 20-year-old primigravida, reports that she has been a strict vegetarian for the past 3 years. IDENTIFY two major guidelines that the nurse should follow when planning menus with Marie.

22. Evaluation of nutritional status is an essential part of a thorough physical assessment of pregnant women. CITE four signs of good nutrition and four signs of inadequate nutrition that the nurse should observe for during the assessment of a pregnant woman.

23. Calculate the body mass index (BMI) for each of the following women, and then determine the recommended weight gain and pattern for each based on her BMI.

WOMAN	BMI	WEIGHT GAIN (TOTAL; PATTERN)
A. June: 1.60 m, 55 kg		
B. Alice: 1.65 m, 82 kg		
C. Ann: 1.70 m, 50 kg		

MULTIPLE CHOICE QUESTIONS: Circle the correct option(s) and state the rationale for the option(s) chosen.

24. A nurse teaching a pregnant woman about the importance of iron in her diet would tell her to consume which foods as good sources of iron? (Circle all that apply.)
    A. Whole-grain breads and cereals
    B. Oranges
    C. Salmon
    D. Raisins
    E. Spinach
    F. Tomatoes

25. A 30-year-old pregnant woman with a BMI of 31 asks the nurse about recommendations for diet and weight gain during pregnancy. What should the nurse tell this woman?
    A. Counsel her to begin a lifestyle change for weight reduction
    B. Recommend a total weight gain goal of 4 kg during pregnancy
    C. Set a weight gain goal of 0.2 kg per week during the second and third trimesters
    D. Limit her third-trimester calorie increase to no more than 600 kcal more than prepregnant needs

26. A 25-year-old pregnant woman is at 10 weeks of gestation. Her BMI is calculated to be 24. Regarding weight gain during pregnancy, the nurse should recommend:
    A. A total weight gain of 18 kg
    B. First-trimester weight gain of 1 to 2 kg
    C. Weight gain of 0.4 kg each week for 40 weeks
    D. Weight gain of 3 kg per month during the second and third trimesters

27. A pregnant woman at 6 weeks of gestation tells her nurse-midwife that she has been experiencing nausea with occasional vomiting every day. As an effective relief measure, the nurse should recommend:
    A. Eating starchy foods such as buttered popcorn or peanut butter with crackers in the morning before getting out of bed
    B. Avoiding eating before going to bed at night
    C. Altering eating patterns to small meals every 2 to 3 hours
    D. Skipping a meal if nausea is experienced

28. A woman demonstrates an understanding of the importance of increasing her intake of foods that are good sources of folic acid (50 mcg or more) when she includes which foods in her diet? (Circle all that apply.)
    A. Baked haddock
    B. Lentil soup
    C. Scrambled eggs
    D. Fruit salad of papaya and oranges
    E. Steamed asparagus
    F. Corn on the cob

29. A nurse taught a pregnant woman about the importance of iron and taking her iron supplement daily. Which statement by the woman indicates the need for further instruction?
    A. "I take my iron supplement at bedtime with a cup of tea."
    B. "I include a lot of citrus fruit and tomatoes in my diet."
    C. "My stools can turn black or dark green."
    D. "I need to keep track of my bowel movements because taking iron can lead to constipation."

30. A 30-year-old woman at 16 weeks of gestation comes for a routine prenatal visit. Her 24-hour dietary recall is evaluated by the nurse. Which entry indicates that this woman needs further instructions regarding nutrient needs during pregnancy?
    A. Eight ounces total from the meat, poultry, fish, dry beans, eggs, and nuts group
    B. Three cups of vegetables and two cups of fruit
    C. Seven ounces of grains, including whole-grain bread and bran cereal
    D. Three cups from the milk, yogurt, and cheese group

III. THINKING CRITICALLY

1. Nutrition and weight gain are important areas of consideration for nurses who care for pregnant women. In addition, weight gain is often a source of stress and body image alteration for the pregnant woman. DISCUSS the approach you would use in each of the following situations.
    A. Kelly (150 cm and 55 kg) complains to you that her physician recommended a weight gain of approximately 30 pounds (14 kg) during her pregnancy. She states: "Babies only weigh about 7 pounds when they are born. Why do I have to gain much more than that?"

B. Kate (160 cm and 57 kg) has just found out that she is pregnant. She states: "I am so glad to be pregnant. I love to eat, and now I can start eating for two. It will be great not to have to watch the scale or what I eat."

C. June tells you that she does not have to worry about her nutrient intake during her pregnancy. "I take plenty of vitamins—everything from A to Z."

D. Mary, a primigravida beginning her second month of pregnancy, asks you why she needs to increase her intake of so many nutrients during pregnancy and states: "I work every weekday and rely on fast foods to get through the week, though I try to eat better over the weekends."

E. Sara (BMI = 28.7) is 1 month pregnant. She asks you for dietary guidance, including a weight reduction diet because she does not want to gain too much weight with this pregnancy.

F. Beth is 2 months pregnant. She states: "I have cut down on my water intake. I do get a little thirsty but it's worth it because I don't have to urinate as often."

G. Hedy is 2 months pregnant and has come for her second prenatal visit. During a discussion about nutritional needs during pregnancy she states: "I know I will never get enough calcium because I get sick when I drink milk."

H. Lara is 36 weeks pregnant. She states that she would like to breastfeed her baby but is concerned about getting back into shape and losing weight after the baby is born. "My friends told me that I will lose weight more slowly since I will not be able to start on a weight reduction diet as long as I am breastfeeding."

I. Jean intends to breastfeed her infant until she returns to work in 6 months. She asks you what guidelines she should follow so that she makes good breast milk for her baby.

2. Yvonne's hemoglobin is 13 g/dL and her hematocrit is 37% at the onset of her pregnancy. She asks the nurse if she will have to take iron during her pregnancy if she tries to follow a good diet. "My friend took iron when she was pregnant and it made her sick to her stomach." DISCUSS the appropriate response by the nurse.

3. IDENTIFY three nursing measures appropriate for each of the following nursing diagnoses.
   A. Imbalanced nutrition: less than body requirements related to inadequate intake associated with moderate nausea and vomiting (morning sickness) associated with pregnancy.

   B. Constipation related to decreased intestinal motility associated with increased progesterone levels during pregnancy.

   C. Pain related to reflux of gastric contents into the esophagus following dinner.

4. Gloria is an 18-year-old Native American (165 cm and 45 kg) who has just been diagnosed as 8 weeks pregnant. In her discussions with you at her first prenatal visit, she expresses a lack of knowledge regarding the nutritional requirements of pregnancy and an interest in learning about what to eat because she wants to have a healthy baby.
   A. OUTLINE the approach that you would use to help Gloria learn about and meet the nutritional requirements of her pregnancy.

   B. PLAN a 1-day menu that incorporates Gloria's nutritional needs and reflects the traditions of her culture.

16 Labor and Birth Processes

I. REVIEWING KEY TERMS

FILL IN THE BLANKS: Insert the term that corresponds to each of the following descriptions.

1. _____, _____, _____,
_____, and _____. The five factors (5 Ps) affecting the
process of labor and birth.

2. _____ Membrane-filled spaces that are located where the sutures in the fetal/neonatal
skull intersect.

3. _____ Overlapping of the bones of the fetal skull that occurs during childbirth, thereby
temporarily changing its shape and facilitating the skull's passage through the birth canal.

4. _____ Part of the fetus that enters the pelvic inlet first and leads through the birth
canal during labor. The three main types are _____ (head first), _____
_____ (buttocks, feet, or both first), and _____.

5. _____ Part of the fetus that lies closest to the internal os of the cervix and is first
felt by the examiner's finger during a vaginal examination. The four types are _____,
_____, _____, and _____.

6. _____ Presentation that occurs when the fetal head is fully flexed, making the fetal
occiput the part first felt by the examining finger.

7. _____ Relationship of the fetal spine (long axis) to the maternal spine (long axis).
_____ Term used when the spines are parallel. _____
Term used when the fetal spine is at a right angle or diagonal to the maternal spine.

8. _____ Relationship of the fetal body parts to one another. _____
_____ The most common type of relationship.

9. _____ Largest transverse diameter of the fetal skull.

10. _____ Smallest anteroposterior diameter of the fetal skull to enter the maternal pelvis
when the fetal head is in complete flexion.

11. _____ Relationship of a reference point on the fetal presenting part (occiput, mentum/
chin, sacrum, scapula) to the four quadrants of the maternal pelvis.

12. _____ This is said to have occurred when the largest transverse diameter of the
presenting part has passed through the pelvic inlet and into the true pelvis, reaching the level of the ischial spines.

115

13. _____ Relationship of the fetal presenting part to an imaginary line drawn between the ischial spines. It is measured in _____ above or below the ischial spines, thereby serving as a method of determining the progress of fetal _____.

14. _____ Process of shortening and thinning of the cervix during the first stage of labor. Progress is expressed in percentages from 0% to 100%.

15. _____ Enlargement and widening of the cervical opening (os) and the cervical canal that occurs during labor. Progress is expressed in centimeters from less than 1 cm to 10 cm when complete.

16. _____ Descent of the fetal presenting part into the true pelvis approximately 2 weeks before term in the primigravida and in the multiparous woman once true labor is in progress.

17. _____ Primary powers of labor. They are responsible for _____ _____ and _____ of the cervix and _____ of the fetus.

18. _____ Term used to designate the time from the beginning of one contraction to the beginning of the next. _____ Term used to designate the length of a contraction. _____ Term used to designate the strength of a contraction at its peak.

19. _____ Secondary powers of labor accomplished when the woman bears down or pushes.

20. _____ Brownish or blood-tinged cervical mucoid discharge representing the passage of the mucous plug as the cervix ripens in preparation for labor.

21. _____ Term used to refer to the movements of the fetus in a vertex presentation as it turns and adjusts its head to facilitate passage through the maternal birth canal. These seven movements are

_____, _____, _____,

_____, _____, _____, and

_____.

22. _____ Term used to refer to the maternal urge to bear down, which occurs when the fetal presenting part reaches the perineal floor, stimulating stretch receptors and causing release of oxytocin.

23. The first stage of labor begins with the onset of _____ and ends with full _____ _____. It is divided into three phases, namely, _____, _____ _____, and _____.

24. The second stage of labor lasts from the time the _____ to the _____ _____.

25. The third stage of labor lasts from the _____ until the _____.

26. The fourth stage of labor is the period of _____ when homeostasis is reestablished.

27. _____, _____, _____, and _____ Four factors that affect fetal circulation during labor.

28. LABEL the following illustrations of the fetal skull and the maternal pelvis with the appropriate landmarks and diameters.

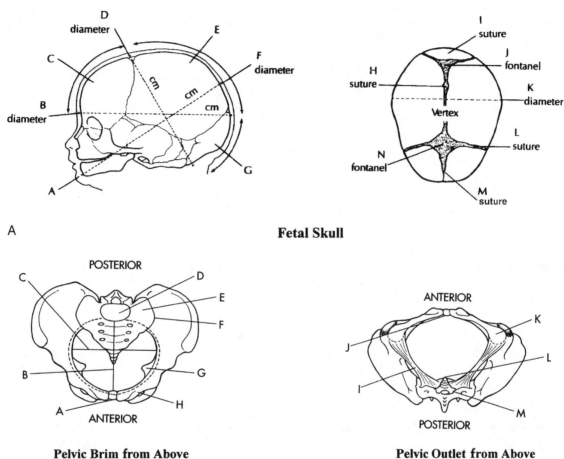

Fetal Skull

A

Pelvic Brim from Above

B

Pelvic Outlet from Above

Maternal Pelvis

29. INDICATE the presentation, presenting part, position, lie, and attitude of the fetus in each of the following illustrations.

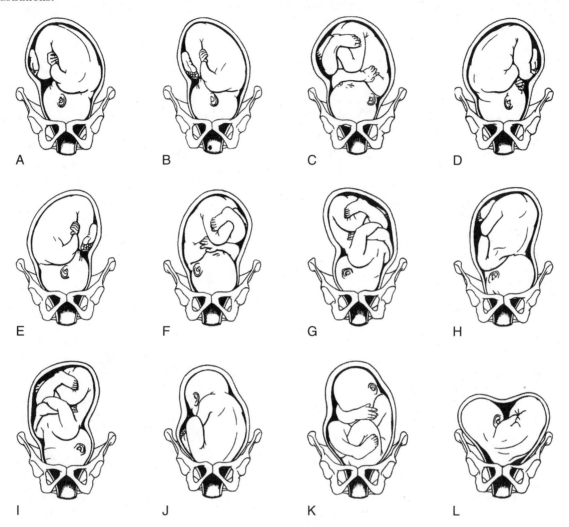

A   B   C   D

E   F   G   H

I   J   K   L

MULTIPLE CHOICE: Circle the correct option(s) and state the rationale for the option(s) chosen.

30. A vaginal examination during labor reveals the following information: LOA, −1, 75%, 3 cm. An accurate interpretation of these data include: (Circle all that apply.)
    A. Attitude: flexed
    B. Station: 3 cm below the ischial spines
    C. Presentation: cephalic
    D. Lie: longitudinal
    E. Effacement: 75% complete
    F. Dilation: 9 cm more to reach full dilation

31. Changes occur as a woman progresses through labor. What maternal adaptations are expected during labor? (Circle all that apply.)
    A. Increase in both systolic and diastolic blood pressure during uterine contractions
    B. Decrease in white blood cell count
    C. Slight increase in baseline pulse and respiratory rates
    D. Decrease in gastric motility leading to nausea and vomiting, especially during the transition phase.
    E. Proteinuria 2+
    F. Hyperglycemia

32. When instructing a group of primigravida women about the onset of labor, the nurse tells them to be alert for:
    A. Urinary retention
    B. Weight gain of 2 kg
    C. Quickening
    D. Energy surge

III. THINKING CRITICALLY

1. During a prenatal class you are going to teach the women and their partners about the process of labor and how it progresses. You decide that the best approach is to use models and illustrations representing the 5 Ps of labor and the cardinal movements to describe the labor process.
   A. OUTLINE what you will present related to the 5 Ps. IDENTIFY the visual aids you will use.

   B. OUTLINE what you will present related to the cardinal movements. IDENTIFY the visual aids you will use.

2. As part of their care of the laboring woman, nurses perform vaginal examinations and interpret the results. STATE the meaning of each of the following vaginal examination findings.

EXAM I	EXAM II	EXAM III	EXAM IV
ROP	RMA	LST	OA
−1	0	+1	+3
50%	25%	75%	100%
3 cm	2 cm	6 cm	10 cm

3. Brooke is a primigravida. During a prenatal visit at 34 weeks of gestation, she asks you the following questions regarding her approaching labor. DESCRIBE how you would respond.

A. "What gets labor to start?"

B. "Are there things I should watch for that will tell me my labor is getting closer to starting?"

C. "My friend just had a baby and she told me that the nurses kept helping her to change her position, to get in and out of bed, and to walk! Isn't that dangerous for the baby and painful for the mom?"

17 Maximizing Comfort for the Laboring Woman

MATCHING: Match the description in Column I with the appropriate pharmacologic method for pain management during childbirth in Column II.

COLUMN I

1. _____ Abolition of pain perception by interrupting nerve impulses to the brain. Loss of sensation (partial or complete) and sometimes loss of consciousness occurs.

2. _____ Method used to repair a tear or hole in the dura mater around the spinal cord as a result of spinal anesthesia; the goal is to prevent or treat postdural puncture headache (PDPH).

3. _____ Single-injection, subarachnoid anesthesia useful for pain control during vaginal or cesarean birth but not for labor.

4. _____ Systemic analgesic, such as nalbuphine and butorphanol, that relieves pain without causing significant maternal or neonatal respiratory depression and is less likely to cause nausea and vomiting.

5. _____ Provides rapid perineal anesthesia for performing and repairing an episiotomy or lacerations.

6. _____ Anesthetic gas mixed with oxygen, which is inhaled beginning 30 seconds before the onset of a contraction to reduce but not eliminate pain during the first and second stages of labor.

7. _____ Injection of an opioid agonist analgesic into the spinal fluid to relieve pain associated with labor and following cesarean birth.

8. _____ Class of drug used to decrease anxiety, increase sedation, and reduce nausea and vomiting but that may impair the analgesic efficacy of opioids.

9. _____ Drug that promptly reverses the effects of opioids, including maternal and neonatal central nervous system (CNS) depression, especially respiratory depression.

10. _____ Systemic analgesic such as meperidine or fentanyl that relieves pain and creates a feeling of well-being but can result in respiratory depression, nausea, and vomiting.

11. _____ Alleviation of pain sensation or raising of the threshold for pain perception without loss of consciousness.

12. _____ Relief from pain of uterine contractions and birth by injecting a local anesthetic agent and/or an opioid agonist analgesic into the peridural space.

13. _____ Relief from pain in the lower vagina, vulva, and perineum, making it useful if an episiotomy is to be performed or forceps or vacuum assistance is required to facilitate birth.

COLUMN II

A. Opioid agonist-antagonist analgesic
B. Anesthesia
C. Analgesia
D. Phenothiazine
E. Epidural analgesia/anesthesia (block)
F. Autologous epidural blood patch
G. Local perineal infiltration anesthesia
H. Spinal anesthesia (block)
I. Opioid antagonist
J. Nitrous oxide
K. Pudendal nerve block
L. Opioid agonist analgesic
M. Intrathecal analgesia

FILL IN THE BLANKS: Insert the term that corresponds to each of the following descriptions.

14. _____ Type of pain that predominates during the first stage of labor and is located over the lower abdomen; it results from cervical changes, distention of the lower uterine segment, uterine ischemia, and pressure and traction on adjacent structures.

15. _____ Type of intense, sharp, burning pain that predominates during the second stage of labor; it results from stretching and distention of perineal tissues and the pelvic floor to allow passage of the fetus, from distention and traction on the peritoneal and uterocervical supports during contractions, from lacerations of soft tissues, and from pressure against bladder and rectum.

16. _____ Type of pain felt in areas of the body other than the area of pain origin. During labor and birth, pain originating in the uterus radiates to the abdominal wall, lumbosacral area of the back, iliac crests, gluteal area, and down the thighs.

17. _____ Point beyond which pain is perceived.

18. _____ Level of pain a laboring woman is willing to endure.

19. _____ Theory of pain based on the principle that certain nerve cell groupings within the spinal cord, brainstem, and cerebral cortex have the ability to modulate the pain impulse through a blocking mechanism. According to this theory, pain sensations travel along sensory nerve pathways to the brain but only a limited number of sensations or messages can travel through these nerve pathways at one time.

20. _____ Endogenous opioids secreted by the pituitary gland that act on the central and peripheral nervous systems to reduce pain.

21. _____ Paced breathing technique during which the woman breathes at approximately half her normal rate (6 to 8 breaths per minute). It is usually the first technique used in early labor when the woman can no longer talk or walk her way through a contraction.

22. _____ Paced breathing technique during which the woman breathes at an accelerated rate, which should not exceed twice her resting respiratory rate (32 to 40 breaths per minute).

23. _____ Full breath taken at the beginning of each contraction to greet it and at the end of each contraction to blow it away.

24. _____ Paced breathing technique that combines breaths and puffs in a ratio (e.g., 3:1 or 4:1) as a means to enhance concentration during the transition phase of the first stage of labor.

25. _____ Rapid, deep breathing that can be an undesirable outcome of the more rapid and more shallow types of paced breathing techniques; it can result in_____.

26. _____ Light stroking of the abdomen or other body part in rhythm with breathing during contractions.

27. _____ Steady pressure applied against the laboring woman's sacrum by the nurse or coach using the fist or heel of the hand or a firm object (e.g., tennis ball); it is especially helpful during back labor.

28. _____ Nonpharmacologic comfort measure that uses the buoyancy of the warm water to provide support for tense muscles, relief from discomfort, and general body relaxation.

29. _____ Nonpharmacologic pain control technique that involves placing two pairs of electrodes on either side of the woman's thoracic and sacral spine to provide continuous low-intensity electrical impulses or stimuli that can be increased during a contraction.

30. _____ Nonpharmacologic pain control technique that is based on the application of pressure, heat, or cold on specific body points called tsubos.

31. _____ Nonpharmacologic pain control technique that involves the insertion of fine needles into specific areas of the body to restore the flow of qi (energy) and to decrease pain.

32. _____ Technique that uses the concept of energy fields within the body called prana that are thought to be deficient in some people who are in pain. It involves the laying on of hands by a specially trained person to redirect energy fields associated with pain.

33. _____ Form of deep relaxation, similar to daydreaming or meditation; the person enters a state of focused concentration and the subconscious mind can be more easily accessed.

34. _____ Nonpharmacologic pain control technique based on the premise that a person can recognize his or her body's physical signals and use mental processes to change or control certain internal physiologic events.

35. _____ Use of essential oils distilled from plants, flowers, herbs, and trees to promote health and well-being, enhance relaxation, and restore balance of mind, body, and spirit.

36. _____ Injection of small amounts of sterile water using a fine needle into four locations on the lower back to relieve low back pain.

II. REVIEWING KEY CONCEPTS

37. EXPLAIN the theoretic basis for using such techniques as massage, stroking, music, and imagery to reduce the sensation of pain during childbirth.

38. Nurses working on childbirth units must be knowledgeable regarding the use of a variety of nerve block analgesia and anesthesia methods to ensure that they manage them in a safe and effective manner. COMPLETE the following table by listing the effects, criteria and timing for use, and care management for each of the analgesic and anesthetic methods.

METHOD	EFFECTS	CRITERIA/TIMING	CARE MANAGEMENT
Local perineal infiltration anesthesia			
Pudendal nerve block			
Spinal anesthesia (block)			
Epidural anesthesia or analgesia (block)			
Combined spinal-epidural analgesia			
Epidural and intrathecal opioids			

MULTIPLE CHOICE: Circle the correct option(s) and state the rationale for the option(s) chosen.

39. In her birth plan, a woman requests that she be allowed to use the new whirlpool bath during labor. When implementing this woman's request, the nurse should:
    A. Assist the woman to maintain a reclining position when in the tub
    B. Tell the woman she will need to leave the tub as soon as her membranes rupture
    C. Begin hydrotherapy when the woman is in active labor (approximately 5 cm)
    D. Limit her to no longer than 1 hour in the tub

40. A variety of medications may be administered to women during labor. Which medication is used to reduce anxiety, potentiate the effects of analgesics, and relieve nausea?
    A. naloxone (Narcan)
    B. metoclopramide (Reglan)
    C. promethazine (Phenergan)
    D. fentanyl citrate (Sublimaze)

41. The physician has ordered nalbuphine hydrochloride (Nubain) 10 mg IV every 3 to 4 hours as needed for pain associated with labor. In fulfilling this order, the nurse knows that:
    A. This medication is a potent opioid agonist analgesic
    B. The dosage of the analgesic is too high for IV administration, necessitating a new order
    C. This is the analgesic of choice if the laboring woman is opioid dependent
    D. This analgesic is unlikely to cause significant maternal or fetal/neonatal respiratory depression

42. Following administration of fentanyl (Sublimaze) IV for pain associated with uterine contractions, a woman's labor progresses more rapidly than expected. The physician orders that a stat dose of naloxone (Narcan) 1 mg IV be administered to the woman to reverse respiratory depression in the newborn after its birth. In fulfilling this order, the nurse knows to:
    A. Question the route, because this medication should be administered orally
    B. Recognize that the dose is too low
    C. Assess the woman's level of pain, because it will return abruptly
    D. Observe the maternal pulse for bradycardia

43. An anesthesiologist is preparing to begin a continuous epidural block using a combination local anesthetic and opioid analgesic as a pain relief measure for a laboring woman. Nursing measures related to this type of nerve block include: (Circle all that apply.)
    A. Assist the woman into a modified Sims position or upright position with back curved for administration of the block
    B. Alternate her position from side to side every hour
    C. Assess the woman for headaches, because they commonly occur in the postpartum period if an epidural is used for labor
    D. Assist the woman to urinate at least every 2 hours during labor to prevent bladder distention
    E. Prepare the woman for use of forceps- or vacuum-assisted birth, because she will be unable to bear down
    F. Assess blood pressure frequently, because severe hypotension can occur

44. Administering an opioid antagonist to a woman who is opioid dependent will result in the opioid abstinence syndrome. The nurse would recognize which clinical manifestations as evidence that this syndrome is occurring? (Circle all that apply.)
    A. Yawning
    B. Coughing
    C. Piloerection
    D. Anorexia
    E. Dry skin, eyes, and nose
    F. Miosis

45. After induction of a spinal block in preparation for an elective cesarean birth, a woman's blood pressure decreases from 124/76 to 96/60. The nurse's initial action is to:
    A. Administer a vasopressor intravenously to raise the blood pressure
    B. Change the woman's position from supine to lateral
    C. Begin to administer oxygen by mask at 10 to 12 L/min
    D. Notify the woman's health care provider

III. THINKING CRITICALLY

1. You are caring for Latisha, a primigravida in active labor, and her partner. Her primary nursing diagnosis at this time is acute pain related to the processes involved in labor and birth. IDENTIFY the factors that you feel could influence this nursing diagnosis and DESCRIBE how these factors influence Latisha's pain experience.

2. Martina is a primigravida in labor. She tells her nurse that she needs something for pain "NOW!"
   A. DESCRIBE the approach that Martina's nurse should use in responding to her request.

   B. The nurse prepares to administer meperidine hydrochloride (Demerol) 25 mg IV as ordered by Martina's primary health care provider. The nurse knows that this medication not only will affect Martina but also will cross her placenta and affect the fetus.
      1. IDENTIFY the maternal reactions to this medication for which the nurse must be alert when assessing Martina after the meperidine is administered.

      2. LIST three factors that influence the effect that systemic analgesics have on the fetus/newborn.

      3. IDENTIFY the fetal/newborn effects that can occur after administration of meperidine.

3. A woman in labor asks the nurse why the pain medication she is getting is put into her IV tubing instead of into her buttocks like the last time she was in labor.
   A. EXPLAIN what the nurse should tell this woman about why the IV route is preferred to the IM route for the administration of systemic analgesics during labor.

   B. STATE the guidelines that the nurse should follow when administering an opioid agonist analgesic intravenously to this patient.

4. A nurse working with a group of expectant fathers is asked if there really is "a physical reason for all the pain women say they feel when they are in labor." DESCRIBE the response that this nurse should give.

5. Nurses working on childbirth units must be sensitive to their clients' pain experiences.
   A. DESCRIBE how women experience pain during childbirth and how they will express it. CREATE a pain assessment guide that you can use in the clinical setting when caring for clients in pain, including women in labor.

   B. DESCRIBE specific measures that nurses can use to alter the laboring woman's perception of pain.

6. On admission to the labor unit in the latent phase of labor, Kimberly (2-0-0-1-0) and her husband, Maurice, tell you that they are so glad they took Lamaze classes and did so much reading about childbirth. "We will not need any medication now that we know what to do. But most importantly, our baby will be safe!" DESCRIBE how you would respond if you were their primary nurse for childbirth.

7. IMAGINE that you are the nurse manager of a labor and birth unit. Major renovations are being planned for your unit and your input is required. You and your staff nurses believe that water therapy, including the use of showers and whirlpool baths, is a beneficial nonpharmacologic method to relieve pain and discomfort and to enhance the progress of labor. DISCUSS the rationale you would use to convince planners that installation of a shower and a whirlpool bath in each birthing room is cost effective.

8. Tara has been in labor for 4 hours. Her blood pressure had been stable, averaging 130/80 mm Hg when assessed between contractions, and the fetal heart rate (FHR) pattern consistently exhibited criteria of a reassuring pattern. An epidural block was initiated. Shortly afterward, during assessment of maternal vital signs and FHR, Tara's blood pressure decreased to 102/60 mm Hg and the FHR pattern began to exhibit a decrease in rate and variability.
   A. STATE what Tara is experiencing. SUPPORT your answer and EXPLAIN the physiologic basis for what is happening to Tara.

   B. WRITE a nursing diagnosis that reflects this occurrence.

C. LIST the immediate nursing actions.

9. Moira, a primigravida, has elected to receive a continuous epidural block as her pharmacologic method of choice during childbirth.
    A. IDENTIFY the assessment procedures that should be used to determine Moira's readiness for the initiation of the epidural block.

    B. DESCRIBE the preparation methods that should be implemented.

    C. DESCRIBE two positions you could help Moira to assume for the induction of the epidural block.

    D. OUTLINE the nursing care management interventions recommended while Moira is receiving the epidural block to ensure her well-being and that of her fetus.

18 Fetal Assessment During Labor

I. LEARNING KEY TERMS

MATCHING: Match the definition in Column I with the appropriate term related to fetal heart rate (FHR) pattern in Column II.

COLUMN I

1. _____ Average FHR range of 110 to 160 beats/minute at term as assessed during a 10-minute segment that excludes periodic or episodic changes and periods of marked variability.

2. _____ Persistent (10 minutes or longer) baseline FHR below 110 beats/minute.

3. _____ Visually apparent abrupt or gradual decrease in the FHR of 15 beats/minute or more below the baseline that lasts more than 2 minutes but less than 10 minutes.

4. _____ Changes from baseline patterns in FHR that occur with uterine contractions.

5. _____ Persistent (10 minutes or longer) baseline FHR greater than 160 beats/minute.

6. _____ Expected irregular fluctuations in the baseline FHR of 2 cycles per minute or greater as a result of the interaction of the sympathetic and parasympathetic nervous systems.

7. _____ Visually apparent gradual FHR decrease starting with the onset of a contraction in response to fetal head compression.

8. _____ Visually apparent gradual FHR decrease after the start of a uterine contraction, usually in response to uteroplacental insufficiency; the lowest point occurs after the peak of the contraction and baseline rate is not usually regained until the uterine contraction is over.

9. _____ Visually abrupt FHR decrease any time during a contraction in response to umbilical cord compression.

10. _____ Visually apparent abrupt increase in the FHR of at least 15 beats/minute above the baseline rate that lasts 15 seconds or more with return to baseline less than 2 minutes from the beginning of the increase.

11. _____ Changes in FHR from baseline that are not associated with uterine contractions.

COLUMN II

A. Acceleration
B. Early deceleration
C. Variability
D. Late deceleration
E. Variable deceleration
F. Tachycardia
G. Prolonged deceleration
H. Bradycardia
I. Baseline FHR
J. Periodic changes
K. Episodic changes

FILL IN THE BLANKS: Insert the term that corresponds to each of the following descriptions related to fetal assessment.

12. _____ Deficiency of oxygen in the arterial blood.

13. _____ Inadequate supply of oxygen at the cellular level.

14. _____ Method of listening to fetal heart sounds at periodic intervals to assess the FHR using a Pinard stethoscope, DeLee-Hillis fetoscope, or ultrasound stethoscope.

15. _____ External monitoring instrument that works by reflecting high-frequency sound waves off of the fetal heart and valves to assess and record the FHR pattern. It is placed over the area of _____ after conductive gel is applied to its surface.

16. _____ External monitoring instrument that measures uterine activity (e.g., frequency, regularity, and approximate duration of uterine contractions) transabdominally. It is placed over the

_____ .

17. _____ Internal monitoring instrument that is attached to the fetal presenting part to assess FHR pattern.

18. _____ Internal monitoring instrument that is solid or fluid filled; it is inserted into the intrauterine cavity to measure uterine activity (e.g., frequency, duration, and intensity of uterine contractions and resting tone).

19. _____ and _____ Methods of assessment that use digital, sound, or light stimulation to determine the reaction of the FHR.

20. _____ Instillation of room-temperature isotonic fluid (e.g., normal saline or lactated Ringer) into the uterine cavity if the volume of amniotic fluid is low to relieve intermittent cord compression that results in variable decelerations and transient fetal hypoxemia.

21. _____ An abnormally small amount of amniotic fluid.

22. _____ Absence of amniotic fluid.

23. _____ Relaxation of the uterus that can be achieved through the administration of drugs that inhibit uterine contractions. The most commonly used drug for this purpose is _____ .

24. _____ Assessment method used immediately after birth as an adjunct to the Apgar score; it measures pH, pO_2, pCO_2, and base deficit or excess of the newborn's blood.

25. _____ Group of interventions initiated when an abnormal (nonreassuring) FHR pattern is noted to improve uteroplacental perfusion and increase maternal oxygenation and cardiac output. Basic corrective measures include _____ , _____ , and

_____ .

II. REVIEWING KEY CONCEPTS

26. It is critical that a nurse working on a labor unit be knowledgeable concerning factors associated with a reduction in fetal oxygen supply, characteristics of normal (reassuring) and abnormal (nonreassuring) FHR patterns, and the characteristics of normal uterine activity.
    A. DESCRIBE the factors associated with a reduction in fetal oxygen supply.

    B. STATE the characteristics of normal (reassuring) FHR patterns (Category I).

    C. STATE the characteristics of indeterminate FHR patterns (Category II).

D. STATE the characteristics of abnormal (nonreassuring) FHR patterns (Category III).

E. STATE the characteristics of normal uterine activity during labor.

FILL IN THE BLANKS: In general, the recommended frequency for evaluation of FHR pattern and uterine activity depends on the risk status of the mother and the stage of labor. Insert the appropriate time for each of the following assessment recommendations made by the American Academy of Pediatrics and American College of Obstetricians and Gynecologists.

27. Low-risk client (risk factors are absent during labor): Evaluate FHR pattern and uterine activity every

_____ in the first stage of labor and every _____ in the second stage of labor.

28. High-risk client (risk factors are present during labor): Evaluate FHR pattern and uterine activity every

_____ in the first stage of labor and every _____ in the second stage of labor.

29. The five essential components of an FHR tracing that must be evaluated at the recommended frequency for the

maternal risk status are _____, _____, _____

_____, _____, and _____.

30. STATE the legal responsibilities related to fetal monitoring for nurses who care for women during childbirth.

MULTIPLE CHOICE: Circle the correct option(s) and state the rationale for the option(s) chosen.

31. A laboring woman's uterine contractions are being internally monitored. When evaluating the monitor tracing, which finding is a source of concern and requires further assessment?
    A. Frequency every 2½ to 3 minutes
    B. Duration of 80 to 85 seconds
    C. Intensity during a uterine contraction of 85 to 90 mm Hg
    D. Average resting pressure of 20 to 25 mm Hg

32. External electronic fetal monitoring will be used for a woman just admitted to the labor unit in active labor. Guidelines that the nurse should follow when implementing this form of monitoring are to: (Circle all that apply.)
    A. Use Leopold maneuvers to determine correct placement of the tocotransducer
    B. Assist the woman to maintain a dorsal recumbent position to ensure accurate monitor tracings that can be evaluated easily
    C. Apply contact gel to the ultrasound transducer prior to application over the point of maximum intensity of the FHR
    D. Reposition the tocotransducer when the fetus changes its position
    E. Caution the woman to avoid effleurage when the transducers are in place
    F. Palpate the fundus periodically to estimate the intensity of the uterine contractions

33. A nurse caring for women in labor should be aware of signs characterizing normal (reassuring) and abnormal (nonreassuring) FHR patterns. What would be characteristic of abnormal patterns? (Circle all that apply.)
    A. Moderate baseline variability
    B. Average baseline FHR of 100 beats/minute
    C. Acceleration of the FHR with movement
    D. Late deceleration patterns approximately every three or four contractions
    E. FHR of 170 beats/minute between contractions
    F. Early deceleration patterns when the cervix is dilated to 7 cm

34. A laboring woman's temperature is elevated as a result of an upper respiratory infection. The FHR pattern that reflects maternal fever is:
    A. Diminished variability
    B. Variable decelerations
    C. Tachycardia
    D. Early decelerations

35. A nulliparous woman is in the active phase of labor and her cervix has progressed to 6 cm dilation. The nurse caring for this woman evaluates the external monitor tracing and notes the following: decrease in FHR shortly after onset of several uterine contractions returning to baseline rate by the end of the contraction; shape is uniform. Based on these findings, the nurse should:
    A. Change the woman's position to her left side
    B. Document the finding on the woman's chart
    C. Notify the physician
    D. Perform a vaginal examination to check for cord prolapse

36. When evaluating the external fetal monitor tracing of a woman whose labor is being induced, the nurse identifies signs of persistent late deceleration patterns and begins intrauterine resuscitation interventions. Which choice indicates that the following appropriate interventions were implemented in the recommended order of priority?
    1. Increase rate of maintenance IV solution.
    2. Palpate uterus for tachysystole.
    3. Discontinue oxytocin (Pitocin) infusion.
    4. Change maternal position to a lateral position, and then elevate her legs if woman is hypotensive.
    5. Administer oxygen at 8 to 10 L/minute by nonrebreather face mask.
       A. 2, 1, 5, 4, 3
       B. 4, 1, 2, 3, 5
       C. 5, 3, 4, 1, 2
       D. 4, 5, 1, 2, 3

III. THINKING CRITICALLY

1. Nurses working on a childbirth unit at a small rural hospital primarily use intermittent auscultation with an ultrasound fetoscope to assess fetal health and well-being during the labors of low-risk women.
    A. STATE the advantages and disadvantages of intermittent auscultation as a method of fetal assessment during childbirth.

    B. CREATE a protocol that these nurses could follow when monitoring the fetus using the intermittent auscultation method.

2. A nurse caring for a laboring woman in active labor notes an abnormal (nonreassuring) FHR pattern when evaluating the monitor tracing. DESCRIBE the action the nurse should take based on this finding.

3. Darlene, a primigravida in active labor, has just been admitted to the labor unit. She becomes very anxious when external electronic fetal monitoring (EFM) equipment is set up. She tells the nurse that her father had a heart attack 2 months ago. "He was so sick they had to put him on a monitor, too. Does this mean that my baby has a heart problem just like my father?"
   A. DESCRIBE the response the nurse should make to address Darlene's expressed concern.

   B. OUTLINE the care measures that the nurse should implement to ensure that the EFM is used in an effective manner to provide accurate data and to ensure that Darlene remains comfortable during this assessment technique.

4. Terry is a primigravida at 43 weeks of gestation. Her labor is being stimulated with oxytocin administered intravenously. Her contractions have been increasing in intensity with a frequency of every 2 to 2½ minutes and a duration of 80 to 85 seconds. She is currently in a supine position with a 30-degree elevation of her head. On observation of the monitor tracing, you note that during the last two contractions the FHR decreased after the contraction peaked and did not return to baseline until about 10 seconds into the rest period. A slight decrease in variability and baseline rate was observed.
   A. IDENTIFY the pattern described and the possible factors responsible for it.

   B. DESCRIBE the actions you would take. STATE the rationale for each action.

5. Taisha is a multiparous client in active labor. Her membranes rupture and the nursing caring for her immediately evaluates the EFM tracing.
   A. What type of periodic FHR pattern would the nurse be alert for when evaluating the tracing? EXPLAIN the rationale for your answer.

   B. STATE the actions the nurse should take in order of priority if the pattern is noted.

19 Nursing Care of the Family During Labor and Birth

FILL IN THE BLANKS: Insert the term that corresponds to each of the following descriptions related to the process of labor.

1. The first stage of labor begins with the onset of _____ and ends with complete cervical _____ and _____. A blood-tinged mucous discharge (bloody show) from the vagina usually indicates the passage of the _____.

2. During the latent phase of the first stage of labor the cervix dilates up to _____ cm in approximately _____ to _____ hours. Cervical dilation progresses from _____ to _____ cm in about _____ _____ to _____ hours during the active phase of the first stage of labor. The duration of the transition phase is approximately _____ to _____ _____ minutes and the cervix dilates from _____ to _____ _____ cm.

3. The second stage of labor is the stage in which the _____. It begins with full cervical _____ and complete _____. It ends with the _____ _____. This stage is divided into the _____ phase, a period of rest and calm (laboring down), and the phase of _____ (descent). The only certain objective sign that the second stage has begun is the inability to feel the _____ during a vaginal examination.

4. The third stage of labor lasts from the _____ until the _____. Detachment of the placenta from the wall of the uterus or separation is indicated by a firmly contracting _____ _____, change in the shape of the uterus from _____ to _____ _____, a sudden _____ from the introitus, apparent _____ _____, and the finding of _____ or of _____ at the introitus.

5. The fourth stage of labor is considered to be the first _____ after birth. During this stage the mother and newborn recover from the physical process of childbirth and get to know each other.

6. _____ Federal regulation enacted to ensure that pregnant women obtain the care they require during emergencies and when in labor regardless of their insurance status or ability to pay.

7. _____ Graphic chart on which cervical dilation and station are plotted to assist in early identification of deviations from expected labor patterns.

8. _____ Trained and experienced female labor attendant who provides a continuous one-on-one caring presence throughout the labor and birth of the woman she is attending.

9. _____ Traditional labor position in which the woman lies on her back with her legs raised in stirrups.

MATCHING: Match the description in Column I with the appropriate term in Column II.

COLUMN I

10. _____ Appearance of fetal intestinal contents in the amniotic fluid, giving it a greenish color.

11. _____ Prolonged holding of breath while bearing down (closed-glottis pushing).

12. _____ Burning sensation of acute pain as vagina stretches and crowning occurs.

13. _____ Artificial rupture of membranes (AROM, ARM).

14. _____ Occurs when widest part of the head (biparietal diameter) distends the vulva just before birth.

15. _____ Incision into perineum to enlarge the vaginal outlet.

16. _____ Test to determine if membranes have ruptured by assessing pH of the fluid.

17. _____ Technique used to control birth of fetal head and protect perineal musculature.

18. _____ Method of breathing during bearing-down efforts characterized by a strong expiratory grunt or groan.

19. _____ Expulsion of placenta with fetal side emerging first.

20. _____ Cord encircles the fetal neck.

21. _____ Method used to palpate fetus through abdomen.

22. _____ Occurs when pressure of presenting part against pelvic floor stretch receptors results in a woman's perception of an urge to bear down.

23. _____ Frondlike crystalline pattern created by amniotic fluid when it is placed on a glass slide.

24. _____ Classification of medication that stimulates the uterus to contract (a uterotonic).

25. _____ Expulsion of placenta with maternal surface emerging first.

26. _____ Application of a gentle yet steady force with hands pressed against the uterus.

27. _____ Protrusion of umbilical cord in advance of the presenting part.

COLUMN II

A. Modified Ritgen maneuver
B. Episiotomy
C. Oxytocic
D. Ferguson reflex
E. Shultz mechanism
F. Valsalva maneuver
G. Ring of fire
H. Crowning
I. Duncan mechanism
J. Amniotomy
K. Nuchal cord
L. Prolapse of umbilical cord
M. Nitrazine test
N. Leopold maneuvers
O. Ferning
P. Meconium staining
Q. Open-glottis pushing
R. Fundal pressure

FILL IN THE BLANKS: Insert the term that corresponds to each of the following descriptions related to the characteristics of the powers of labor.

28. _____ The primary powers of labor that act involuntarily to expel the fetus and the placenta from the uterus.

29. _____ "Building up" of a contraction from its onset.

30. _____ The peak of a contraction with an intrauterine pressure less than 80 mm Hg.

31. _____ "Letting down" of a contraction.

136

32. _____ How often uterine contractions occur; the time that elapses from the beginning of one contraction to the beginning of the next contraction.

33. _____ The strength of a contraction at its peak.

34. _____ The time that elapses between the onset and the end of a contraction.

35. _____ The tension of the uterine muscle between contractions.

36. _____ Period of rest between contractions.

37. _____ An involuntary urge to push in response to the Ferguson reflex.

II. REVIEWING KEY CONCEPTS

38. When caring for women in labor, a nurse should periodically palpate the uterus during and between contractions. DESCRIBE how the nurse should assess frequency, duration, intensity, and relaxation using palpation.

39. Laura (3-1-1-0-1) has just been admitted in the latent phase of the first stage of labor. As part of the admission procedure, you review her prenatal record and interview her regarding what she has observed regarding her labor and discuss her current health status.
    A. LIST the essential data you would need to obtain from Laura's prenatal record to plan appropriate care for her.

    B. IDENTIFY the information required regarding the status of Laura's labor.

    C. STATE the information required regarding Laura's current health status.

40. A nurse caring for a laboring woman needs to be alert for signs indicative of potential complications. IDENTIFY the signs for which the nurse must be alert when assessing her labor patients.

41. IDENTIFY two advantages associated with each of the following labor positions.
    Semirecumbent

Upright

Lateral

Hands and knees

42. OUTLINE the critical factors to be included in the physical assessment of the maternal-fetal unit during the first stage of labor.

43. INDICATE the laboratory and diagnostic tests that are recommended during labor. STATE the purpose of each.

44. IDENTIFY the factors that can influence the duration of the second stage of labor.

45. DESCRIBE the maternal positions recommended to enhance the effectiveness of a woman's bearing-down efforts during the second stage of labor. STATE the basis for each position's effectiveness in facilitating the descent and birth of the fetus.

46. EXPLAIN why the nurse should encourage a woman planning to breastfeed to begin breastfeeding during the fourth stage of labor.

MULTIPLE CHOICE: Circle the correct option(s) and state the rationale for the option(s) chosen.

47. A primigravida calls the hospital and tells a nurse on the labor unit that she knows she is in labor. The nurse's initial response is:
    A. "Tell me why you know that you are in labor."
    B. "How far do you live from the hospital?"
    C. "When is your expected date of birth?"
    D. "Have your membranes ruptured?"

48. A woman's amniotic membranes have apparently ruptured. The nurse assesses the fluid to determine its characteristics and confirm membrane rupture. An expected assessment finding of membrane rupture is:
    A. pH 5.5
    B. Absence of ferning
    C. Pale, clear fluid with white flecks
    D. Strong odor

49. When admitting a primigravida to the labor unit, the nurse observes for signs that indicate that the woman is in true labor and should be admitted. The nurse recognizes which of the following signs as indicative of true labor? (Circle all that apply.)
    A. Woman reports that her contractions seem stronger since she walked from the car to her room on the labor unit.
    B. Cervix feels soft and is 50% effaced.
    C. Woman perceives pain to be in her back or abdomen above the level of the navel.
    D. Fetus is engaged in the pelvis at zero station.
    E. Cervix is in the posterior position.
    F. Woman continues to feel her contractions intensify following a back rub and with use of effleurage.

50. A vaginal examination is performed on a multiparous woman who is in labor. The results of the examination were documented as 4 cm, 75%, +1, ROA. An accurate interpretation of these data is:
    A. Woman is in the latent phase of the first stage of labor
    B. Station is 1 cm above the ischial spines
    C. Presentation is cephalic
    D. Lie is transverse

51. A physical care measure for a laboring woman that has been identified as unlikely to be beneficial and may even be harmful is:
    A. Allowing the laboring woman to drink fluids and eat light solids as tolerated
    B. Administering a Fleet enema at admission
    C. Ambulating periodically throughout labor as tolerated
    D. Using a whirlpool bath once active labor is established

III. THINKING CRITICALLY

1. Alice, a primigravida, calls the labor unit. She tells the nurse that she thinks she is in labor. "I have had some pains for about 2 hours. Should my husband bring me to the hospital now?"
    A. DESCRIBE how the nurse should approach this situation.

    B. WRITE several questions the nurse could use to elicit the appropriate information required to determine the course of action required.

C. Based on the data collected during the telephone interview, the nurse determines that Alice is in very early labor. Because she lives fairly close to the hospital, she is instructed to stay home until her labor progresses. OUTLINE the instructions and recommendations for care that Alice and her husband should be given.

2. Analyze the assessment findings documented for each of the following **women**.

Denise (2-0-0-1-0)	Teresa (4-3-0-0-3)	Danielle (2-1-0-0-1)
5 cm	9 cm	2 cm
Moderate	Very strong	Mild
q4 min	q2–3 min	q6–8 min
40–55 sec	65–75 sec	30–35 sec
0	+2	−1

A. IDENTIFY the phase of labor being experienced by each woman.

B. DESCRIBE the behavior and appearance you would expect to be exhibited by each woman.

C. SPECIFY the physical care and emotional support measures you would implement if you were caring for each of these women.

D. Denise's husband, Sam, is her major support person during labor. The nurse observes that he is beginning to appear fatigued and "stressed" after being with Denise since her admission 5 hours ago. DESCRIBE the actions the nurse can take to support Sam and his efforts to care for Denise.

3. DESCRIBE the procedure that should be followed before auscultating the FHR or applying an ultrasound transducer to the abdomen of a laboring woman. EXPLAIN the rationale for using this procedure.

4. Tonya, a client in active labor, begins to cry during a vaginal examination to assess her status. "Why not watch the monitor to see how I am progressing instead of doing these vaginal exams? They really hurt and they are embarrassing!"

   A. DESCRIBE the response the nurse should make to Tonya's concern.

   B. DISCUSS the measures the nurse could use to meet Tonya's safety and comfort needs during a vaginal examination.

5. Tasha is dilated 6 cm. Her coach comes to tell you that her "water just broke with a gush!" IDENTIFY each action you would take in this situation, in order of priority. STATE the rationale for the actions you have identified.

6. Sara, a 17-year-old primigravida, is admitted in the latent phase of labor. Her boyfriend, Dan, is with her as her only support. They appear committed to each other. During the admission interview Sara tells you that they did not go to any classes because she was embarrassed about not being married. Both Sara and Dan appear very nervous and assessment indicates that they know little about what is happening, what to expect, and how to work together with the process of labor. IDENTIFY the nursing diagnosis reflected in these data. STATE one expected outcome and list nursing measures appropriate for the diagnosis you identified.

Nursing Diagnosis	Expected Outcome	Nursing Measures

7. Identifying a laboring couple's cultural and religious beliefs and practices regarding childbirth is a critical factor in providing culturally sensitive care that enhances the couple's sense of control and eventual satisfaction with their childbirth experience.

   A. LIST the questions you would ask when assessing a couple's cultural and religious preferences for childbirth.

   B. DISCUSS the importance of considering the couple's cultural and religious preferences when planning and implementing care.

8. Cori (4-3-0-0-3) is in latent labor. She and her husband are being oriented to the birthing room. Their last birth occurred in a delivery room 10 years ago. Both she and her husband are amazed by the birthing room and the birthing bed that will allow her to give birth in an upright position. They are also informed that changes in bearing-down efforts now allow a woman to follow her own body feelings and even to vocalize with pushing. Both Cori and her husband state that with every other birth they put her legs in stirrups, she held her breath for as long as she could, and she pushed quietly. "Everything turned out okay, so why should we change?" DESCRIBE the response the primary nurse caring for this couple should make to their concerns.

9. A nurse living in a rural area is called to her neighbor's home to assist his wife, who is in labor. "Everything is happening so fast. She says she is ready to deliver!"
   A. IDENTIFY the measures the nurse can use to reassure and comfort the woman.

   B. Shortly after the nurse arrives, crowning begins. STATE what the nurse should do.

   C. DESCRIBE the action the nurse should take after the birth of the head.

   D. LIST the measures the nurse should use to prevent excessive neonatal heat loss after the birth.

   E. IDENTIFY the infection control measures that should be implemented during a home birth.

   F. SPECIFY the measures the nurse should use to prevent excessive maternal blood loss or hemorrhage until the ambulance arrives.

   G. OUTLINE the information the nurse should document regarding the childbirth.

10. Beth is in the descent phase of the second stage of labor. She is actively pushing and bearing down to facilitate birth. INDICATE the criteria a nurse would use to evaluate the correctness of Beth's technique.

11. Imagine that you are participating in a panel discussion on childbirth practices. Your topic is "Episiotomy: Is it needed to ensure the safety and well-being of the laboring woman and her fetus?" OUTLINE the information you would include in your presentation.

12. Imagine that you are a staff nurse on a childbirth unit. Your hospital is instituting a change in policy that would allow the participation of children in the labor and birth process of their mother. You are asked to be a part of the committee that will formulate the guidelines regarding sibling participation during childbirth. DISCUSS the suggestions you would make to help ensure a positive outcome for parents, children, and health care providers.

13. Annie is a primipara in the fourth stage of labor following a long and difficult childbirth process.
    A. IDENTIFY the essential nursing assessment and care measures required to insure Annie's safety and recovery during this stage of her labor.

    B. As she performs the first assessment, the nurse notes that Annie seems disinterested in her baby. She looks him over quickly and then asks the nurse to take him back to the nursery. IDENTIFY the factors that could be accounting for Annie's behavior.

    C. DISCUSS the nursing measures you would use to encourage future maternal-newborn interactions and facilitate the attachment process.

14. Felisha is a primipara who gave birth to a baby girl 15 minutes ago. Her baby is very alert and interacting well with both parents. The nurse encourages Felisha to attempt to breastfeed her baby but she asks why she needs to breastfeed now because she feels a little tired and is unsure about what to do. DESCRIBE the approach this nurse should take to assist Felisha to breastfeed comfortably. INCLUDE a response to her question about why breastfeeding her newborn during the fourth stage of labor is beneficial to both her and her baby.

20 Postpartum Physiologic Changes

I. LEARNING KEY TERMS

FILL IN THE BLANKS: Insert the term that corresponds to each of the following descriptions.

1. _____ Profuse sweating that occurs after birth, especially at night, to rid the body of fluid retained during pregnancy.

2. _____ Uncomfortable uterine cramping that occurs during the early postpartum period as a result of periodic relaxation and vigorous contractions.

3. _____ The lactogenic hormone secreted by the pituitary gland of lactating women.

   _____ is another pituitary hormone that is responsible for uterine contraction and the let-down reflex.

4. _____ Surgical incision of the perineum to facilitate vaginal birth.

5. _____ Failure of the uterine muscle to contract firmly, making the fundus soft or boggy. It is the most frequent cause of excessive postpartum bleeding.

6. _____ An anal varicosity.

7. _____ Return of the uterus to a nonpregnant state.

8. _____ The self-destruction of excess hypertrophied uterine tissue as a result of the decrease in estrogen and progesterone levels following birth.

9. _____ ; _____ Terms used interchangeably with *postpartum* to refer to the period of recovery after childbirth that lasts approximately 6 weeks, although the time can vary from woman to woman.

10. _____ Separation of the abdominal wall muscles related to the effect of the enlargement of the uterus on the abdominal musculature.

11. _____ Postchildbirth uterine discharge or flow.

12. _____ The bright red, bloody uterine discharge that occurs for the first few days following birth; it consists primarily of blood and decidual tissue and trophoblastic debris and may contain small clots.

13. _____ The pink to brownish uterine discharge that begins about 3 to 4 days after birth; it consists of old blood, serum, leukocytes, and tissue debris and continues for 10 to 14 days (for some, 22 to 27 days).

14. _____ The yellowish white flow that begins about 10 days after birth and continues for 2 to 6 weeks or even longer; it consists of leukocytes, decidua, epithelial cells, mucous, serum, and bacteria.

15. _____ Term used to describe distended, firm, tender, and warm breasts during the postpartum period.

16. _____ Failure of the uterus to return to a nonpregnant state. The most common causes for this failure are retained _____ and _____.

17. _____ Medication usually administered intravenously (IV) or intramuscularly (IM) immediately after expulsion of the placenta to ensure that the uterus remains firm and well contracted.

18. _____ Discomfort or pain with intercourse.

19. _____ Exercises that help to strengthen perineal muscles and encourage healing.

20. _____ Clear, yellowish fluid produced in the breasts before lactation.

21. _____ Increased production of urine that occurs in the postpartum period to rid the body of excess tissue fluid retained during pregnancy.

22. _____ Lengthening and weakening of the fascial supports of pelvic structures, which include the uterus, vagina, urethra, bladder, and rectum.

II. REVIEWING KEY CONCEPTS

23. When caring for a woman following vaginal birth, it is of critical importance for the nurse to assess the woman's bladder for distention.
    A. EXPLAIN why bladder distention is more likely to occur during the immediate postpartum period.

    B. IDENTIFY the problems that can occur if the bladder is allowed to become distended.

24. CITE the factors that can interfere with bowel elimination in the postpartum period.

25. EXPLAIN why hypovolemic shock is less likely to occur in the postpartum woman experiencing a normal or average blood loss.

26. INDICATE the factors that place a postpartum woman at increased risk for the development of thrombophlebitis.

27. COMPARE and CONTRAST the characteristics of lochial bleeding and nonlochial bleeding.

MULTIPLE CHOICE: Circle the correct option(s) and state the rationale for the option(s) chosen.

28. A nurse has assessed a woman who gave birth vaginally 12 hours ago. Which findings would require further assessment?
    A. Bright to dark red uterine discharge
    B. Midline episiotomy—approximated, moderate edema, slight erythema, absence of ecchymosis
    C. Protrusion of abdomen with sight separation of abdominal wall muscles
    D. Fundus firm at 2 cm above the umbilicus and to the right of midline

29. A woman, 24 hours after giving birth, complains to the nurse that her sleep was interrupted the night before because of sweating and the need to have her gown and bed linens changed. The nurse's first action is to:
    A. Assess this woman for signs of infection
    B. Explain to the woman that the sweating represents her body's attempt to eliminate the fluid that was accumulated during pregnancy
    C. Notify her physician of the finding
    D. Document the finding as postpartum diaphoresis

30. Which woman at 24 hours following birth is least likely to experience afterpains?
    A. Primipara who is breastfeeding her twins, who were born at 38 weeks of gestation
    B. Multipara who is breastfeeding her 10-pound full-term baby girl
    C. Multipara who is bottle-feeding her 8-pound baby boy
    D. Primipara who is bottle-feeding her 7-pound baby girl

III. THINKING CRITICALLY

1. DESCRIBE how you would respond to each of the following typical questions and concerns of postpartum women.
    A. Mary is a primipara who is breastfeeding. "Why am I experiencing so many painful cramps in my uterus? I thought this happens only in women who have had babies before."

    B. Susan is being discharged after giving birth 20 hours ago. "For how many days should I be able to palpate my uterus to make sure it is firm?"

    C. June is a primipara. "My friend, who had a baby last year, said that she had a flow for 6 weeks. Isn't that a long time to bleed after having a baby?"

    D. Jean is 24 hours postpartum. "I cannot believe it—I look as if I am still pregnant! How can this be?"

Chapter **20** **Postpartum Physiologic Changes**

E. Marion is 1 day postpartum. "It seems like I am urinating all the time and sweating a lot, too. Do you think that I have a bladder infection?"

F. Joan is a primipara who is breastfeeding her baby. "My friend told me that I cannot get pregnant as long as I continue to breastfeed. This is great because I do not like to use birth control."

G. Alice, a multipara, is concerned. She states: "My doctor is not going to give me a drug to dry up my breasts like I had with my first baby. How will my breasts ever get back to normal now?"

H. Andrea, a primipara, is 1 day postpartum. While breastfeeding her baby she confides to the nurse that she does not know how long she will continue to breastfeed. "My husband and I have always had a satisfying sex life but my friend told me that as long as I breastfeed, intercourse is painful."

21 Nursing Care of the Family During the Postpartum Period

I. LEARNING KEY TERMS

FILL IN THE BLANKS: Insert the term that corresponds to each of the following descriptions regarding the postpartum period.

1. _____ First three months after childbirth.

2. _____ Nursing care management approach in which one nurse cares for both the mother and her infant. It is also called _____.

3. _____ Term used for the decreasing length of hospital stays of mothers and their babies after low-risk births. Other terms used are _____ and _____.

4. _____ Classification of medications that stimulate contraction of the uterine smooth muscle.

5. _____ Failure of the uterine muscle to contract firmly. It is the most frequent cause for excessive bleeding following childbirth.

6. _____ Perineal treatment that involves sitting in warm water for approximately 20 minutes to soothe and cleanse the site and to increase blood flow, thereby enhancing healing.

7. _____ Menstrual-like cramps experienced by many women as the uterus contracts after childbirth.

8. _____ Dilation of the blood vessels supplying the intestines as a result of the rapid decease in intraabdominal pressure after birth. It causes blood to pool in the viscera and thereby contributes to a drop in blood pressure called _____ when the woman who has recently given birth sits or stands, first ambulates, or takes a warm shower.

9. _____ Complaint of pain in calf muscles when the foot is sharply dorsiflexed; it could signal the presence of a deep vein thrombosis (DVT).

10. _____ Exercises that can assist women to regain muscle tone that is often lost when pelvic tissues are stretched and torn during pregnancy and birth.

11. _____ Swelling of breast tissue caused by increased blood and lymph supply to the breasts as the body begins the process of lactation; it occurs about 72 to 96 hours after birth.

12. _____ Vaccine that can be given to postpartum women whose antibody titer is less than 1:8 or whose EIA level is less than 0.8. It is used to prevent nonimmune women from contracting this TORCH infection during a subsequent pregnancy.

13. _____ Blood product that is administered to Rh-negative, antibody (Coombs)-negative women who give birth to Rh-positive newborns. It is administered at 28 weeks of gestation and again within 72 hours after birth.

14. _____ Telephone-based postpartum consultation service that can provide information and support; it is not a crisis intervention line to be used for emergencies.

II. REVIEWING KEY CONCEPTS

15. A postpartum woman at 6 hours after a vaginal birth is having difficulty voiding. LIST the measures that you would try to help this woman void spontaneously.

16. IDENTIFY the measures the nurse should teach a postpartum woman in an effort to prevent the development of thrombophlebitis.

17. STATE the two most important interventions that can be used to prevent excessive postpartum bleeding in the early postpartum period. INDICATE the rationale for the effectiveness of each intervention you identified.

18. A nurse is planning a home visit to a woman who gave birth 5 days ago. LIST the signs, if exhibited by the woman, that indicate the potential for postpartum psychosocial complications.

MULTIPLE CHOICE: Circle the correct option(s) and state the rationale for the option(s) chosen.

19. A nurse is prepared to assess a postpartum woman's fundus. To facilitate the accuracy and comfort of the examination, the nurse should tell the woman to:
    A. Elevate the head of her bed
    B. Place her hands under her head
    C. Flex her knees
    D. Lie flat with legs extended and toes pointed

20. The expected outcome for care when an oxytocic is administered to a postpartum woman is that the woman will:
    A. Demonstrate expected lochial characteristics
    B. Achieve relief of pain associated with uterine cramping
    C. Remain free from infection
    D. Void spontaneously within 4 hours of birth

21. A nurse is preparing to administer RhoGAM to a postpartum woman. Before implementing this care measure the nurse should:
    A. Ensure that medication is given within 12 hours after the birth
    B. Verify that the indirect and direct Coombs test results are negative
    C. Make sure that the newborn is Rh negative
    D. Cancel the administration of the RhoGAM if it was given to the woman during her pregnancy

22. When teaching a postpartum woman with an episiotomy about using a sitz bath, the nurse should emphasize:
    A. Using sterile equipment
    B. Filling the sitz bath basin with hot water (at least 42°C)
    C. Taking a sitz bath once a day for 10 minutes
    D. Squeezing her buttocks together before sitting down, then relaxing them

23. Before discharge at 2 days postpartum, the nurse evaluates a woman's level of knowledge regarding the care of her second degree perineal laceration. Which statements made by the woman indicate the need for further instruction before she goes home? (Circle all that apply.)
    A. "I will wash my stitches at least once a day with mild soap and warm water."
    B. "I will change my pad every time I go to the bathroom—at least four times each day."
    C. "I will position my squeeze bottle upward so that the warm water can remove lochia from my vagina."
    D. "I will use my squeeze bottle filled with warm water to cleanse my stitches after I urinate."
    E. "I will wear a pair of clean, disposable gloves when I wash my stitches and change my pad just like the nurses did."
    F. "I will apply the anesthetic cream to my stitches at least six times per day."

24. When assessing postpartum women during the first 24 hours after birth, the nurse must be alert for signs that could indicate the development of postpartum physiologic complications. Which signs are of concern to the nurse? (Circle all that apply.)
    A. Temperature—38°C
    B. Fundus—midline, boggy
    C. Lochia—three quarters of pad saturated in 3 hours
    D. Positive Homans sign in right leg
    E. Anorexia
    F. Voids approximately 150 to 200 mL of urine in each of the first three voidings after birth

III. THINKING CRITICALLY

1. Marie just gave birth to her second child. She plans to bottle-feed her baby just as she did with her first child, who was born 12 years ago. She asks the nurse what medication her doctor ordered to "dry up her milk." DESCRIBE how the nurse should respond to Marie's question and assist her with the process of lactation suppression.

2. Tara is breastfeeding at 12 hours postpartum. She requests medication for pain. DESCRIBE the approach that you would take when fulfilling Tara's request.

3. When caring for a woman who gave birth 4 hours earlier, the nurse notes an excessive rubra flow and early signs of hypovolemic shock.
    A. STATE the criteria that the nurse should have used to determine that the flow is rubra and excessive and that the early signs of hypovolemic shock are being exhibited.

    B. IDENTIFY the nurse's priority action in response to these assessment findings.

    C. IDENTIFY additional interventions that a nurse may need to implement to ensure this woman's safety and to prevent the development of further complications.

4. Carrie is a postpartum client awaiting discharge. Because her rubella titer indicates that she is not immune, a rubella vaccination has been ordered before discharge. STATE what you would tell Carrie regarding this vaccination.

5. A physician has written the following order for a postpartum woman: "Administer RhoGAM [Rh immunoglobulin] if indicated." DESCRIBE the actions the nurse should take in fulfilling this order.

6. Susan, a postpartum breastfeeding client, confides to the nurse: "My partner and I have always had a very satisfying sex life even when I was pregnant. My sister told me that this will definitely change now that I have had a baby." DESCRIBE what the nurse should tell Susan regarding sexual changes and activity after birth.

7. IDENTIFY the priority nursing diagnosis as well as one expected outcome and appropriate nursing management for each of the following situations.
   A. Tina is 2 days postpartum. During a home visit the nurse notes that Tina's episiotomy is edematous and slightly reddened, with approximated wound edges and no drainage. A distinct odor is noted and there is a buildup of secretions and the HurriCaine gel that Tina uses for discomfort. During the interview Tina reveals that she is afraid to wash the area. "I rinse with a little water in my peribottle in the morning and again at night. I also apply plenty of my gel."

Nursing Diagnosis	Expected Outcome	Nursing Measures

   B. Erin, who gave birth 3 days ago, has not had a bowel movement since a day or two before labor. She tells the visiting nurse during the interview that she has been avoiding "fiber" foods for fear that the baby will get diarrhea. Her activity level is low. "My family is taking good care of me. I do not have to lift a finger! Besides, I would prefer to wait until my episiotomy is less sore before trying to have a bowel movement."

Nursing Diagnosis	Expected Outcome	Nursing Measures

C. Mary gave birth 24 hours ago. She complains of perineal discomfort. "My hemorrhoids and stitches are killing me but I do not want to take any medication because it will get into my breast milk and hurt my baby."

Nursing Diagnosis	Expected Outcome	Nursing Measures

8. Dawn gave birth 8 hours ago. On palpation, her fundus was found to be two fingerbreadths above the umbilicus and deviated to the right of midline. It was also assessed to be less firm than previously noted.
   A. STATE the most likely basis for these findings.

   B. DESCRIBE the action that the nurse should take based on these assessment findings.

9. Jill gave birth 3 hours ago. During labor, epidural anesthesia was used for pain relief. Jill's primary health care provider has written the following order: "Out of bed and ambulating when able." DISCUSS the approach the nurse should take in safely fulfilling this order.

10. Taisha and her husband, Raushaun, are expecting their first baby. They have been given the option by their nurse-midwife of early postpartum discharge but are unsure of what to do.
    A. DESCRIBE the approach that the nurse-midwife could take to help this couple make a decision that is right for them.

    B. Taisha and Raushaun decide to take the option of early discharge within 12 hours of birth. DESCRIBE the nurse's legal responsibility as she prepares this couple for discharge following the birth of their daughter.

C. LIST the criteria for discharge that Taisha and her newborn must meet before discharge from the hospital to home.

D. OUTLINE the essential content that must be taught before discharge. A home visit by a nurse is planned for Taisha's third postpartum day.

11. Cultural beliefs and practices must be considered when planning and implementing care in the postpartum period.
   A. DISCUSS the importance of using a culturally sensitive approach when providing care to postpartum women and their families.

   B. Kim, a Korean American, has just given birth. Assessment reveals that she and her family are guided by beliefs and practices based on a balance of heat and cold. DESCRIBE how the nurse would adjust typical postpartum care to respect and accommodate Kim's cultural beliefs and practices.

   C. A Muslim woman has been admitted to the postpartum unit following the birth of her second son. DESCRIBE the approach you would use in managing this woman's care in a culturally sensitive manner.

12. Tamara delivered vaginally 8 hours ago. She has a midline episiotomy.
   A. DESCRIBE the position that Tamara should assume to facilitate palpation of her fundus.

   B. IDENTIFY the characteristics of Tamara's fundus that should be assessed.

   C. DESCRIBE the position Tamara should assume to facilitate the examination of her episiotomy.

D. IDENTIFY the characteristics that should be assessed to determine progress of healing and adequacy of Tamara's perineal self-care measures.

E. STATE the characteristics of Tamara's uterine flow that should be assessed.

13. Imagine that you are the nurse who cared for a woman during her labor and birth and her recovery during the fourth stage of labor. OUTLINE the information that you would report to the mother-baby nurse when you transfer the new mother and her baby to her room on the postpartum unit.

14. Infection control measures should guide the practice of nurses working on a postpartum unit.
A. DISCUSS the measures designed to prevent transmission of infection from person to person.

B. DISCUSS measures that a postpartum woman should be taught to reduce her risk of infection.

22 Transition to Parenthood

I. LEARNING KEY TERMS

FILL IN THE BLANKS: Insert the appropriate term for each of the following descriptions regarding parent-infant interaction and parenting.

1. _____ Process by which a parent comes to love and accept a child and a child comes to love and accept a parent. The term _____ is often used to refer to this process.

2. _____ Process that occurs as parents interact with their newborn and maintain close proximity as they identify the infant as an individual and claim him or her as a member of the family.

3. _____ Infant behaviors and characteristics call forth a corresponding set of parental behaviors and characteristics.

4. _____ Infant behaviors such as crying, smiling, and cooing that initiate contact and bring the caregiver to the child.

5. _____ Infant behaviors such as rooting, grasping, and postural adjustments that maintain contact.

6. _____ Process in which parents identify the new baby, first in terms of likeness to other family members, then in terms of differences, and finally in terms of uniqueness.

7. _____ Position used for mutual gazing in which the parent's face and the infant's face are approximately 20 cm apart and are on the same plane.

8. _____ Newborns move in time with the structure of adult speech by waving their arms, lifting their heads, and kicking their legs, seemingly "dancing in tune" to a parent's voice.

9. _____ Personal biorhythm developed by the infant; parents facilitate this process by giving consistent loving care and using their infant's alert state to develop responsive behavior and thereby increase social interaction and opportunities for learning.

10. _____ Type of body movement or behavior that provides the observer with cues. The observer or receiver interprets those cues and responds to them.

11. _____ The "fit" between the infant's cues and the parents' response.

12. _____ Period from the decision to conceive through the first months of having a child.

13. _____ Phase of maternal adjustment that occurs during the first 24 hours (range of 1 to 2 days) when the woman focuses on herself and meeting basic needs with a reliance on others for comfort, rest, closeness, and nourishment. She is often talkative and desires to discuss her childbirth experience.

14. _____ Phase of maternal adjustment that begins on the second or third day postpartum and lasts for about 10 days to several weeks, during which the woman focuses on caring for her baby and becoming competent as a mother; she is eager to learn and to practice and may experience baby blues.

15. _____ Phase of maternal adjustment during which the woman reasserts her relationship with her partner and resumes sexual intimacy.

16. _____ Process of transformation and growth of the mother identity during which the woman learns new skills and increases her confidence in herself as she meets new challenges in caring for her child(ren).

17. _____ The quality of a mother's sensitive behaviors that are based on her awareness, perception, and responsiveness to infant cues and behaviors.

18. _____ Period surrounding the first day or two of birth, characterized by heightened joy and feelings of well-being. _____ Period following birth that is characterized by emotional lability, depression, a let-down feeling, restlessness, fatigue, insomnia, anxiety, sadness, and anger. Lability peaks around the fifth day postpartum and subsides by the tenth day.

19. _____ Father's absorption, preoccupation, and interest in his infant.

II. REVIEWING KEY CONCEPTS

20. Attachment of the newborn to parents and family is critical for optimum growth and development.
    A. LIST conditions that must be present for the parent-newborn attachment process to begin favorably.

    B. DISCUSS how nurses should assess the progress of attachment between parents and their new baby.

    C. IDENTIFY what nurses can do to facilitate the process of attachment in the immediate postbirth period.

21. DESCRIBE three parental tasks and responsibilities that are part of parental adjustment to a new baby.

22. DISCUSS how each of the following forms of parent-infant contact can facilitate attachment and promote the family as a focus of care.
    A. Early contact

    B. Extended contact

23. DESCRIBE how a mother's touching of her newborn progresses in the immediate postbirth period.

24. DESCRIBE how each of the following factors influences the manner in which parents respond to the birth of their child. State two nursing implications or actions related to each factor.
Parental age

Parenting in same-sex couples

Social support

Culture

Socioeconomic conditions

Personal aspirations

Sensory impairment

25. COMPARE and CONTRAST Rubin's *Maternal Role Attainment Model of Maternal Adjustment After Birth* and Mercer's *Becoming a Mother Model.*

MULTIPLE CHOICE: Circle the correct option(s) and state the rationale for the option(s) chosen.

26. During the final phase of the claiming process of a newborn, a mother might say:
    A. "She has her grandfather's nose."
    B. "His ears lie nice and flat against his head, not like mine and his sister's, which stick out."
    C. "She gave me nothing but trouble during pregnancy and now she is so stubborn she won't wake up to breastfeed."
    D. "He has such a sweet disposition and pleasant expression. I have never seen a baby quite like him before."

27. Which nursing action is least effective in facilitating parental attachment to the new infant?
    A. Referring the couple to a lactation consultant to ensure continuing success with breastfeeding
    B. Keeping the baby in the nursery as much as possible for the first 24 hours after birth so the mother can rest
    C. Extending visiting hours for the woman's partner or significant other as the couple desires
    D. Providing guidance and support as the parents care for their baby's nutrition and hygiene needs

28. Which behavior illustrates engrossment?
    A. A father is sitting in a rocking chair, holding his new baby boy, touching his toes, and making eye contact.
    B. A mother tells her friends that her baby's eyes and nose are just like hers.
    C. A mother picks up and cuddles her baby girl when she begins to cry.
    D. A grandmother gazes into her new grandson's face, which she holds about 8 inches away from her own; she and the baby make eye-to-eye contact.

29. A woman expresses a need to review her labor and birth experience with the nurse who cared for her while in labor. This behavior is most characteristic of which phase of maternal postpartum adjustment?
    A. Taking-hold (dependent-independent phase)
    B. Taking-in (dependent phase)
    C. Letting-go (interdependent)
    D. Postpartum blues (baby blues)

30. Before discharge, a postpartum woman and her partner ask the nurse about the baby blues. "Our friend said she felt so let down after she had her baby and we have heard that some women actually become very depressed. Is there anything we can do to prevent this from happening to us or at least to cope with the blues if they occur?" The nurse could tell this couple:
    A. "Postpartum blues usually happen in pregnancies that are high risk or unplanned, so there is no need for you to worry."
    B. "Try to become skillful in breastfeeding and caring for your baby as quickly as you can."
    C. "Get as much rest as you can and sleep when the baby sleeps, because fatigue can precipitate the blues or make them worse."
    D. "I will call your doctor before you leave to get you a prescription for an antidepressant to prevent the blues from happening."

III. THINKING CRITICALLY

1. Jane and Andrew are parents of a newborn girl. DESCRIBE what you would teach them regarding the communication process as it relates to their newborn.
    A. Techniques they can use to communicate effectively with their newborn.

    B. The manner in which the baby is able to communicate with them.

2. Allison had a difficult labor that resulted in an emergency cesarean birth under general anesthesia. She did not see her baby until 12 hours after her birth. Allison tells the nurse who brings the baby to her room: "I am so disappointed. I had planned to breastfeed my baby and hold her close, skin to skin, right after her birth, just like all the books say. I know that this is so important for our relationship." DESCRIBE how the nurse should respond to Allison's concern.

3. Angela is the mother of a 1-day-old boy and a 3-year-old girl. As you prepare Angela for discharge, she states: "My little girl just saw her brother. She says she loves him and cannot wait for him to come home. I am so glad that I do not have to worry about any of that sibling rivalry business!" INDICATE how you would respond to Angela's comments.

4. Sara and Ben have just experienced the birth of their first baby. They are very happy with their baby boy but appear very unsure of themselves and are obviously anxious about how to tell what their baby needs. Sara is trying very hard to breastfeed and is having some success but not as much as she had hoped. Both parents express self-doubt about their ability to succeed at the "most important role in our lives."
   A. STATE the nursing diagnosis that is most appropriate for this couple.

   B. DESCRIBE what the nurse caring for this family can do to facilitate the attachment process.

5. Mary and Jim are the parents of three sons. They very much wanted to have a girl this time but after a long and difficult birth they had another son who weighed 10 pounds. His appearance reflects the difficult birth process: occipital molding, caput succedaneum, and forceps marks on each cheek. Mary and Jim express their disappointment not only in the appearance of their son but also about the fact that they had another boy. "This was supposed to be our last child. Now we just do not know what we will do." DISCUSS how you would facilitate Mary and Jim's attachment to their son and reconcile their fantasy ("dream") child with the reality of their actual child.

6. Dawn and Matthew have just given birth to their first baby. This is the first grandchild for both sets of grandparents. The grandmothers approach the nurse to ask how they can help the new family, stating: "We want to help Dawn and Matthew but at the same time not interfere with what they want to do." DISCUSS the role of the nurse in helping these grandparents to recognize their importance to the new family and develop a mutually satisfying relationship with Dawn, Matthew, and the new baby.

7. Jane is 2 days postpartum. When the nurse makes a home visit, Jane is found crying. Jane states: "I have such a let-down feeling. I cannot understand why I feel this way when I should be so happy about the healthy outcome for myself and my baby." Jane's husband confirms her behavior and expresses confusion as well, stating: "I wish I knew what to do to help her." IDENTIFY the priority nursing diagnosis and one expected outcome for this situation. DESCRIBE the recommended nursing management for the nursing diagnosis you have identified.

Nursing Diagnosis	Expected Outcome	Care Measures

8. Adam has just become a father with the birth of his first child, a baby boy.
   A. DESCRIBE the process Adam will follow as he adjusts to fatherhood.

   B. IDENTIFY several measures that the nurse caring for Adam's wife and baby boy can use to facilitate his adjustment to fatherhood and attachment to his baby.

23 Physiologic and Behavioral Adaptations of the Newborn

I. LEARNING KEY TERMS

FILL IN THE BLANKS: Insert the term that corresponds to each of the following descriptions related to newborn characteristics and care.

1. _____ Protein manufactured in type II cells of the lungs that reduces surface tension, thereby decreasing the pressure required to keep alveoli open with inspiration and preventing total alveolar collapse on exhalation; alveolar stability is maintained.

2. _____ Maintenance of balance between heat loss and heat production.

3. _____ Generation of heat.

4. _____ Heat production process unique to the newborn accomplished primarily by brown fat metabolism and secondarily by increased metabolic activity in the brain, heart, and liver.

5. _____ Environment in which heat balance for the newborn is maintained; it is at the temperature that allows the newborn to maintain a normal body temperature to minimize oxygen and glucose consumption.

6. _____ Flow of heat from the body surface to cooler ambient air. Two measures to reduce heat loss using this method are to keep the ambient air at 24°C and wrap the infant who is in an open bassinet.

7. _____ Loss of heat from the body surface to a cooler, solid surface not in direct contact but in relative proximity. To prevent this type of heat loss, cribs and examining tables are placed away from outside windows and care is taken to avoid direct air drafts.

8. _____ Loss of heat that occurs when a liquid is converted to vapor; in the newborn, heat loss occurs when moisture from the skin is vaporized. This heat loss can be intensified by failure to dry the newborn directly after birth or by drying the newborn too slowly after a bath.

9. _____ Loss of heat from the body surface to cooler surfaces in direct contact. When admitted to the nursery, the newborn is placed in a warmed crib to minimize heat loss. Placing a protective cover on the scale when weighing the newborn will also minimize heat lost by this method.

10. _____ High body temperature (>37.5°C) that develops more rapidly in the newborn than in the adult. The newborn has a decreased ability to increase evaporative skin water losses because of a relatively large body surface and sweat glands that do not function sufficiently to allow the newborn to sweat; it can cause neurologic injury and increased risk of seizures and, if severe, heat stroke and death.

11. _____ Pinkish, easily blanched areas on the upper eyelids, nose, upper lip, back of the head, and nape of the neck. They are also known as "stork bites," "angel kisses," or "salmon patches."

12. _____ Overlapping of cranial bones to facilitate passage of the fetal head through the maternal pelvis during the process of labor and birth.

13. _____ Generalized, easily identifiable edematous area of the scalp usually over the occiput.

14. _____ Collection of blood between skull bone and its periosteum as a result of pressure during birth; it does not cross a suture line.

15. _____ Bluish-black pigmented areas usually found on back and buttocks.

16. _____ Bluish discoloration of the hands and feet, especially when chilled; it is a normal intermittent finding over the first 10 days after birth related to vasomotor instability and capillary stasis.

17. _____ White cheeselike substance that coats and protects the fetus's skin while in utero.

18. _____ White facial pimples caused by distended sebaceous glands.

19. _____ Yellowish skin discoloration caused by elevated serum levels of unconjugated (indirect) bilirubin.

20. _____ Nonpathologic unconjugated hyperbilirubinemia that occurs in approximately 60% of term newborns and 80% of preterm newborns. It appears after 24 hours of age and usually resolves without treatment.

21. _____ Acute manifestations of bilirubin toxicity that occur during the first weeks after birth; these can include lethargy, hypotonia, irritability, seizures, coma, and death.

22. _____ Irreversible, long-term consequences of bilirubin toxicity such as hypotonia, delayed motor skills, hearing loss, cerebral palsy, and gaze abnormalities.

23. _____ Hyperbilirubinemia that can be manifested by breastfed newborns. Early onset, which begins in the first 2 to 4 days of age, is associated with ineffective breastfeeding. The etiology of the late-onset form, which can begin at age 5 or 10 days and persist for up to 12 weeks, is uncertain but could be related to factors found naturally in breast milk.

24. _____ Thick, dark green–black stool formed during fetal life and usually passed within 24 hours of birth.

25. _____ Sudden, transient newborn rash characterized by erythematous macules, papules, and small vesicles found anywhere on the body.

26. _____ Condition in which the urethral opening is located on the ventral side of the surface of the penis. _____ Condition in which the urethral opening is located on the dorsal side of the surface of the penis.

27. _____ Accumulation of fluid in the scrotum, around the testes.

28. _____ Small whitish areas found on the gum margins and at the juncture of the hard and soft palates.

29. _____ Membranous area formed where skull bones join.

30. _____ Soft, downy hair on face, shoulders, and back.

31. _____ Bruise.

32. _____ Peeling of the skin that occurs in the term infant a few days after birth as vernix caseosa is removed; if present at birth, it may be an indication of postmaturity.

33. _____ Vascular lesion visible at birth as pink and flat but darkens with time, becoming red or purple and pebbly in consistency; it varies in size, shape, and location but is usually found on the neck and face. It does not blanch under pressure or disappear.

34. _____ Birthmark consisting of dilated, newly formed capillaries occupying the entire dermal and subdermal layers with associated connective tissue hypertrophy; it is typically a raised, sharply demarcated bright or dark red, rough-surfaced swelling, usually found as a single lesion on the head.

35. _____ Slightly blood-tinged mucoid vaginal discharge associated with an estrogen decrease after birth.

36. _____ Foreskin.

37. _____ Skeletal abnormality resulting in a hip that dislocates easily.

38. _____ Small, white, firm cysts seen at the tip of the foreskin.

39. _____ Missing digits.

40. _____ Extra digits.

41. _____ Fused fingers or toes.

FILL IN THE BLANKS: Insert the term that corresponds to each of the following descriptions related to newborn behavioral adaptations and characteristics.

42. _____ Variations in the state of consciousness of newborn infants.

43. _____ and _____ The two sleep states. The newborn sleeps about

_____ hours a day, with periods of wakefulness gradually _____.

44. _____, _____, _____, and

_____ The four wake states.

45. _____ The optimum state of arousal in which the infant can be observed smiling, responding to voices, watching faces, vocalizing, and moving in synchrony with speech.

46. _____ Ability of the newborn to respond to internal and external environmental factors by controlling sensory input and regulating the sleep-wake states, thereby making smooth transitions between states.

47. _____ Protective mechanism that allows the infant to become accustomed to environmental stimuli. It is a psychologic and physiologic phenomenon in which the response to a constant or repetitive stimulus is decreased.

48. _____ Quality of alert states and ability to attend to visual and auditory stimuli while alert.

49. _____ Individual variations in a newborn's primary reaction pattern.

MATCHING: Match the description in Column I with the appropriate newborn reflex in Column II.

COLUMN I

50. _____ Place infant in a supine position and apply pressure to soles of the feet with fingers when the lower limbs are semi-flexed; legs extend against examiner's pressure.

51. _____ Place infant supine on flat surface and make a loud abrupt noise; symmetric abduction and extension of arms, fingers fan out, thumb and forefinger form a C; arms are then adducted into an embracing motion and return to relaxed flexion and movement.

52. _____ Place finger in palm of hand or at base of toes; infant's fingers curl around examiner's finger or toes curl downward.

53. _____ Place infant prone on flat surface, run finger down side of back first on one side and then down the other side 4 to 5 cm lateral to spine; trunk flexes and pelvis swings toward stimulated side.

54. _____ Tap over forehead, bridge of nose, or maxilla when eyes are open; blinks for first four or five taps.

55. _____ Use finger to stroke sole of foot beginning at heel, upward along lateral aspect of sole, then across ball of foot; all toes hyperextend, with dorsiflexion of big toe ("positive response").

56. _____ Anal sphincter responds to touch by opening and closing.

57. _____ Testes retract when infant is chilled.

58. _____ Touch infant's lip, cheek, or corner of mouth with nipple or finger; turns head toward stimulus and opens mouth ready to take hold and suck.

59. _____ Place sleepy infant in a supine position, then turn head quickly to one side; arm and leg on side to which head is turned extend while opposite arm and leg flex.

60. _____ Hold infant vertically, allowing one foot to touch table surface; infant alternates flexion and extension of feet.

61. _____ Touch or depress tip of tongue; tongue is forced outward.

62. _____ Place infant in a supine position. Then extend one leg, press knee downward, and stimulate bottom of foot; opposite leg flexes, adducts, and then extends.

COLUMN II

A. Rooting
B. Grasp
C. Extrusion
D. Glabellar (Myerson sign)
E. Tonic neck (fencing)
F. Moro
G. Stepping (walking)
H. Wink reflex
I. Babinski (plantar)
J. Truncal incurvation (Galant)
K. Magnet
L. Cremasteric
M. Crossed extension

II. REVIEWING KEY CONCEPTS

63. The most critical adjustment that a newborn must make at birth is the establishment of respirations. LIST the factors that are responsible for the initiation of breathing after birth.

64. During the first 6 to 8 hours after birth, newborns experience a transitional period characterized by three phases of instability. INDICATE the timing, duration, and typical behaviors for each phase of this transitional period.
First period of reactivity

Period of decreased responsiveness

Second period of reactivity

65. EXPLAIN how each of the following factors influences newborn behavior.
   ■ Gestational age

   ■ Time

   ■ Stimuli

   ■ Medication

MULTIPLE CHOICE: Circle the correct option(s) and state the rationale for the option(s) chosen.

66. A newborn, at 5 hours old, wakes from a sound sleep and becomes very active and begins to cry. Which signs, if exhibited by this newborn, indicate expected adaptation to extrauterine life? (Circle all that apply.)
   A. Increased mucus production
   B. Passage of meconium
   C. Heart rate of 160 beats/minute
   D. Respiratory rate of 24 breaths/minute and irregular
   E. Fine crackles on auscultation
   F. Expiratory grunting with nasal flaring

67. When assessing a newborn boy at 12 hours of age, the nurse notes a rash on his abdomen and thighs. The rash appears as irregular reddish blotches with scattered papules. The nurse:
   A. Documents the finding as erythema toxicum
   B. Isolates the newborn and his mother until infection is ruled out
   C. Applies an antiseptic ointment to each lesion
   D. Requests nonallergenic linens from the laundry

68. A breast-fed full-term newborn girl is 12 hours old and being prepared for early discharge. If present, which assessment findings could delay discharge? (Circle all that apply.)
   A. Dark green–black stool, thick consistency
   B. Yellowish tinge in sclera and on face
   C. Swollen breasts with a scant amount of thin discharge
   D. Blood-tinged mucoid vaginal discharge
   E. Blood glucose level of 35 mg/dL
   F. Acrocyanosis

Chapter **23** **Physiologic and Behavioral Adaptations of the Newborn**

69. As part of a thorough assessment of a newborn, the pediatric nurse practitioner (PNP) should check for hip dislocation and dysplasia. Which technique does the PNP use?
A. Check for syndactyly bilaterally
B. Stepping or walking reflex
C. Magnet reflex
D. Ortolani maneuver

70. When assessing a newborn after birth, the nurse notes flat, irregular, pinkish marks on the bridge of the nose, nape of the neck, and over the eyelids. The areas blanch when pressed with a finger. The nurse documents this finding as:
A. Milia
B. Nevus vasculosus
C. Telangiectatic nevi
D. Nevus flammeus

III. THINKING CRITICALLY

1. When caring for newborns, especially during the transition period following birth, the nurse recognizes that newborns are at increased risk for cold stress.
A. EXPLAIN the basis for this risk.

B. STATE the dangers that cold stress poses for the newborn.

C. IDENTIFY one nursing diagnosis and one expected outcome related to this danger.

D. DESCRIBE care measures the nurse should implement to prevent cold stress from occurring.

2. After a long and difficult labor, baby boy James was born with a caput succedaneum, significant molding over the occipital area, and a small cephalhematoma over the right parietal bone. Low forceps were used for the birth, resulting in ecchymotic areas on both cheeks. James's parents tell the nurse that they are very concerned that James may have experienced brain damage. DESCRIBE what the nurse should tell the parents about these assessment findings.

3. Mary and Jim are concerned that their baby boy, born 2 days ago via a cesarean birth, appears to look a little "yellow," especially in his eyes. They ask the nurse if there is something wrong with their baby's liver. After examination of the baby, a diagnosis of physiologic jaundice is made.

A. LIST the criteria used to make this diagnosis.

B. EXPLAIN to Mary and Jim what caused their baby to appear yellow.

4. Susan and Allen are first-time parents of a baby girl. They ask the nurse about their baby's ability to see and hear things around her and to interact with them.

A. SPECIFY what the nurse should tell these parents about the sensory capabilities of their healthy full-term newborn.

B. NAME four stimuli that Susan and Allen can provide for their baby that would help to foster her development.

C. DESCRIBE what the nurse should tell the parents about the best time to interact with their newborn.

5. Tonya and Sam, an African-American couple, express concern that their new baby girl has several bruises on her back and buttocks. They ask if their baby was injured during birth or in the nursery. DESCRIBE the appropriate response of the nurse to this couple's concern.

24 Nursing Care of the Newborn and Family

I. LEARNING KEY TERMS

FILL IN THE BLANKS: Insert the term that corresponds to each of the following descriptions of newborns and their care.

1. _____ Tool used to rapidly assess the newborn's transition to extrauterine life at 1 and 5 minutes after birth; it is based on five signs that indicate the newborn's physiologic state, namely

   _____, _____, _____,

   _____, and _____.

2. _____ Device used to suction mucus and secretions from the newborn's mouth and nose immediately after birth and when needed.

3. _____ Automatic sensor usually placed on the upper quadrant of the abdomen immediately below the right or left costal margin; it is attached to the radiant warmer and monitors the newborn's skin temperature.

4. _____ Instillation of antibiotic ointment into the eyes of a newborn after birth to prevent infection.

5. _____ Inflammation of the newborn's eyes caused by sexually transmitted bacteria (e.g., gonorrhea, chlamydia) acquired by the newborn during passage through the mother's birth canal.

   _____ or _____ ointment is usually instilled into the newborn's eyes within 1 to 2 hours after birth to prevent this infection.

6. _____ Medication administered intramuscularly to the newborn to prevent neonatal hemorrhagic disease; it is administered in a dose of 0.5 to 1 mg.

7. _____ Tool used to assess and estimate a newborn's gestational age after birth; it involves assessment of the degree of the newborn's physical and neurologic maturity.

8. _____ Term used to describe an infant whose birth weight falls between the 10th and 90th percentiles as a result of growing at a normal rate during fetal life regardless of length of gestation.

9. _____ Term used to describe an infant whose birth weight falls above the 90th percentile as a result of growing at an accelerated rate during fetal life, regardless of length of gestation.

10. _____ Term used to describe an infant whose birth weight falls below the 10th percentile as a result of growing at a restricted rate during fetal life, regardless of length of gestation.

11. _____ Infant born before the completion of 37 weeks of gestation, regardless of birth weight.

12. _____ Infant born at 34 to 36 weeks of gestation; this infant has risk factors due to his or her physiologic immaturity that require close attention by nurses. _____ Infant born between 37 and 38 weeks of gestation; they are at greater risk than full-term infants for both short-term and long-term health problems.

13. _____ Infant born between the beginning of week 39 and the end of week 40 of gestation. _____ Infant born during the 41st week of gestation.

14. _____ Infant born at 42 weeks of gestation and beyond.

15. _____ Infant born after the completion of 42 weeks of gestation and showing the effects of progressive placental insufficiency.

16. _____ Pinpoint hemorrhagic areas acquired during birth that may extend over the upper trunk and face; they are benign if they disappear within 2 to 3 days of birth and no new lesions appear.

17. _____ One of the products derived from the hemoglobin released with the breakdown of red blood cells and the myoglobin in muscle cells; accumulation of the unconjugated form in the blood results in a yellowish discoloration of the skin, sclera, and oral mucous membranes.

18. _____ Yellowish discoloration of the integument and sclera that appears after the first 24 hours of life, peaks at 3 to 5 days, and resolves in 1 to 2 weeks, usually without the need for treatment.

19. _____ Test performed to distinguish cutaneous jaundice of the skin from normal skin color. It is performed by applying pressure with a finger over a bony area such as the nose, forehead, or sternum for several seconds to empty all capillaries in the spot. The area will appear yellow when the finger is removed if jaundice is present.

20. _____ Device used for noninvasive monitoring of bilirubin via cutaneous reflectance measurements; it allows for repetitive estimation of bilirubin and works well on both dark-skinned and light-skinned newborns.

21. _____ Infection characterized by white plaques on cheeks or tongue that bleed if touched.

22. _____ Blood glucose concentration less than adequate to support neurologic, organ, and tissue function during the early newborn period; the precise level at which this occurs in every neonate is not known, though intervention is usually required if the blood glucose level falls below 40 to 45 mg/dL.

23. _____ Serum calcium level less than 7.8 to 8 mg/dL in the term infant and slightly lower than 7 mg/dL in the preterm infant.

24. _____ Newborn respiratory rate of 30 breaths/minute or less.

25. _____ Newborn respiratory rate of 60 breaths/minute or more.

26. _____ The most important single measure in the prevention of neonatal infection.

27. _____ Use of light energy to treat hyperbilirubinemia by converting unconjugated bilirubin to a conjugated form that can be excreted through the urine or feces.

28. _____ Surgical procedure that involves removing all or part of the prepuce (foreskin) of the penis.

29. _____ Pain assessment tool for newborns. A score is determined by evaluating five signs, namely, _____, _____, _____, _____, and _____.

II. REVIEWING KEY CONCEPTS

Neonatal nurses are responsible for the assessment of the physiologic integrity of newborns. As part of this responsibility, the nurse must be aware of the significance of data collected. LABEL each of the following assessment findings, if present, in a group of three full-term 12-hour-old newborns who are all in the quiet-alert state as "N" (reflective of normal adaptation or acceptable variation to extrauterine life) or "P" (reflective of potential problems with adaptation to extrauterine life).

_____ 30. Crackles on auscultation of the lungs

_____ 31. Respirations: 36 breaths/minute, irregular, shallow

_____ 32. Episodic apnea lasting 5 to 10 seconds

_____ 33. Nasal flaring and sternal retractions

_____ 34. Slight bluish discoloration of hands and feet

_____ 35. Blood pressure 76/44 mm Hg

_____ 36. Apical heart rate: 126 beats/minute with murmurs

_____ 37. Temperature 36°C

_____ 38. Pink-tinged stains on diaper with first two voidings

_____ 39. Two small white cysts at gum margins and on palate

_____ 40. Boggy, edematous swelling over occiput

_____ 41. Overlapping of parietal bones

_____ 42. White pimplelike spots on nose and chin

_____ 43. Jaundice on face

_____ 44. Regurgitation of small amount of milk following first two feedings

_____ 45. Liver palpated at 1 cm below right costal margin

_____ 46. Absence of bowel elimination since birth

_____ 47. Spine straight with dimple and small tuft of hair at the base

_____ 48. Adhesion of prepuce—unable to fully retract foreskin

_____ 49. Edema of labia majora

_____ 50. Flaring of toes and hyperextension of big toe when sole is stroked upward

_____ 51. Hematocrit 36% and hemoglobin 12 g/dL

_____ 52. White blood cell count (WBC) 20,000/mm^3

_____ 53. Blood glucose 48 mg/dL

54. OUTLINE the specific measures that nurses should use when caring for newborns to ensure a safe and protective environment.

55. When assessing newborns, nurses should be alert for evidence of physical injuries sustained by the newborn during the labor and birth process. IDENTIFY the predisposing factors for birth trauma and the types of injuries that can occur.

56. Preparing parents for the discharge of their newborn requires informing them about the essential aspects of newborn care. IDENTIFY three points that you would emphasize when teaching parents about each of the following aspects of newborn characteristics and care. Include teaching methodologies you would use.

A. Vital signs: temperature and respirations

B. Elimination: urinary and bowel

C. Positioning and holding

D. Safety

E. Hygiene: bathing, cord care, and skin care

57. A nurse is measuring a full-term newborn boy 1 hour after his birth. SPECIFY the guidelines that this nurse should follow to ensure accuracy of the findings and safety of the newborn when measuring him. INDICATE the expected range for the term newborn.

Weight

Head circumference

Chest circumference

Abdominal circumference

Length

58. Nurses caring for newborns are often required to collect blood and urine specimens for laboratory testing. OUTLINE the guidelines that nurses should use for each of the following specimen collection techniques.
Heelstick

Venipuncture

Collection bag for specimen collection

59. Maintaining a patent airway and supporting respirations to ensure an adequate oxygen supply in the newborn are essential focuses of nursing care management of the newborn, especially in the early postbirth period.
A. STATE the four conditions that are essential for maintaining an adequate oxygen supply in the newborn.

B. LIST four signs that the nurse who is assessing a newborn would recognize as indicative of abnormal breathing.

C. DESCRIBE the bulb syringe method of relieving airway obstruction in an infant.

60. Nurses must educate new parents regarding the dangers of shaking a baby.
    A. EXPLAIN the purpose of the Period of PURPLE Crying program.

    B. IDENTIFY the meaning of each letter in the acronym PURPLE.

MULTIPLE CHOICE: Circle the correct option(s) and state the rationale for the option(s) chosen.

61. A newborn male is estimated to be at 40 weeks of gestation following an assessment using the New Ballard Scale. New Ballard Scale findings consistent with this newborn's full-term status are: (Circle all that apply.)
    A. Apical pulse rate of 120 beats/minute, regular, and strong
    B. Popliteal angle of 160 degrees
    C. Weight of 3200 g, placing him at the 50th percentile
    D. Thinning of lanugo with some bald areas
    E. Testes descended into the scrotum
    F. Elbow does not pass midline when arm is pulled across the chest

62. The nurse evaluates the laboratory test results of a newborn who is 4 hours old. Which results require notification of the pediatrician? (Circle all that apply.)
    A. Hemoglobin 20 g/dL
    B. Hematocrit 54%
    C. Glucose 34 mg/dL
    D. White blood cell count 24,000/mm³
    E. Calcium 7 mg/dL

63. A newborn male has been designated as large for gestational age. His mother was diagnosed with gestational diabetes late in her pregnancy. The nurse should be alert for signs of hypoglycemia. Which assessment finding is consistent with a diagnosis of hypoglycemia?
    A. High-pitched cry
    B. Jitteriness
    C. Hyperthermia
    D. Laryngospasm

64. A radiant warmer will be used to help a newborn girl to stabilize her temperature. The nurse implementing this care measure should:
    A. Undress and dry the infant before placing her under the warmer
    B. Set the control panel between 35°C and 38°C
    C. Place the thermistor probe on her abdomen just below her umbilical cord
    D. Assess her rectal temperature every hour until her temperature stabilizes

65. A newborn male has been scheduled for a circumcision. Essential nursing care measures following this surgical procedure include:
    A. Use the New Ballard Score to determine if the newborn is in pain
    B. Applying petroleum ointment to the site with every diaper change until the site is healed
    C. Checking the penis for bleeding every 15 minutes for the first 4 hours
    D. Teaching the parents to remove the yellowish exudate that forms over the glans using a diaper wipe

66. A physician has ordered that a newborn receive a hepatitis B vaccination prior to discharge. In fulfilling this order the nurse should: (Circle all that apply.)
    A. Confirm that the mother is hepatitis B positive before the injection is given
    B. Obtain parental consent prior to administering the vaccination
    C. Inform the parents that the next vaccine in the series needs to be given at 1 to 2 months
    D. Administer the injection into the vastus lateralis muscle
    E. Use a 1-inch 23-gauge needle
    F. Insert the needle at a 45-degree angle

67. A nurse is preparing to administer erythromycin ophthalmic ointment 0.5% to a newborn after birth. Which nursing actions are appropriate? (Circle all that apply.)
    A. Administer the ointment within 30 minutes of the birth
    B. Wear gloves
    C. Cleanse the eyes if secretions are present
    D. Squeeze an ointment ribbon of 3 cm into the lower conjunctival sac
    E. Wipe away excess ointment after 1 minute
    F. Apply the ointment from the inner to outer canthus

III. THINKING CRITICALLY

1. Apgar scoring is a method of newborn assessment used in the immediate postbirth period, at 1 and 5 minutes. INDICATE the Apgar score for each of the following newborns.
   A. Baby boy Smith at 1 minute after birth:
      Heart rate—160 beats/minute
      Respiratory effort—good, crying vigorously
      Muscle tone—active movement, well flexed
      Reflex irritability—cries with stimulus to soles of feet
      Color—body pink, feet and hands cyanotic
         Score: _____
         Interpretation:

   B. Baby girl Doe at 5 minutes after birth:
      Heart rate—102 beats/minute
      Respiratory effort—slow, irregular with weak cry
      Muscle tone—some flexion of extremities
      Reflex irritability—grimace with stimulus to soles of feet
      Color—pale
         Score: _____
         Interpretation:

2. Baby girl June was just born.
   A. OUTLINE the protocol that the nurse should follow when assessing June's physical status during the first 2 hours after her birth.

   B. STATE the nurse's legal responsibility regarding identification of June and her mother after birth.

   C. IDENTIFY the priority nursing diagnosis for the first 2 hours after birth.

D. CITE the priority nursing care measures that the nurse must implement to ensure June's well-being and safety during the first 2 hours after birth.

E. DESCRIBE the emotional and physiologic benefits of early contact between the mother and her newborn.

3. Baby boy Tim is 24 hours old. The nurse is preparing to perform a physical examination of this newborn before his discharge.
   A. LIST the actions the nurse should take to ensure safety and accuracy. Include the rationale for the actions identified.

   B. IDENTIFY the major points that should be assessed as part of this physical examination.

   C. SUPPORT the premise that Tim's parents should be present during this examination.

4. Baby girl Susan has an accumulation of mucus in her nasal passages and mouth, making breathing difficult.
   A. STATE the nursing diagnosis represented by the assessment findings.

   B. LIST the steps that the nurse should follow when clearing Susan's airway using a bulb syringe.

5. Susan and James are taking their newly circumcised (6 hours postprocedure) baby home. This is their first baby and they express anxiety concerning care of both the circumcision and the umbilical cord.
   A. STATE one nursing diagnosis related to this situation.

B. STATE one expected outcome related to the nursing diagnosis identified.

C. SPECIFY the instructions that the nurse should give to Susan and James regarding assessment of both sites and the care measures required to facilitate healing.

6. Andrew and Marion are parents of a newborn, 30 hours old, who has developed hyperbilirubinemia. They are very concerned about the color of their baby and the need to put the baby under special lights. "A relative was yellow just like our baby and later died of liver cancer!"
A. DESCRIBE how the nurse should respond to Andrew and Marion's concern.

B. DESCRIBE the blanch test as a method of assessment for jaundice.

C. IDENTIFY the expected assessment findings and physiologic effects related to hyperbilirubinemia.

D. LIST the precautions and care measures required for the newborn undergoing phototherapy to prevent injury to the newborn yet maintain the effectiveness of the treatment. State the rationale for each action identified.

7. A newborn is scheduled for a circumcision. The nurse caring for this newborn is aware that he will experience pain as a result of this procedure.
A. DESCRIBE the most common newborn behavioral responses to pain.

B. INDICATE how a newborn's vital signs and integument will change when he or she experiences pain.

C. EXPLAIN how the CRIES assessment can be used to monitor a newborn's pain during circumcision.

D. OUTLINE the nonpharmacologic and pharmacologic measures that the nurse could use or suggest to be used to minimize the pain experience and its effects and maximize the newborn's ability to cope with the pain and recover.

8. You are caring for a newborn girl born vaginally 30 minutes ago. As part of your care of this newborn, you are required to administer two medications as listed below. STATE the purpose for each of the medications and the guidelines you would follow to ensure their safe and effective administration.
   A. erythromycin ophthalmic ointment 0.5%

   B. vitamin K (AquaMEPHYTON) 0.5 mg IM

9. Mary and Jim are concerned because their breastfed baby boy, who weighed 8 lb, 6 oz at birth, now "weighs only 7 lb, 14 oz" at 2 days of age. They wonder if Mary should stop breastfeeding as a result of this continuing weight loss. Mary states: "Maybe my breast milk is just not good enough to help my baby grow." DESCRIBE how you would respond to their concern.

25 Newborn Nutrition and Feeding

I. LEARNING KEY TERMS

FILL IN THE BLANKS: Insert the term that corresponds to the following descriptions of breast structures and the breastfeeding process.

1. _____ Structures in the breast that contain alveoli surrounded by myoepithelial cells. There are approximately 15 to 20 of these structures embedded in the fat and connective tissue in each female breast.

2. _____ Milk-producing cells.

3. _____ Breast structures that transport milk from the milk-producing cells to the nipple; they form a complex intertwining network.

4. _____ Cells that surround the alveoli; these cells contract in response to oxytocin, resulting in the milk ejection reflex or let-down.

5. _____ Rounded, pigmented section of tissue surrounding the nipple.

6. _____ The process of milk production.

7. _____ The lactogenic hormone secreted by the anterior pituitary gland in response to the infant's suck and emptying of the breast.

8. _____ Posterior pituitary hormone that triggers the let-down reflex.

9. _____ Reflex response of the nipple when the infant cries, suckles, or rubs against the breast; this response aides in propelling milk through the milk ducts to the nipple pores.

10. _____ Nipple type that becomes hard, erect, and protrudes on stimulation, thereby facilitating latch-on. _____ Nipple type that remains flat and soft and does not protrude even when stimulated.

11. _____ Plastic device that can be placed over the nipple and areola to keep clothing off the nipple and put pressure around its base to promote protrusion of the nipple.

12. _____ Clear yellowish, high-protein, antibody-rich fluid present in the breasts before the formation of milk.

13. _____ Difficulty in knowing how to latch on to the breast after having taken a bottle or artificial nipple (pacifier).

14. _____ Newborn behaviors that indicate hunger and a desire to eat, such as hand-to-mouth movements, rooting, and mouth and tongue movements.

15. _____ or _____ Reflex triggered by the contraction of myoepithelial cells as a result of oxytocin stimulation. Colostrum, and later milk, is transported to the nipple.

16. _____ Reflex stimulated when the area around a hungry baby's mouth is touched. The baby opens its mouth and begins to suck.

17. _____ Placement of the infant's mouth over the nipple, areola, and breast, making a seal between the mouth and the breast to create adequate suction for milk removal.

18. _____ Breast response that occurs around the third to fifth day, when the "milk comes in" and blood supply to the breasts increases. The breasts become tender, swollen, hot and hard, and even shiny and red.

19. _____ Breastfeeding position in which the mother holds the baby's head and shoulders in her hand with the baby's back and body tucked under her arm.

20. _____ Breastfeeding position in which the baby's head is positioned in the crook of the mother's arm and the mother and baby are "tummy to tummy."

21. _____ Health care professional who specializes in breastfeeding and may be available to assist a new mother with breastfeeding while in the hospital or after discharge.

22. _____ Infection of the breast manifested by a swollen, tender breast and sudden onset of influenza-like symptoms.

23. _____ Oral infection caused by a fungus or yeast.

24. _____ Short or tight frenulum, which interferes with extrusion and effective sucking.

25. _____ Process whereby the infant is gradually introduced to drinking from a cup and eating solid food while breastfeeding and bottle-feeding is reduced by gradually decreasing the number of feedings.

26. _____ Milk that is initially released with breastfeeding; it is bluish white, is composed of part skim milk and part whole milk, and provides primarily lactose, protein, and water-soluble vitamins.

27. _____ Milk that is let down 10 to 20 minutes into the feeding; often called the cream, it is denser in calories from fat necessary for optimal growth and contentment between feedings.

28. _____ and _____ The "mothering" hormones.

29. _____ Medications or substances that are believed to increase milk production.

II. REVIEWING KEY CONCEPTS

30. A nurse has been asked to participate in a women's health seminar for women of childbearing age in the community. Her topic is "Breastfeeding: The Goals for *Healthy People 2020* and Beyond." OUTLINE the points that this nurse should emphasize to help women appreciate the benefits of breastfeeding and seriously consider breastfeeding when they have a baby.

31. It is important that a breastfeeding woman alter the position she uses for breastfeeding as one means of preserving nipple and areolar integrity. DESCRIBE four positions that the nurse should demonstrate to a woman who is breast-feeding her newborn.

32. Infants exhibit feeding cues as they recognize and express their hunger.
    A. IDENTIFY feeding cues of the infant.

    B. STATE why the new mother should be guided by these cues when determining the timing of feeding sessions.

33. A proper latch-on is essential for effective breastfeeding and preservation of nipple and areolar integrity.
    A. INDICATE the steps that the nurse should teach a breastfeeding woman to follow to ensure a proper latch-on.

    B. When observing a woman breastfeeding, it is essential that the nurse determine the effectiveness of the latch-on. STATE the signs a nurse should look for that would indicate a proper latch-on.

    C. DESCRIBE the way in which a woman should remove her baby from her breast after feeding is completed.

MULTIPLE CHOICE: Circle the correct option(s) and state the rationale for the option(s) chosen.

34. During a home visit, the mother of a 1-week-old infant son tells the nurse that she is very concerned about whether her baby is getting enough breast milk. The nurse should tell this mother that at 1 week of age a well-nourished newborn should exhibit:
    A. Weight gain sufficient to reach his birth weight
    B. A minimum of three bowel movements each day of soft, yellow, seedy stools
    C. Approximately 10 to 12 wet diapers each day
    D. Breastfeeding at a frequency of every 4 hours, or about 6 times each day

35. A woman is trying to calm her fussy baby daughter in preparation for feeding. She exhibits a need for further instruction if she:
    A. Removes all clothing from the infant except the diaper
    B. Dims the lights in the room and turns off the television
    C. Gently rocks the baby and talks to her in a low voice
    D. Allows the baby to suck on her finger

36. The nurse should teach breastfeeding mothers about breast care measures to preserve the integrity of the nipples and areola. What should the nurse include in these instructions?
    A. Cleanse nipples and areola twice a day with mild soap and water.
    B. Apply vitamin E cream to nipples and areola at least four times each day before a feeding.
    C. Insert plastic-lined pads into the bra to absorb leakage and protect clothing.
    D. Apply modified lanolin to both dry and sore nipples.

Chapter **25** **Newborn Nutrition and Feeding**

37. A breastfeeding woman asks the nurse about a reliable and safe method of birth control she should use during the postpartum period. The best recommendation for a safe yet effective method during the first 6 weeks after birth is:
   A. Combination oral contraceptive that she used before she was pregnant
   B. Barrier method using a combination of a condom and spermicide foam
   C. The diaphragm she used prior to getting pregnant
   D. Complete breastfeeding—baby only receives breast milk for nourishment

38. A woman has determined that bottle-feeding is the best feeding method for her. Instructions that the woman should receive regarding this feeding method include:
   A. Check nipple before feeding to ensure that it allows passage of formula in a slow stream.
   B. Sterilize water by boiling; then cool and mix with formula powder or concentrate.
   C. Expect a 2-week-old newborn to drink approximately 90 to 150 mL of formula at each feeding.
   D. Microwave refrigerated formula for about 2 minutes before feeding the newborn.

39. At a home visit 1 week after birth, a nurse is evaluating a woman's breastfeeding technique. Which actions indicate that the woman needs further instruction regarding breastfeeding to ensure success? (Circle all that apply.)
   A. Waits to feed her baby until he wakes up and begins to cry.
   B. Massages a small amount of breast milk into her nipple and areola before and after each feeding.
   C. Squeezes her nipple and areola between her thumb and forefinger and then inserts her nipple into the baby's mouth.
   D. Positions her baby, supporting back and shoulders securely, and then brings her breast toward the baby, putting the nipple in the baby's mouth.
   E. Inserts her finger into the corner of her baby's mouth between the gums before removing the baby from the breast.

40. A new breastfeeding mother asks the nurse how to prevent nipple soreness. The nurse tells this woman that the key to preventing sore nipples is:
   A. Limiting the length of breastfeeding to no more than 10 minutes on each breast until the milk comes in
   B. Applying lanolin to each nipple and areola after each feeding
   C. Using correct technique for latch-on and removal from the breast
   D. Using breast shells to protect the nipples and areola between feedings

III. THINKING CRITICALLY

1. Tonya is bottle-feeding her baby. She expresses concern to the nurse at the well-baby clinic about heart disease and cholesterol levels as they relate to her 2-month-old baby. She tells the nurse that her family has a history of cardiac disease and hypertension and she has already changed her diet and wants to do the same for her baby. Tonya asks, "When should I start giving my baby skim milk instead of the prepared formula that I am using, which seems to contain quite a bit of fat?" DISCUSS how the nurse should respond to Tonya's question.

2. Elise and her husband, Mark, are experiencing their first pregnancy. During one of their prenatal visits they tell the nurse that they are as yet unsure about the method they want to use for feeding their baby. "Everyone has an opinion—some say breastfeeding is best yet others tell us that bottle-feeding is more convenient, especially because the father can help. What should we do?"
   A. IDENTIFY one nursing diagnosis and one expected outcome appropriate for this situation.

   B. DISCUSS why it is important for the pregnant couple to make this decision together.

C. INDICATE why is it preferable to make this decision during the prenatal period rather than waiting until the baby is born.

D. DESCRIBE how the nurse could use the decision-making process to assist Elise and Mark to choose the method that is best for them.

3. Mary, as a first-time breastfeeding mother, has many questions. DESCRIBE how you would respond to the following questions and comments.
   A. "I am so afraid that I will not make enough milk for my baby. My breasts are not as large as some of my friends who breastfeed."

   B. "Everyone keeps talking about this let-down that is supposed to happen. What is it and how will I know I have it?"

   C. "How can I possibly know if breastfeeding is going well and my baby is getting enough if I cannot tell how many ounces he gets with each feeding?"

   D. "It is only the first day that I am breastfeeding and my nipples already feel sore. What can I do to relieve this soreness and prevent it from getting worse?"

   E. "My friends all told me to watch out for the fourth day and engorgement. What can I do to keep it from being too bad and to take care of myself when it occurs?"

   F. "Every time I breastfeed, I get cramps and my flow seems to get heavier. Is there something wrong with me?"

G. "I am so glad I do not have to worry about getting pregnant again as long as I am breastfeeding. I hate using birth control and my friend told me I do not have to use it as long as I am breastfeeding."

H. "What should I do when I am ready to stop breastfeeding my baby?"

4. Susan is 2 days old. She last fed 5 hours ago. Her mother tells the nurse that Susan is so sleepy that she just does not have the heart to wake her.
   A. IDENTIFY one nursing diagnosis and one expected outcome appropriate for this newborn.

   B. DISCUSS the approach the nurse should take with regard to this situation.

5. Alice has decided that for personal and professional reasons, bottle-feeding with a commercially prepared formula is the feeding method that is best for her. She tells the nurse that she hopes she made a good decision for her baby. "I hope she will be well nourished and feel that I love her even though I am bottle-feeding."
   A. DESCRIBE how the nurse should respond to Alice's concern.

   B. STATE three guidelines for bottle-feeding technique that the nurse should teach Alice to ensure the safety and health of her baby.

6. Prior to discharge, a nurse is evaluating a woman's ability to breastfeed and her newborn's response to breastfeeding.
   A. IDENTIFY the factors that the nurse should assess before and during breastfeeding to ensure that the mother and newborn are ready to breastfeed at home.

   B. After determining that breastfeeding is progressing well, the woman is discharged. One week later the nurse calls the woman to discuss breastfeeding. WRITE several questions that this nurse should ask to determine if breast-feeding is continuing to progress normally.

26 Assessment of High Risk Pregnancy

I. LEARNING KEY TERMS

FILL IN THE BLANKS: Insert the term that corresponds to each of the following descriptions.

1. _____ A pregnancy in which the life or health of the mother or her fetus is jeopardized by circumstances coincidental with or unique to the pregnancy.

2. _____ Assessment of fetal activity by the mother; it is a simple yet valuable method for monitoring the condition of the fetus. The _____ refers to the cessation of fetal movements entirely for 12 hours.

3. _____ Diagnostic test that involves the use of sound having a frequency higher than that detectable by humans to examine structures inside the body. During pregnancy it can be performed by using either the _____ or the _____ approach.

4. _____ Decreased or deficient amount of amniotic fluid.

5. _____ Increased or excessive amount of amniotic fluid.

6. _____ Prenatal screening method that uses ultrasound measurement of fluid in the nape of the fetal neck between 10 and 14 weeks of gestation to identify possible fetal abnormalities.

7. _____ Noninvasive study of blood flow in the fetus and placenta.

8. _____ Noninvasive dynamic assessment of the fetus and its environment that is based on acute and chronic markers of fetal disease. It uses both real-time _____ and external _____. This test includes assessment of five variables, namely _____, _____, _____, _____, and _____.

9. _____ Noninvasive radiologic technique used for obstetric and gynecologic diagnosis by providing excellent pictures of soft tissue without the use of ionizing radiation.

10. _____ Prenatal diagnostic test performed to obtain amniotic fluid to examine the fetal cells it contains.

11. _____ Prenatal diagnostic test that provides direct access to the fetal circulation during the second and third trimesters.

12. _____ Procedure that involves the removal of a small tissue specimen from the fetal portion of the placenta. Because this tissue originates from the zygote, it reflects the genetic makeup of the fetus; it is performed between 10 and 13 weeks of gestation, either transcervically or transabdominally.

13. _____ Test used as a screening tool for neural tube defects in pregnancy. The test is ideally performed between _____ and _____ weeks of gestation.

14. _____ Test used to screen for Down syndrome. It is performed between _____ and _____ weeks of gestation. The levels of three markers, namely, _____, _____, and _____, in combination with maternal _____ are used to determine risk. The _____ test adds an additional marker called inhibin A to increase the accuracy of screening for Down syndrome in women more than 35 years of age.

15. _____ Screening test for Rh incompatibility by examining the serum of Rh-negative women for Rh antibodies.

16. _____ Test that provides a definitive diagnosis noninvasively for fetal Rh status, fetal gender, and certain paternally transmitted single gene disorders.

17. _____ Test based on the fact that a healthy awake fetus with an intact central nervous system produces characteristic heart rate patterns in response to its own movements, uterine contractions, or stimulation.

18. _____ Test used to determine fetal response to sound or vibration; the expected response is acceleration of the fetal heart rate.

19. _____ Test used to identify the jeopardized fetus who is stable at rest but shows evidence of compromise when exposed to the stress of uterine contractions. If the resultant hypoxia of the fetus is sufficient, a deceleration of the fetal heart rate (FHR) will result. Two methods used for this test are the _____ test and the _____ test.

20. _____ Goal of antepartal assessment during the first and second trimesters.

21. _____ and _____ Two major goals of antepartal assessment during the third trimester.

II. REVIEWING KEY CONCEPTS

22. EXPLAIN how risk factors in each of the following categories could place the maternal-fetal unit in jeopardy. IDENTIFY several strategies that a nurse could use to eliminate or reduce the risk.
Biophysical factors:

Psychosocial factors:

Sociodemographic factors:

Environmental factors:

23. DISCUSS the role of the nurse when caring for high risk pregnant women who are required to undergo antepartal assessment testing to determine fetal well-being.

24. STATE two risk factors for each of the following pregnancy-related problems:
Polyhydramnios

Intrauterine growth restriction

Oligohydramnios

Chromosomal abnormalities

MULTIPLE CHOICE: Circle the correct option(s) and state the rationale for the option(s) chosen.

25. A 34-year-old woman at 36 weeks of gestation has been scheduled for a biophysical profile. She asks the nurse why the test needs to be performed. The nurse tells her that the test is performed because it:
    A. Determines how well her baby will breathe after it is born
    B. Evaluates the response of her baby's heart to uterine contractions
    C. Measures her baby's head and length
    D. Observes her baby's activities in utero to ensure that her baby is getting enough oxygen

26. As part of preparing a 24-year-old woman at 42 weeks of gestation for a nonstress test, the nurse should:
    A. Tell the woman to fast for 8 hours before the test
    B. Explain that the test will evaluate how well her baby is moving inside her uterus
    C. Show her how to indicate when her baby moves
    D. Attach a spiral electrode to the presenting part to determine FHR patterns

27. A 40-year-old woman at 18 weeks of gestation is having a quad marker test performed. She is obese, and her health history reveals that she is Rh negative. The primary purpose of this test is to screen for:
    A. Spina bifida
    B. Down syndrome
    C. Gestational diabetes
    D. Rh antibodies

28. During a contraction stress test, four contractions lasting 45 to 55 seconds each were recorded in a 10-minute period. A late deceleration was noted during the third contraction. The nurse conducting the test documents the result as:
    A. Negative
    B. Positive
    C. Equivocal or suspicious
    D. Unsatisfactory

29. A pregnant woman is scheduled for a transvaginal ultrasound test to establish gestational age. In preparing this woman for the test the nurse should:
    A. Place the woman in a supine position with her hips elevated on a folded pillow
    B. Instruct her the woman to come for the test with a full bladder
    C. Administer an analgesic 30 minutes before the test
    D. Lubricate the vaginal probe with transmission gel

30. A pregnant woman at 42 weeks of gestation is undergoing a nonstress test. During the test an evaluation of the monitor tracing indicated that two accelerations of the fetal heart rate occurred within a 20-minute period. The first acceleration of 18 beats/minute lasted 20 seconds and the second acceleration of 20 beats/minute lasted 16 seconds. The nurse conducting the test records the test result as:
    A. Reactive
    B. Positive
    C. Nonreactive
    D. Equivocal hyperstimulatory

III. THINKING CRITICALLY

1. Annie is a primigravida who is at 10 weeks of gestation. Her prenatal history reveals that she was treated for pelvic inflammatory disease (PID) 2 years ago. She describes irregular menstrual cycles and is therefore unsure about the first day of her last menstrual period (LMP). Annie is scheduled for a transvaginal ultrasound.
   A. CITE the likely reasons for the performance of this test.

   B. DESCRIBE how the nurse should prepare Annie for this test.

2. Latisha, pregnant at 20 weeks of gestation, is scheduled for a series of transabdominal ultrasounds to monitor the growth of her fetus. DESCRIBE the nursing role as it applies to Latisha and transabdominal ultrasound examinations.

3. Mary is at 42 weeks of gestation. Her physician has ordered a biophysical profile (BPP). She is very upset and tells the nurse: "All my doctor told me is that this test will see if my baby is okay. I do not know what is going to happen and if it will be painful to me or possibly harmful for my baby."
   A. STATE a nursing diagnosis that reflects this situation.

   B. DESCRIBE how the nurse should respond to Mary's concerns.

   C. Mary receives a score of 8 on the BPP. LIST the factors that were evaluated to obtain this score, and specify the meaning of Mary's test result of 8.

4. Jan, age 42 years, is 18 weeks pregnant. Because of her age, Jan's fetus is at risk for genetic anomalies. Jan's blood type is A negative and her partner's, the father of her baby, is B positive. Her primary health care provider has suggested an amniocentesis. DESCRIBE the nurse's role in terms of each of the following:
   A. Preparing Jan for the amniocentesis.

Chapter **26** **Assessment of High Risk Pregnancy**

B. Supporting Jan during the procedure.

C. Providing Jan with postprocedure care and instructions.

5. Susan, who has diabetes and is in week 36 of pregnancy, has been scheduled for a nonstress test.
   A. DISCUSS what you would tell Susan about the purpose of this test and what will be learned about her baby's well-being.

   B. DESCRIBE how you would prepare Susan for this test.

   C. DISCUSS how you would conduct the test.

   D. INDICATE the criteria you would use to determine if the result of the test was:
   Reactive

   Nonreactive

6. Beth is scheduled for a contraction stress test following a nonreactive result on a nonstress test. Nipple stimulation will be used to induce the required contraction pattern.
   A. DISCUSS what you would tell Beth about the purpose of this test and what will be learned about the well-being of her fetus.

B. DESCRIBE how you would prepare Beth for the test.

C. INDICATE how you would conduct the test.

D. STATE how you would conduct the test differently if exogenous oxytocin (Pitocin) is used instead of nipple stimulation.

E. INDICATE the criteria you would use to determine if the result of the test is:
Negative

Positive

Equivocal suspicious

Equivocal hyperstimulatory

Unsatisfactory

27 Hypertensive Disorders

I. LEARNING KEY TERMS

MATCHING: Match the client description in Column I with the appropriate diagnosis in Column II.

COLUMN I

1. _____ During a prenatal visit at 30 weeks of gestation, Angela's blood pressure (BP) was 156/98 mm Hg; it has ranged between 142/92 and 150/90 mm Hg since the 28th week of her pregnancy; her urinalysis indicated a protein level of 2+ using a dipstick; her biceps and patellar reflexes are 2+.

2. _____ At 37 weeks of gestation, Mary's BP rose from a prepregnant baseline of 118/66 mm Hg to 142/88 mm Hg. No other problematic signs and symptoms, including proteinuria, were noted.

3. _____ Susan, a 34-year-old pregnant client, has had a consistently high BP ranging from 148/92 mm Hg to 160/98 mm Hg since she was 28 years old. Her weight gain has followed normal patterns and urinalysis remains normal as well.

4. _____ At 32 weeks of gestation, Maria—with hypertension since 28 weeks, hyperactive deep tendon reflexes (DTRs) with clonus, and proteinuria of 4+—has a convulsion.

5. _____ Shawna is a primigravida at 28 weeks of gestation. Her BP has risen to 160/110 mm Hg and higher. Proteinuria is at 3+. She has been complaining of a headache and states that she needs to wear sunglasses even indoors because light hurts her eyes. She reports that she has been using two pillows at night instead of one to breathe more easily when she sleeps.

6. _____ Dawn has been hypertensive since her 24th week of pregnancy. Urinalysis indicates a protein content of 3+. Further testing reveals a platelet count of 95,000 and elevated aspartate aminotransferase (AST) and alanine aminotransferase (ALT) levels; she has begun to experience nausea with some vomiting and epigastric pain.

COLUMN II

A. Eclampsia
B. Chronic hypertension
C. Gestational hypertension
D. HELLP syndrome
E. Preeclampsia (mild) without severe features
F. Preeclampsia (severe) with severe features

FILL IN THE BLANKS: Insert the term that corresponds to each of the following descriptions of hypertensive disorders during pregnancy.

7. _____ Onset of hypertension without proteinuria after the 20th week of pregnancy; it does not persist longer than 12 weeks postpartum, usually resolving during the first postpartum week.

8. _____ Hypertension that is present before pregnancy.

9. _____ Pregnancy-specific condition in which hypertension develops after 20 weeks of gestation or in the early postpartum period in a previously normotensive woman; the presence of thrombocytopenia, impaired liver function, newly developed renal insufficiency, pulmonary edema, or new onset cerebral or visual disturbances confirms the diagnosis.

10. _____ A systolic blood pressure greater than 140 mm Hg or a diastolic blood pressure greater than 90 mm Hg. The elevated values must be present on _____ separate occasions at least _____ hours apart but within a maximum of a _____ -week period.

11. _____ A protein concentration at or greater than 300 mg/dL in a 24-hour urine collection.

12. _____ Accumulation of fluid in the tissues of the lowest or most dependent parts of the body, where hydrostatic pressure is the greatest. For ambulating women it is first evident in _____; if the pregnant woman is confined to bed, it occurs in the _____.

13. _____ Onset of seizure activity or coma in the woman diagnosed with preeclampsia, with no history of preexisting pathology that can result in seizure activity.

14. _____ A laboratory diagnosis for a variant of severe preeclampsia that involves hepatic dysfunction; it is characterized by _____, elevated _____, and low _____.

15. _____ Activity in blood vessels that diminishes their diameter, thereby impeding tissue perfusion in all organ systems, increasing peripheral vascular resistance and blood pressure, and increasing endothelial cell permeability.

II. REVIEWING KEY CONCEPTS

16. DESCRIBE the assessment technique used to determine if the following findings are present in women with preeclampsia. (Note: You may wish to review this information in a physical assessment textbook for a complete explanation of each technique.)
Hyperreflexia

Ankle clonus

Proteinuria (24-hour method; dipstick method)

Pitting edema

MULTIPLE CHOICE: Circle the correct option(s) and state the rationale for the option(s) chosen.

17. When measuring the blood pressure to ensure consistency and to facilitate early detection of blood pressure changes consistent with preeclampsia, the nurse should:
    A. Place the woman in a sitting position with feet flat on the floor
    B. Allow the woman to rest for 5 minutes after positioning her before measuring her blood pressure
    C. Record Korotkoff phase IV (muffled sound) as the diastolic pressure
    D. Use a proper-sized cuff that covers at least 50% of her upper arm

18. When caring for a woman with preeclampsia without severe features, it is critical that during assessment the nurse be alert for signs of progress to preeclampsia with severe features. Progress to preeclampsia with severe features is indicated by which of the following assessment findings?
    A. Serum creatinine 0.9 mg/dL
    B. Platelet count of 180,000/mm^3
    C. Positive ankle clonus response with DTRs 4+ bilaterally
    D. Blood pressure of 150/88 and 154/96 mm Hg, 6 hours apart

19. A woman with preeclampsia is admitted to the hospital and her primary health care provider has ordered that an infusion of magnesium sulfate be started. In implementing this order, the nurse should: (Circle all that apply.)
    A. Prepare a solution of 20 g of magnesium sulfate in 100 mL of 5% glucose in water
    B. Monitor maternal vital signs, fetal heart rate (FHR) patterns, and uterine contractions every hour
    C. Expect the maintenance dose to be approximately 1 to 3 g/hour
    D. Administer a loading dose of 4 to 6 g over 15 to 30 minutes
    E. Prepare to administer hydralazine (Apresoline) if signs of magnesium toxicity occur
    F. Report a respiratory rate of less than 12 breaths/minute to the primary health care provider immediately

20. The primary expected outcome for nursing care associated with the administration of magnesium sulfate would be met if which assessment finding is present?
    A. The woman exhibits a decrease in both systolic and diastolic blood pressure.
    B. The woman experiences no seizures.
    C. The woman states that she feels more relaxed and calm.
    D. The woman urinates more frequently, resulting in a decrease in pathologic edema.

21. A woman has been diagnosed with preeclampsia without severe features and will be treated at home. In teaching this woman about her treatment regimen for preeclampsia, the nurse should tell her to: (Circle all that apply.)
    A. Follow a low-salt diet
    B. Use a dipstick to check a clean catch specimen of her urine for protein
    C. Maintain a fluid intake of six to eight 8-ounce glasses of water each day
    D. Increase the roughage in her diet
    E. Perform gentle range-of-motion exercises of her upper and lower extremities
    F. Ask her friends to avoid visiting or calling her because she needs to rest

22. A woman with preeclampsia with severe features is receiving nifedipine (Procardia). She asks the nurse what this medication is for. The nurse should tell her that nifedipine is used to:
    A. Prevent seizures
    B. Relieve the headaches she is starting to have
    C. Decrease her blood pressure
    D. Reduce the edema in her hands and legs

23. A woman with preeclampsia gave birth by cesarean section 1 hour ago. She is still receiving a magnesium sulfate infusion at 1 g/hour. A major concern regarding the administration of magnesium sulfate at this time is:
    A. Increased risk for seizures
    B. Central nervous system depression
    C. Hypotension
    D. Diuresis

24. Following vaginal birth 2 hours ago a woman with preeclampsia is experiencing a heavy flow as a result of a boggy uterus. It is determined that she will require medication to reduce the amount of blood loss. Which medication would the nurse anticipate administering?
   A. Methergine (methylergonovine)
   B. Calcium gluconate
   C. Pitocin (oxytocin)
   D. Normodyne (labetalol)

25. A woman, who is at 35 weeks of gestation with preeclampsia, has a seizure. Immediately after the seizure the nurse's priority action is to:
   A. Evaluate fetal heart rate and pattern for signs of decreasing variability, late decelerations, or bradycardia
   B. Assess status of the maternal airway, respiratory effort, and pulse
   C. Determine if membranes have ruptured and if the amniotic fluid contains meconium
   D. Prepare to increase the amount of magnesium sulfate being infused from 1 g/hour to 2 g/hour

III. THINKING CRITICALLY

1. Hypertension during pregnancy can result in serious health problems for the woman and her fetus. As a result, nurses working with pregnant women need to be consistent in the technique they use to monitor blood pressure changes. DEVELOP a protocol that nurses could follow to ensure the accuracy of blood pressure measurement during pregnancy.

2. Preeclampsia is a serious complication of pregnancy. CREATE a profile of two women who, when pregnant, are at risk for preeclampsia (use different risk factors for each profile you create). EXPLAIN how nurses working with these women could identify the risks these women present.

3. Amber, a primigravida at 30 weeks of gestation, is diagnosed with preeclampsia without severe features. The nurse caring for Amber recognizes that preeclampsia and eclampsia can affect both maternal and fetal well-being.
   A. DESCRIBE how preeclampsia and eclampsia can adversely affect the health and well-being of Amber's fetus.

   B. Amber is concerned about her diagnosis, stating, "I know this can have an effect on my baby, so I will do whatever is necessary to keep both of us safe. But how will you and I know my baby is doing okay?" INDICATE the fetal surveillance measures recommended for women experiencing preeclampsia that the nurse should discuss with Amber.

4. Jean (2-1-0-0-1) is at 30 weeks of gestation and has been diagnosed with preeclampsia without severe features. The treatment plan includes home care with limited activity consisting of bed rest with bathroom privileges and being out of bed twice a day for meals, appropriate nutrition, and stress reduction. Jean and her husband are very anxious about the diagnosis and are also concerned about how they will manage the care of their active 3-year-old daughter, Anne.

A. INDICATE the clinical manifestations that support this diagnosis.

B. LIST three priority nursing diagnoses for Jean and her family.

C. DESCRIBE how you would help this couple to organize their home care routine.

D. SPECIFY what you would teach this couple regarding assessment of Jean's status in terms of each of the following:

Blood pressure

Weight

Protein in urine

Fetal well-being

Signs of a worsening condition

E. DESCRIBE the instructions you would give to Jean regarding her nutrient and fluid intake.

F. DISCUSS the measures Jean can use to cope with the boredom and alteration in circulation and muscle tone that accompany activity restrictions including bed rest.

G. Limited activity can lead to a nursing diagnosis of risk for constipation related to changes in bowel function associated with pregnancy and limited activity. CITE two measures that Jean can use to enhance bowel elimination and prevent constipation.

5. Ellen, pregnant at 37 weeks of gestation, is admitted to the hospital with a diagnosis of preeclampsia with severe features.
   A. INDICATE the signs and symptoms that support this diagnosis.

   B. LIST three priority nursing diagnoses for Ellen.

   C. SPECIFY the measures that should be taken to protect Ellen and her fetus from injury.

   D. Ellen's physician orders magnesium sulfate to be infused at 4 g in 20 minutes as a loading dose and then a maintenance intravenous infusion of 2 g/hour.
      1. CREATE a protocol that will be a guide nurses can follow when administering the magnesium sulfate infusion.

      2. WRITE one nursing diagnosis related to the treatment with magnesium sulfate.

3. EXPLAIN the expected therapeutic effect of magnesium sulfate to Ellen and her family.

4. LIST the maternal and fetal assessments that should be accomplished on a regular basis during the infusion of magnesium sulfate.

5. IDENTIFY the progressive signs of magnesium sulfate toxicity.

6. STATE the interventions that must be instituted immediately if magnesium sulfate toxicity occurs.

E. Despite all prevention efforts, Ellen has a convulsion.
   1. SPECIFY the nursing measures that should be implemented at the onset of the convulsion and immediately afterward.

   2. LIST the problems that can occur as a result of the convulsion that Ellen experienced.

F. Ellen successfully gave birth vaginally despite her high-risk status. DESCRIBE Ellen's care management during the first 48 hours of her postpartum recovery period.

28 Hemorrhagic Disorders

I. LEARNING KEY TERMS

FILL IN THE BLANKS: Insert the appropriate term for each description of antepartal bleeding.

1. _____, _____, _____, and
_____ The common bleeding disorders of early pregnancy.

2. _____ and _____ The common bleeding disorders of
late pregnancy.

3. _____ Pregnancy that ends as a result of natural causes before 20 weeks of gestation,
the point of viability when the fetus may survive outside the uterus. The five types are _____,
_____, _____, _____, and
_____.

4. _____ Term used to refer to three or more spontaneous pregnancy losses prior to
20 weeks of gestation.

5. _____ Placental hormone used in the diagnosis of pregnancy and pregnancy loss.

6. _____ Surgical procedure in which the cervix is widened and an instrument is inserted
to scrape the uterine walls and remove uterine contents.

7. _____ A cause of late miscarriage; it is traditionally defined as passive and painless
dilation of the cervix during the second trimester.

8. _____ Procedure in which a suture is placed around the cervix beneath the mucosa to
constrict the internal os of the cervix.

9. _____ Pregnancy in which the fertilized ovum is implanted outside the uterine cavity,
usually in the ampulla or largest part of the uterine tube.

10. _____ An ecchymotic blueness around the umbilicus indicating hematoperitoneum; it
may develop in an undiagnosed intraabdominal ectopic pregnancy.

11. _____ A gestational trophoblastic disease (GTD); it is a benign proliferative growth of
the placental trophoblast.

12. _____ A group of pregnancy-related trophoblastic proliferative disorders without a
viable fetus; they are caused by abnormal fertilization.

13. _____ Term used to refer to the result of fertilization of an egg with a lost or inacti-
vated nucleus; it resembles a bunch of white grapes; there is an increased risk for persistent GTD.

14. _____ Term used to refer to the result of two or more sperm fertilizing an apparently
normal ovum; embryonic or fetal parts and an amniotic sac are often present in the uterus.

15. _____ Implantation of the placenta in the lower uterine segment such that it completely or partially covers the cervix or is close enough to the cervix to cause bleeding when dilation or effacement occurs.

16. _____, _____, and _____ Major placental complications involving abnormal attachment to the uterus that inhibits the placental separation process after birth and can result in hemorrhage.

17. _____ Detachment of part or all of a normally implanted placenta from the uterus.

18. _____ Disorder of the uterus in which blood accumulates between a separating placenta and the uterine wall; the uterus appears purple or blue and contractility is lost.

19. _____ Type of vasa previa when the cord vessels begin to branch at the membranes and then course into the placenta.

20. _____ Marginal insertion of the cord into the placenta.

21. _____ Type of vasa previa when the placenta is divided into two or more separate lobes; fetal vessels run between the lobes.

22. _____ Pathologic form of clotting that is diffuse and consumes large amounts of clotting factors, causing widespread external bleeding, internal bleeding, or both, and clotting.

II. REVIEWING KEY CONCEPTS

23. Disseminated intravascular coagulation (DIC) is an acute, life-threatening disorder that can occur during pregnancy.
    A. IDENTIFY the obstetric risk factors for the development of DIC. EXPLAIN how these risk factors can lead to DIC.

    B. DESCRIBE the pathophysiology that leads to DIC.

    C. INDICATE the clinical manifestations of DIC that would be noted during physical examination and with laboratory testing.

    D. DESCRIBE four priority nursing measures that should be used when caring for a woman experiencing DIC.

24. DESCRIBE the effect that bleeding during pregnancy can have on maternal and fetal well-being.

MULTIPLE CHOICE: Circle the correct option(s) and state the rationale for the option(s) chosen.

25. A primigravida at 10 weeks of gestation reports mild uterine cramping and slight vaginal spotting without passage of tissue. When she is examined, no cervical dilation is noted. The nurse caring for this woman should:
    A. Anticipate that the woman will be sent home with instructions to limit her activity and to avoid stress or orgasm
    B. Prepare the woman for a dilation and curettage
    C. Notify a grief counselor to assist the woman with the imminent loss of her fetus
    D. Tell the woman that the doctor will most likely perform a cerclage to help her maintain her pregnancy

26. A woman is admitted through the emergency department with a medical diagnosis of ruptured ectopic pregnancy. The primary nursing diagnosis at this time is:
    A. Acute pain related to irritation of the peritoneum with blood
    B. Risk for infection related to tissue trauma
    C. Deficient fluid volume related to blood loss associated with rupture of the uterine tube
    D. Anticipatory grieving related to unexpected pregnancy outcome

27. A woman diagnosed with an ectopic pregnancy is to receive methotrexate. The nurse should explain to the woman that: (Circle all that apply.)
    A. Methotrexate is an analgesic that will relieve the dull abdominal pain she is experiencing.
    B. She should double-flush the toilet with the lid down for 72 hours after receiving methotrexate.
    C. She will receive the medication intramuscularly.
    D. She must stop taking folic acid supplements as long as she is on methotrexate.
    E. Her partner should use a condom during intercourse.
    F. She must return weekly for a measurement of her progesterone level to determine if the methotrexate therapy has been effective.

28. A pregnant woman at 32 weeks of gestation comes to the emergency department because she has begun to experience bright red vaginal bleeding. She reports that she has no pain. The admission nurse suspects that the woman is experiencing:
    A. Abruptio placentae
    B. Disseminated intravascular coagulation
    C. Placenta previa
    D. Preterm labor

29. A pregnant woman at 38 weeks of gestation and diagnosed with marginal placenta previa has just given birth to a healthy newborn male. The nurse recognizes that the immediate focus for the care of this woman is:
    A. Preventing hemorrhage
    B. Relieving acute pain
    C. Preventing infection
    D. Fostering attachment of the woman with her new son

III. THINKING CRITICALLY

1. Andrea is admitted to the hospital, where a diagnosis of acute ruptured ectopic pregnancy in her fallopian tube is made.
    A. STATE the risk factors associated with ectopic pregnancy.

B. DESCRIBE the findings that were most likely experienced and exhibited by Andrea as her ectopic pregnancy progressed and then ruptured.

C. IDENTIFY the other health problems that share the same or similar clinical manifestations as ectopic pregnancy.

D. STATE the major care management problem at this time. SUPPORT your answer.

E. IDENTIFY two priority nursing diagnoses appropriate for Andrea.

F. OUTLINE the nursing measures Andrea will require during the preoperative and postoperative period.

2. Janet is 10 weeks pregnant. She comes to the clinic and states that she has been experiencing slight bleeding with mild cramping for about 4 hours. No tissue has been passed and pelvic examination reveals that the cervical os is closed.
   A. INDICATE the most likely basis for Janet's signs and symptoms.

   B. OUTLINE the expected care management of Janet's problem.

3. Denise, a primigravida, calls the clinic. She is crying while she tells the nurse that she has noted "a lot of bleeding" and that she is sure she is losing her baby.
   A. WRITE several questions the nurse should ask Denise to obtain a more definitive picture of the bleeding she is experiencing.

B. Denise is admitted to the hospital for further evaluation. A medical diagnosis of incomplete miscarriage is made. DESCRIBE the assessment findings that indicate the diagnosis of incomplete miscarriage.

C. STATE the nursing diagnosis that takes priority at this time.

D. OUTLINE the nursing measures that are appropriate for the priority nursing diagnosis you identified and for the expected medical management of Denise's health problem.

E. SPECIFY the instructions that Denise should receive prior to her discharge from the hospital.

F. LIST the nursing measures appropriate for a nursing diagnosis of anticipatory grieving related to unexpected outcome of pregnancy.

4. Marsha (5-0-1-4-0) is pregnant and at 12 weeks of gestation. She has a history of early and recurring pregnancy loss. In an attempt to maintain the current pregnancy to term, a prophylactic cerclage has been performed. OUTLINE the discharge care and instructions the nurse should give Marsha to ensure her safe recovery at home.

5. Mary has been diagnosed with hydatidiform mole (complete).
   A. IDENTIFY the typical signs and symptoms Mary most likely exhibits to establish this diagnosis.

   B. SPECIFY the posttreatment care and instructions that the nurse should include in a follow-up management plan with Mary and her family.

6. Two pregnant women are admitted to the labor unit with vaginal bleeding. Sara is at 29 weeks of gestation and is diagnosed with marginal placenta previa. Jane is at 34 weeks of gestation and is diagnosed with a moderate (grade II) premature separation of the placenta (abruptio placentae).

   A. COMPARE the clinical pictures that each of these women is likely to exhibit during assessment.

   B. IDENTIFY two priority nursing diagnoses for both Sara and Jane.

   C. CONTRAST the care management approach required by each of the women as it relates to her diagnosis and the typical medical management.

   D. INDICATE the considerations that must be given top priority following birth for each of these women.

29 Endocrine and Metabolic Disorders

I. LEARNING KEY TERMS

1. EXPLAIN the interrelationship of each of the following clinical manifestations associated with diabetes mellitus.
   Hyperglycemia

   Polyuria

   Glycosuria

   Polydipsia

   Ketoacidosis and acetonuria

   Weight loss

   Polyphagia

FILL IN THE BLANKS: Insert the term that corresponds to each of the following descriptions.

2. _____ Group of metabolic diseases characterized by hyperglycemia resulting from defects in insulin secretion, insulin action, or both.

3. _____ Excretion of large volumes of urine.

4. _____ Excessive thirst.

5. _____ Eating excessive amounts of food.

6. _____ Results when unusable glucose is excreted.

7. _____ Metabolic disease that occurs when pancreatic islet beta cells are destroyed, resulting in an absolute insulin deficiency; an autoimmune process may be involved in its etiology.

8. _____ Metabolic disease resulting in insulin resistance and relative rather than absolute insulin deficiency; it is the most prevalent form of the disease.

9. _____ Label given to type 1 or type 2 diabetes that existed before pregnancy.

10. _____ Carbohydrate intolerance with onset or first recognition occurring during pregnancy.

11. _____ Key to optimal outcome of a diabetic pregnancy before conception and throughout pregnancy.

12. _____ Excessive amount of amniotic fluid.

13. _____ Less than the normal amount of glucose in the blood.

14. _____ Excess glucose in the blood.

15. _____ Accumulation of ketones in the blood resulting from hyperglycemia and leading to metabolic acidosis; it occurs most often during the second and third trimesters when the diabetogenic effect of pregnancy is the greatest.

16. _____ Normal blood glucose level with preprandial range of _____ and 1-hour postprandial range no higher than _____.

17. _____ Result of excessive fetal growth in utero; newborn weighs more than 4000 to 4500 g at birth or greater than the 90th percentile.

18. _____ Blood test that evaluates glycemic control over the previous 4 to 6 weeks.

19. _____ Measurement of blood glucose levels prior to eating. Acceptable results for this test range from _____ to _____ during pregnancy.

20. _____ Measurement of blood glucose levels 1 to 2 hours after eating; acceptable results for 1 hour after meals range from _____ to _____ and for 2 hours after meals it should be _____.

21. _____ Substance in amniotic fluid that is a better predictor of fetal lung maturity than is the lecithin/sphingomyelin (L/S) ratio in pregnancies complicated by diabetes; it should be at a level greater than 3% to confirm adequate lung maturity.

22. _____ Prenatal test performed between 15 and 20 weeks of gestation (ideally 16 and 18 weeks) to screen for neural tube defects, for which the fetus of a diabetic mother is at higher risk.

23. _____ Ultrasound test used along with maternal serum screening between 11 and 14 weeks of gestation to detect fetal heart defects and other anomalies in women with pregestational diabetes.

24. _____ Excessive vomiting during pregnancy resulting in a weight loss of at least 5% of prepregnancy weight and accompanied by dehydration, electrolyte imbalance, ketosis, and acetonuria.

210

25. Women with diabetes mellitus are attending a preconception care class regarding the risks of pregnancy for mother and fetus and how to prevent or minimize the complications that can result. DISCUSS the major maternal and fetal/neonatal risks and complications associated with diabetic pregnancies (pregestational and gestational) that should be included in this class. SUGGEST several measures a nurse could include in the class to reduce the risk for these complications.

26. Rosario, a woman with type 1 diabetes, has just discovered that she is pregnant. She is concerned that pregnancy will affect her diabetes and her diabetes will affect her pregnancy and baby. EXPLAIN to Rosario the metabolic changes that occur during pregnancy, and INDICATE how these changes will affect her care management during the first trimester, the second and third trimesters, and the postpartum period of her pregnancy.

27. DISCUSS how each of the following types of insulin is used during pregnancy to achieve and maintain euglycemia. Give an example of each type of insulin.
    A. Rapid acting

    B. Short acting

    C. Intermediate acting

    D. Long acting

28. Magda, a 28-year-old Hispanic American, is pregnant for the first time. Her body mass index (BMI) is 29. She asks you why she needs to have a glucose test done at 24 weeks into her pregnancy because she does not have diabetes like her mother does.
    A. EXPLAIN to Magda the current recommendations for screening for and diagnosis of gestational diabetes mellitus. Include in your explanation the risk factors Magda presents that make screening especially important and what the glucola screening involves.

B. The result of Magda's test is 145 mg/dL.
   1. EXPLAIN the meaning of this test result.

   2. As step two in the diagnosis process, an oral glucose tolerance test is ordered for Magda. DESCRIBE how you would prepare her for this test.

C. STATE the results that confirm a diagnosis of gestational diabetes.

29. You are part of a health care team caring for two pregnant women. One is Anna, who is hypothyroid, and the other is Tanisha, who is hyperthyroid. DESCRIBE how you anticipate their pregnancies will be affected by their thyroid disorder and COMPARE the management approaches you anticipate.

MULTIPLE CHOICE: Circle the correct option(s) and state the rationale for the option(s) chosen.

30. A pregestational diabetic woman at 20 weeks of gestation exhibits the following: thirst, nausea and vomiting, abdominal pain, drowsiness, and increased urination. Her skin is flushed and dry and her breathing is rapid, with a fruity odor. A priority nursing action when caring for this woman is to:
    A. Provide the woman with a simple carbohydrate immediately
    B. Request an order for an antiemetic
    C. Assist the woman into a lateral position to rest
    D. Administer insulin according to the woman's blood glucose level

31. During her pregnancy a woman with pregestational diabetes has been monitoring her blood glucose level several times a day. Which level requires further assessment?
    A. 85 mg/dL—15 minutes prior to breakfast
    B. 98 mg/dL—prior to lunch
    C. 140 mg/dL—2 hours after lunch
    D. 126 mg/dL—1 hour after supper

32. Specific guidelines should be followed when planning a diet with a pregestational diabetic woman (BMI 24) to ensure a euglycemic state. Which dietary practices does the woman need to modify? (Circle all that apply.)
    A. Follows a diet that reflects 45 kcal per kg daily based on her preconception BMI
    B. Eats three meals a day along with a midmorning, a midafternoon, and a bedtime snack
    C. Drinks a cup of tea and a piece of dry toast as her bedtime snack
    D. Divides her daily carbohydrate intake as 50% simple carbohydrates and 50% complex carbohydrates
    E. Maintains a fat intake of approximately 25% of the total daily kcal recommendation
    F. Monitors the appropriateness of her nutritional intake by checking her blood glucose levels before and after meals

33. An obese pregnant woman with gestational diabetes is learning self-injection of insulin. While evaluating the woman's technique for self-injection of rapid-acting and NPH insulin, the nurse evaluates that the woman understands the instructions when she: (Circle all that apply.)
    A. Washes her hands and puts on a pair of clean gloves
    B. Gently rotates the NPH insulin vial to fully mix the insulin
    C. Draws the NPH insulin into her syringe first when mixing it with regular insulin
    D. Spreads her skin taut and punctures the skin at a 90-degree angle
    E. Cleanses the top of each insulin vial thoroughly with warm water and soap
    F. Wipes the injection site gently with alcohol, waiting until it dries to administer the insulin

34. A woman has just been admitted with a diagnosis of hyperemesis gravidarum. She has been unable to retain any oral intake and as a result has lost weight and is exhibiting signs of dehydration with electrolyte imbalance and acetonuria. The nurse anticipates that the care management of this woman will include:
    A. Administering vitamin K to control nausea and vomiting
    B. Separating liquids from solids, alternating them every 2 to 3 hours once she is able to tolerate oral intake
    C. Avoiding oral hygiene until the woman is able to tolerate oral fluids
    D. Providing three daily meals of bland foods with warm fluids once the woman is able to tolerate oral intake

III. THINKING CRITICALLY

1. Mary is a 24-year-old diabetic client. When Mary informed her gynecologist that she and her husband were trying to get pregnant, she was referred to an endocrinologist for preconception counseling. Mary tells the nurse that she just cannot understand why this is necessary. She says, "I have had diabetes since I was 12 years old and I have not had many problems. All I want to do is get pregnant!" DISCUSS how the nurse should respond to Mary's comments.

2. Luann is a 25-year-old nulliparous client in her first trimester of pregnancy (sixth week of gestation). She has had type 1 diabetes since she was 15 years old. Recently she has been experiencing some nausea and is eating less as a result. She took her usual dose of lispro (Humalog) and NPH (Humulin N) insulin prior to eating a very light breakfast of tea and a piece of toast. Just before her midmorning snack at work, she began to experience nervousness and weakness. She felt dizzy and became diaphoretic and pale.
    A. IDENTIFY the problem that Luann is experiencing. INDICATE the basis for her symptoms.

    B. DESCRIBE the action that Luann should take.

    C. LIST several "glucose boosters" (15 g of simple carbohydrate) that Luann should have on hand should this problem occur again.

    D. STATE what Luann should do after she takes the action described in B.

3. Judy's pregnancy has just been confirmed. She also has type 1 diabetes.
   A. As a result of her high-risk status, a variety of additional assessment measures are emphasized during her prenatal period to evaluate the status of her fetus. IDENTIFY these additional assessment measures and their relevance in a diabetic pregnancy.

   B. DISCUSS the stressors that might confront Judy and her family as a result of her status as a diabetic woman who is pregnant.

   C. WRITE two nursing diagnoses that reflect Judy's health status.

   D. INDICATE the activity and exercise recommendations that Judy should be given.

   E. OUTLINE the required nursing interventions and health teaching for the following major care components at each stage of Judy's pregnancy.
      ■ Diet

      ■ Blood glucose monitoring

      ■ Insulin therapy

   F. After birth, Judy, who will be bottle-feeding, asks the nurse about birth control. DISCUSS the birth control options that would be best for Judy and her partner.

4. Elena (2-1-0-0-1) is a 32-year-old Hispanic American in week 28 of her pregnancy. Her BMI is 30. Her mother, who is 59 years old, was recently diagnosed with type 2 diabetes. Elena's first pregnancy resulted in the birth of a 10 lb, 6 oz daughter who is now 2 years old. A 1-hour, 50-g oral glucose tolerance test last week revealed a glucose level of 152 mg/dL. A 3-hour oral glucose tolerance test was done yesterday, with the following results: fasting—110 mg/dL, 1 hour—192 mg/dL, 2 hours—166 mg/dL, 3 hours—142 mg/dL.

A. IDENTIFY the complication of pregnancy that Elena is exhibiting. STATE the rationale for your answer.

B. LIST the risk factors for this health problem that are present in Elena's assessment data.

C. DESCRIBE the pathophysiology involved in creating Elena's problem.

D. OUTLINE the ongoing assessment measures necessitated by Elena's health problem.

E. STATE two nursing diagnoses for Elena and her fetus.

F. STATE the dietary changes that Elena will have to make to maintain glycemic control during the rest of her pregnancy.

G. Based on blood glucose levels, it was determined that despite Elena's adherence to the prescribed diet, she will need to take insulin. When told, Elena becomes very upset, stating that she is sure she will not be able to give herself shots. DESCRIBE how the nurse should approach this situation.

H. Before discharge after the full-term vaginal birth of her second daughter, who was determined to be appropriate for gestational age (AGA), Elena asks the nurse if the health problem she experienced during this pregnancy will continue now that she has had her baby. She also wonders if it will happen with her next pregnancy, because she wants to get pregnant again soon so she can "try for a son." DISCUSS the response the nurse should give to address Elena's concerns.

5. Marie, a 19-year-old obese primigravida, is diagnosed with hyperemesis gravidarum at 14 weeks of gestation. She is unmarried and lives at home with her parents. The father of Marie's baby recently told her that he wants nothing to do with her or the baby. Marie is in the second semester of her sophomore year in college and is worried about how having a baby will affect her goals of obtaining a college degree and pursuing a career as a teacher. She states that she cannot bear the thought of having an abortion or giving her baby up for adoption. Her parents are upset about the pregnancy but are willing to help her as much as they can, emphasizing that, as the baby's mother, she will be its major caregiver. Marie is admitted to the high risk antepartal unit.

A. IDENTIFY the etiologic factors that may have contributed to Marie's current health problem.

B. LIST the physiologic and psychologic factors that the nurse should be alert for when assessing Marie on her admission.

C. STATE two nursing diagnoses related to Marie's current health status.

D. OUTLINE the nursing care measures appropriate for Marie while she is hospitalized.

E. Once stabilized, Marie is discharged to home care. She is able to tolerate oral food and fluid intake. EXPLAIN the important care measures that the nurse should discuss with Marie and her family before she goes home.

30 Medical-Surgical Disorders

I. LEARNING KEY TERMS

FILL IN THE BLANKS: Insert the term that corresponds to each of the following descriptions.

1. _____ Inability of the heart to maintain a sufficient cardiac output.

2. _____ Classification system for cardiovascular disorders developed by the New York Heart Association. Class I implies _____. Class II implies _____. Class III implies _____. Class IV implies _____.

3. _____ Type of congenital heart defect that results in an abnormal opening between the right and left upper chambers of the heart.

4. _____ Type of congenital heart defect that results in an abnormal opening between the right and left lower chambers of the heart.

5. _____ Type of congenital heart defect that involves failure of the ductus arteriosus to close; it results in a left-to-right shunt.

6. _____ Type of acyanotic congenital heart defect that results in a localized narrowing of the aorta near the insertion of the ductus.

7. _____ Type of cyanotic congenital heart defect that results in an abnormal opening between the ventricles, pulmonary stenosis, overriding aorta, and right ventricular hypertrophy.

8. _____ Narrowing of the opening of the aortic valve leading to an obstruction to left ventricular ejection.

9. _____ Acute ischemic event involving the heart.

10. _____ Development of congestive heart failure with cardiomyopathy in the last month of pregnancy or within the first 5 months postpartum; there is lack of another cause for heart failure and absence of heart disease prior to the last month of pregnancy.

11. _____ Narrowing of the opening of the valve between the left atrium and the left ventricle of the heart by stiffening of the valve leaflets, which obstructs blood flow from the left atrium to the left ventricle. It is the characteristic lesion resulting from rheumatic heart disease.

12. _____ Inflammation of the innermost lining (endocardium) of the heart caused by invasion of microorganisms.

13. _____ Right-to-left or bidirectional shunting at either the atrial or the ventricular level, combined with elevated pulmonary vascular resistance.

14. _____ Common, usually benign cardiac condition that involves the protrusion of the leaflets of the mitral valve back into the left atrium during ventricular systole, allowing some backflow of blood.

15. _____ Autosomal dominant genetic disorder characterized by generalized weakness of the connective tissue, resulting in joint deformities, ocular lens dislocation, and weakness of the aortic wall and root.

16. _____ Disorder characterized by constriction of the arteriolar vessels in the lungs, leading to an increase in the pulmonary artery pressure.

17. _____ Reduction of the oxygen-carrying capacity of the blood primarily caused by an iron deficiency; the heart attempts to compensate by increasing the cardiac output; hemoglobin is less than 11 g/dL in the first and third trimesters and less than 10.5 g/dL in the second trimester.

18. _____ Deficiency is the most common cause of megaloblastic anemia during pregnancy; if present during conception and early pregnancy, it is also associated with an increased incidence of neural tube defects, cleft lip, and cleft palate.

19. _____ Disease caused by the presence of abnormal hemoglobin in the blood. It is a recessive, hereditary, familial hemolytic anemia that affects persons of African-American and Mediterranean ancestry.

20. _____ Anemia in which an insufficient amount of hemoglobin is produced to fill red blood cells; it is a hereditary disorder.

21. _____ Chronic inflammatory disorder involving the tracheobronchial airways with increased airway responsiveness to a variety of stimuli; it is characterized by periods of exacerbations and remissions.

22. _____ Respiratory disorder in which the lungs are unable to maintain levels of oxygen and carbon dioxide within normal limits; it is also known as shock lung.

23. _____ Autosomal recessive genetic disorder in which exocrine glands produce excessive viscous secretions, which cause problems with both respiratory and digestive functions.

24. _____ Generalized itching during pregnancy without the presence of a rash; it is often limited to the abdomen and is usually caused by skin distention and development of striae.

25. _____ Common pregnancy-specific cause of pruritus in pregnancy; it is also termed polymorphic eruption of pregnancy and is most common in primigravidas during the third trimester.

26. _____ Liver disorder unique to pregnancy that is characterized by generalized pruritus most commonly affecting the palms and soles; no skin lesions are present.

27. _____ Disorder of the brain that causes recurrent seizures; it is the most common major neurologic disorder accompanying pregnancy.

28. _____ Patchy demyelinization of the spinal cord and the central nervous system (CNS); it may be a viral disorder.

29. _____ Chronic, multisystemic inflammatory disease that affects the skin, joints, kidneys, lungs, nervous system, liver, and other body organs; it is the most common serious autoimmune disease affecting women of reproductive age.

30. _____ Autoimmune motor (muscle) end-plate disorder that involves acetylcholine use and affects the motor function at the myoneural junction; it results in muscle weakness, particularly of the eyes, face, tongue, neck, limbs, and respiratory muscles.

31. _____ Presence of gallstones in the gallbladder.

32. _____ Inflammation of the gallbladder.

33. _____ Disorder of the intestine, including ulcerative colitis and Crohn disease.

34. _____ Common medical complication of pregnancy, occurring in approximately 20% of all pregnancies and responsible for 10% of all hospitalizations during pregnancy; the most common cause is *Escherichia coli*. This type of infection includes asymptomatic _____, _____, and _____.

35. _____ Most common surgical emergency during pregnancy.

36. _____ Acute idiopathic facial paralysis.

II. REVIEWING KEY CONCEPTS

37. Sara, who has been diagnosed with mitral valve stenosis (MVS) class II heart disease, is considering pregnancy. She and her husband ask the nurse during a preconception care visit to explain the potential risks that Sara and their potential fetus would face as a result of her cardiac status. DESCRIBE how the nurse should approach the question that Sara and her husband have. Include the maternal and fetal complications that are more common among pregnant women who have cardiac problems in your answer.

38. EXPLAIN the modifications that should be made in the protocol used for cardiopulmonary resuscitation (CPR) and the abdominal thrust maneuver when a woman is pregnant.

MULTIPLE CHOICE: Circle the correct option(s) and state the rationale for the option(s) chosen.

39. When assessing a pregnant woman at 28 weeks of gestation who is diagnosed with mitral valve stenosis, it is important that the nurse be alert for signs and symptoms indicating cardiac decompensation. Signs and symptoms of cardiac decompensation include: (Circle all that apply.)
    A. Dry, hacking cough
    B. Orthopnea
    C. Wheezing with inspiration and expiration
    D. Rapid pulse that is irregular and weak
    E. Woman reports that shoes and rings are tight
    F. Supine hypotension

40. A woman at 30 weeks of gestation with a class II cardiac disorder calls her primary health care provider's office and speaks to the nurse practitioner. She tells the nurse that she has been experiencing a frequent moist cough for the past few days. In addition, she has been feeling more tired and is having difficulty completing her routine activities as a result of some difficulty with breathing. The nurse's best response is:
    A. "Have someone bring you to the office so we can assess your cardiac status."
    B. "Try to get more rest during the day, because this is a difficult time for your heart."
    C. "Take an extra diuretic tonight before you go to bed, because you may be developing some fluid in your lungs."
    D. "Ask your family to come over and do your housework for the next few days so you can rest."

41. A pregnant woman with a valvular disorder of her heart requires medication to prevent clot formation. In preparing the woman for this treatment measure, the nurse expects to teach the woman about self-administration of:
    A. furosemide (Lasix)
    B. propranolol (Inderal)
    C. heparin
    D. warfarin (Coumadin)

42. At a previous antepartum visit, the nurse taught a pregnant woman diagnosed with a class II cardiac disorder about measures to use to lower her risk for cardiac decompensation. This woman indicates a need for further instruction if she:
   A. Increases roughage in her diet
   B. Remains on bed rest, getting out of bed only to go to the bathroom
   C. Sleeps 10 hours every night and rests after meals
   D. States that she will call the nurse immediately if she experiences any pain or swelling in her legs

43. A pregnant woman has been diagnosed with cholelithiasis. An important component of her treatment regimen is dietary modification. The nurse helps this woman to plan a diet that:
   A. Reduces dietary fat to approximately 60 g per day
   B. Limits protein to 30% of total calories
   C. Chooses foods that ensure that most calories come from carbohydrates
   D. Avoids putting spices in foods

III. THINKING CRITICALLY

1. Serena, a 30-year-old pregnant client at 24 weeks of gestation, begins to complain of pain in her lower abdomen, nausea with some vomiting, and anorexia. Her husband brings her to the emergency department.
   A. IDENTIFY the factors that will make it difficult for the doctor to diagnose the condition causing Serena's clinical manifestations.

   B. Serena is diagnosed with appendicitis. IDENTIFY the clinical manifestations that Serena most likely exhibited to lead to this diagnosis.

   C. EXPLAIN why it is vital that surgical treatment occur prior to rupture of the appendix.

   D. CITE the major fears that Serena and her husband will have about the impending surgery.

   E. OUTLINE the preoperative and postoperative care that Serena will require.

   F. Serena's surgery was successful and she is discharged to home. IDENTIFY the nursing considerations and topics for teaching related to the discharge planning process for Serena as a pregnant woman who is recovering from surgery.

2. Linda, age 26 years, had rheumatic fever as a child and subsequently developed mitral valve stenosis. She is 6 weeks pregnant. She is classified as class II according to the New York Heart Association functional classification of organic heart disease. This is the first pregnancy for Linda and her husband, Sam.

A. IDENTIFY two nursing diagnoses appropriate for Linda related to her cardiac status and her anticipated care management. STATE an expected outcome for each nursing diagnosis identified.

B. DISCUSS a recommended therapeutic plan for Linda that will reduce her risk for cardiac decompensation in terms of each of the following:
- Rest, sleep, and activity patterns

- Prevention of infection

- Nutrition

- Bowel elimination

C. IDENTIFY several physiologic and psychosocial factors that could increase the stress placed on Linda's heart during her pregnancy.
- Physiologic factors

- Psychosocial factors

D. LIST the subjective symptoms that the nurse should teach Linda and her family to look for as indicators of possible cardiac decompensation.

E. LIST the objective signs that indicate that Linda is experiencing signs of cardiac decompensation and heart failure.

F. Linda is admitted to the labor unit. Her cardiac condition is still classified as class II. OUTLINE the nursing measures designed to assess Linda and promote optimum cardiac function during labor and birth.

G. Linda should be observed carefully during the postpartum period because cardiac risk continues. INDICATE the physiologic events after birth that place Linda at risk for cardiac decompensation.

H. IDENTIFY two nursing diagnoses appropriate for the first 24 to 48 hours of Linda's postpartum period.

I. DISCUSS the measures the nurse can use to reduce the stress placed on Linda's heart during the postpartum period.

J. Linda indicates that she wishes to breastfeed her infant. DESCRIBE the nurse's response.

K. IDENTIFY the important factors to be considered when preparing Linda's discharge plan.

3. Allison is a pregnant woman with a cardiac disorder. As part of her medical regimen, her primary health care provider substituted subcutaneous heparin for the oral warfarin sodium (Coumadin) she had been taking before pregnancy.
   A. Allison states: "I cannot give myself a shot! Why can't I just take the medication orally?" DISCUSS how you would respond as to the purpose of heparin and why it must be used instead of the Coumadin she is used to taking.

   B. INDICATE the information that the nurse should give Allison to ensure safe use of the heparin.

4. Jean is a primigravida at 4 weeks of gestation. She has been an epileptic for several years and her seizures have been controlled with phenytoin (Dilantin). Jean expresses concern regarding how her medication use will affect her pregnancy and her baby. She wants to stop taking the Dilantin. DESCRIBE the approach you would take in addressing Jean's concern and the course of action she is contemplating.

31 Mental Health Disorders and Substance Abuse

I. LEARNING KEY TERMS

FILL IN THE BLANKS: Insert the term that corresponds to each of the following descriptions.

1. _____ Group of mental health disorders that have as their dominant feature a disturbance in the prevailing emotional state (e.g., depression, anxiety).

2. _____ The most common group of mental health disorders; some of these disorders are twice as likely to be diagnosed in women compared to men.

3. _____ Anxiety disorder that is characterized by irrational fears that lead a person to avoid common objects, events, or situations.

4. _____ Anxiety disorder that is characterized by repeated, brief (5- to 15-minute) episodes of intense fear or discomfort that develop without warning and are not related to any specific event; they may be associated with a continuing fear of future attacks.

5. _____ Anxiety disorder characterized by excessive worrying about multiple problems that are realistic but where the level of worry is more intense than is appropriate.

6. _____ Anxiety disorder characterized by recurrent, persistent, and intrusive thoughts that cause anxiety, which a person then tries to control by performing repetitive behaviors.

7. _____ Anxiety disorder that can be precipitated by highly stressful events such as sexual assault and military combat.

8. _____ Postpartum mood disorder characterized by an intense and pervasive sadness with severe and labile mood swings. The woman experiences feelings of intense fear, anxiety, anger, irritability, and despondency that persist past the baby's first few weeks of life.

9. _____ Syndrome most often characterized by depression, delusions, hallucinations, elements of delirium or disorientation, extreme deficits in judgment, and thoughts by the mother of harming the infant, herself, or both.

10. _____ Mood disorder preceded or accompanied by manic episodes and characterized by elevated, expansive, or irritable moods that often alternate with periods of depression.

11. _____ Discrete periods in which there is a sudden onset of intense apprehension, fearfulness, or terror.

II. REVIEWING KEY CONCEPTS

12. Before major depression can be diagnosed, the client must experience at least five specific signs and symptoms nearly every day. DESCRIBE the signs and symptoms used to diagnose major depression.

13. EXPLAIN why diagnostic assessment of pregnant women for depression is difficult. STATE the cues for which the nurse could look in an effort to facilitate a diagnosis of depression.

14. It is essential to screen pregnant women for substance abuse early in pregnancy.
    A. STATE the purpose for the 4 Ps Plus screening tool.

    B. IDENTIFY the questions you would ask when using this screening tool.

15. SPECIFY the harmful effects that use of each of the following substances can have on the pregnant woman and her fetus/newborn.
    ■ Tobacco

    ■ Alcohol

    ■ Marijuana

    ■ Cocaine

    ■ Methamphetamine

■ Opioids

MULTIPLE CHOICE: Circle the correct option(s) and state the rationale for the option(s) chosen.

16. Nurses caring for postpartum women experiencing depression need to be aware of the safety of administering antidepressants. Which antidepressant should be avoided by women who wish to continue breastfeeding?
    A. desipramine (Norpramin)
    B. sertraline (Zoloft)
    C. doxepin (Sinequan)
    D. paroxetine (Paxil)

17. Which measure is least effective in helping a woman to prevent postpartum depression?
    A. Share feelings and emotions with family members and her partner.
    B. Recognize that emotional problems after having a baby are not unusual.
    C. Care for the baby by herself to increase her level of self-confidence and self-esteem.
    D. Ask friends or family members to take care of the baby while she sleeps or has a date with her partner.

18. A pregnant woman being treated for major depression arrives for her first prenatal visit. During the health history interview she shows the nurse the cough medicine that she just bought for a cold. The nurse notes that the cough medicine contains dextromethorphan. The nurse is concerned if the woman reports taking which medication for her depression?
    A. citalopram (Celexa)
    B. desipramine (Norpramin)
    C. clomipramine (Anafranil)
    D. amoxapine (Asendin)

19. A priority question to ask a woman experiencing postpartum depression is:
    A. "Have you thought about hurting yourself?"
    B. "How often do you cry?"
    C. "Have you been feeling insecure, fragile, or vulnerable?"
    D. "Does the responsibility of motherhood seem overwhelming?"

20. The nurse should recognize that a complication of pregnancy associated with the intravenous use of cocaine is:
    A. Prolonged, difficult labor
    B. Premature separation of the placenta
    C. Increased risk for vaginal and urinary tract infections
    D. Severe fetal/neonatal central nervous system (CNS) depression

21. When conducting a health history interview during a pregnant woman's first prenatal visit, the nurse must determine if the woman is substance dependent. The nurse's first question should relate to the woman's use of:
    A. Alcohol
    B. Tobacco
    C. Cocaine
    D. Over-the-counter and prescription medications

III. THINKING CRITICALLY

1. CREATE two profiles of women who, based on the risk factors they exhibit, are at increased risk for postpartum depression. USE different risk factors for each profile.

2. A common nursing diagnosis for a woman with postpartum depression who is hospitalized is impaired parenting related to limited ability of the mother to interact with and care for her infant, secondary to postpartum depression. IDENTIFY the nursing measures appropriate for this nursing diagnosis.

3. IMAGINE that you are a nurse working on a postpartum mother-baby unit. You have been asked to develop a teaching plan regarding postpartum depression that will be incorporated in the standard postpartum discharge instructions presented to postpartum women and their families.
   A. OUTLINE the teaching plan that you would develop regarding postpartum depression—its identification, prevention, and treatment.

   B. CREATE a handout outlining the most critical points covered in your teaching plan that new parents can take home and use as a reference.

4. Julia is a 20-year-old primigravida at 21 weeks of gestation. When the nurse assesses her during her first prenatal visit, she suspects that Julia may be abusing drugs.
   A. IDENTIFY the behaviors Julia may have exhibited that led to this nurse's suspicion.

   B. Julia confirms that she uses cocaine once in a while. How should the nurse respond to Julia's admission?

   C. Julia tells the nurse that she can quit using cocaine on her own, stating: "I know what can happen if you are pregnant and go to a treatment program. My friend went to one and she was put in jail—and they ended up taking her baby away." DISCUSS the legal implications of cocaine use during pregnancy and the barriers women face in seeking and accepting treatment for their addictions.

D. EXPLAIN how you can use the process of change, including the importance of readiness to make a change, in helping Julia.

E. EXPLAIN the considerations that should guide the nurse when planning care and setting expected outcomes for Julia as a pregnant woman who abuses illicit drugs.

F. INDICATE the nursing measures appropriate for Julia, who is addicted to cocaine, during pregnancy, childbirth, and the postpartum period.

5. Mary, a 23-year-old primipara beginning her second week postpartum, is bottle-feeding her baby. Two month ago she and her husband, Tom, moved from Buffalo, where they had lived all of their lives, to Los Angeles to take advantage of a career opportunity for Tom. They live in a community with many other young couples who are also starting families but have not had time to make friends with any of them. Last month they joined the Catholic church near their home so that their baby can be baptized when the time comes. Tom tries to help Mary with the baby but he has to spend long hours at work to establish his position. Mary's prenatal record reveals that she often exhibited anxiety about her well-being and that of her baby. During a home visit by a nurse as part of an early discharge program, Mary tells the nurse that she always wants to sleep and just cannot seem to get enough rest. Mary is very concerned that she is not being a good mother and states: "Sometimes I just do not know what to do to care for my baby the right way. I feel so bad that I am not breastfeeding my baby but I just could not handle it because I heard how hard it is to do successfully. It seems that Tom enjoys spending what little time he has at home with the baby and not with me. I even find myself yelling at him for the silliest things." The nurse recognizes that Mary is exhibiting behaviors strongly suggestive of postpartum depression.
A. INDICATE the signs and symptoms that Mary exhibited that led the nurse to suspect postpartum depression.

B. SPECIFY the predisposing factors for postpartum depression that are present in Mary's situation.

C. EXPLAIN the Two-Item Tool that the nurse could use to screen Mary for postpartum depression.

D. WRITE one nursing diagnosis that is reflective of Mary and Tom's current situation.

E. DESCRIBE the measures that the nurse could use to help Mary and Tom cope with postpartum depression.

6. Imagine that you are an advanced practice nurse who specializes in the treatment of men and women who are alcohol and drug dependent. You have been hired to establish a treatment program specifically designed for pregnant women. OUTLINE the approach you would take to ensure that the program you establish takes into consideration the unique characteristics of women who abuse alcohol and drugs.

32 Labor and Birth Complications

FILL IN THE BLANKS: Insert the term that corresponds to each of the following descriptions.

1. _____ Regular uterine contractions along with cervical changes (dilation) occurring between 20 and 37 weeks of pregnancy.

2. _____ Any birth that occurs between 20 and 37 weeks of gestation.

3. _____ Birth that occurs between 34 and 36 weeks of gestation.

4. _____ Birth that occurs before 32 weeks of gestation; the great majority of deaths and most serious morbidity occur to infants born at this time.

5. _____ Weight at the time of birth of 2500 g or less.

6. _____ Condition of inadequate fetal growth not necessarily correlated with the initiation of labor.

7. _____ Glycoprotein found in plasma and produced during fetal life; its reappearance in the cervical mucus during the late second and early third trimesters of pregnancy may be related to placental inflammation, which is thought to be one possible cause of spontaneous preterm labor.

8. _____ Spontaneous rupture of the amniotic sac and leakage of amniotic fluid before the onset of labor at any gestational age.

9. _____ Spontaneous rupture of the amniotic sac and leakage of fluid before the completion of 37 weeks of gestation most likely occurring as a result of pathogenic weakening of the amniotic membranes by inflammation, stress of uterine contractions, or other factors that cause increased intrauterine pressure.

10. _____ A bacterial infection of the amniotic cavity that is potentially life threatening for the fetus and the woman; it is the most common maternal complication of PROM.

11. _____ Long, difficult, or abnormal labor caused by various conditions associated with the five factors affecting labor.

12. _____ or _____ Abnormal uterine activity often experienced by an anxious first-time mother who is having painful, uncoordinated, and frequent contractions that are ineffective in causing cervical dilation and effacement to progress; they usually occur in the latent phase of the first stage of labor.

13. _____ or _____ Abnormal uterine activity that usually occurs when a woman initially makes normal progress into the active phase of the first stage of labor but then uterine contractions become weak and inefficient or stop altogether.

14. _____ Abnormal labor caused by contractures of the pelvic diameters that reduce the capacity of the bony pelvis, including the inlet, midpelvis, outlet, or any combination of these planes.

15. _____ Abnormal labor caused by obstruction of the birth passage by an anatomic abnormality other than that involving the bony pelvis; the obstruction may result from placenta previa, leiomyomas (uterine fibroid tumors), ovarian tumors, or a full bladder or rectum.

16. _____ Abnormal labor caused by fetal anomalies, excessive fetal size, malpresentation, malposition, or multifetal pregnancy.

17. _____ Excessive fetal size.

18. _____ or _____ Abnormal labor caused by excessive fetal size in relation to the size of the maternal pelvis.

19. _____ The most common fetal malposition.

20. _____ The most common form of malpresentation.

21. _____ Gestation of twins, triplets, quadruplets, or more.

22. _____ Labor pattern defined as a latent phase that exceeds 20 hours in nulliparas and exceeds 14 hours in multiparas.

23. _____ Labor pattern defined as an active phase during which cervical dilation occurs at a rate of less than 1.2 cm/hour in nulliparas and less than 1.5 cm/hour in multiparas.

24. _____ Labor pattern defined as no progress in dilation for 2 hours or more in both nulliparas and multiparas.

25. _____ Labor pattern during which fetal progress through the birth canal occurs at a rate of less than 1 cm/hour in nulliparas and less than 2 cm/hour in multiparas.

26. _____ Labor pattern defined as no progress in fetal descent for 1 hour or more in a nullipara and 30 minutes or more in a multipara.

27. _____ Labor pattern defined as no change in fetal progress through the birth canal during the deceleration phase and second stage of labor.

28. _____ Labor pattern that lasts less than 3 hours from the onset of contractions to the time of birth, often resulting from hypertonic uterine contractions that are tetanic in intensity. For nulliparas, dilation is greater than 5 cm in 1 hour and, for multiparas, dilation is 10 cm in 1 hour.

29. _____ Attempt to turn the fetus from a breech or shoulder presentation to a vertex presentation for birth by exerting gentle, constant pressure on the abdomen.

30. _____ Observance of a woman and her fetus for a reasonable period of spontaneous active labor (e.g., 4 to 6 hours) to assess the safety of a vaginal birth for both.

31. _____ Chemical or mechanical initiation of uterine contractions before their spontaneous onset for the purpose of bringing about the birth.

32. _____ Rating system used to evaluate the inducibility of the cervix. The five characteristics assessed are _____, _____, _____, _____, and _____.

33. _____ Artificial rupture of the membranes often used to induce labor when the cervix is ripe or to augment labor if progress begins to slow.

34. _____ Stimulation of uterine contractions after labor has started spontaneously but progress is unsatisfactory. Common methods include _____ infusion and

_____ .

35. _____ More than five uterine contractions in 10 minutes averaged over a 30-minute window; it can occur during both spontaneous and stimulated labor.

36. _____ Birth method in which an instrument with two curved blades is used to assist the birth of the fetal head.

37. _____ or _____ Birth method involving the attachment of a vacuum cup to the fetal head using negative pressure.

38. _____ Birth of the fetus through a transabdominal incision of the uterus.

39. _____ , _____ , or _____ Pregnancy that extends beyond the end of week 42 of gestation. _____ Syndrome characterized by dry, cracked, peeling skin; long nails; meconium staining of skin, nails, and umbilical cord; and perhaps loss of subcutaneous fat and muscle mass.

40. _____ Uncommon obstetric emergency in which the head of the fetus is born but the anterior shoulder cannot pass under the pubic arch. Two major causes are _____ or maternal _____ .

41. _____ Obstetric emergency in which the umbilical cord lies below the presenting part of the fetus; it may be occult (hidden) or more commonly frank (visible).

42. _____ Nonsurgical disruption of all uterine layers; it is a rare but life-threatening obstetric injury occurring during labor and birth. The major risk factor for its occurrence is _____ and it usually occurs during _____ .

43. _____ or _____ Obstetric emergency in which amniotic fluid enters the maternal circulation triggering a rapid, complex series of pathophysiologic events leading to disseminated intravascular coagulation (DIC), hypotension, and hypoxia.

II. REVIEWING KEY CONCEPTS

44. When caring for pregnant women, IDENTIFY the factors that would alert the nurse to the woman's increased risk for preterm labor and birth.

MATCHING: Match the description of medications used as part of the management of preterm labor in Column I with the appropriate medication listed in Column II.

COLUMN I

45. _____ An antenatal glucocorticoid administered intramuscularly to acceler-
ate fetal lung maturation when there is risk for preterm birth; its use
results in an increase in the production and release of surfactant.

46. _____ Beta$_2$-adrenergic receptor agonist administered subcutaneously; it
relaxes uterine smooth muscles and is used to diagnose preterm
labor, temporarily suppress preterm labor, or treat uterine tachysystole.

47. _____ A calcium channel blocker administered orally; it relaxes smooth
muscles, including those of the contracting uterus; maternal hypotension is a concern.

48. _____ Classification of medications given to arrest labor after uterine contractions and cervical change have occurred.

49. _____ A central nervous system (CNS) depressant used during preterm
labor for its ability to relax smooth muscles, including those of the
uterus; it is administered intravenously.

50. _____ A prostaglandin synthesis inhibitor that relaxes uterine smooth
muscles; it is administered orally.

COLUMN II

A. tocolytic
B. betamethasone
C. terbutaline (Brethine)
D. magnesium sulfate
E. nifedipine (Procardia)
F. indomethacin (Indocin)

MATCHING: Match the description of medications used during the process of stimulating uterine contractions and cervical ripening in Column I with the appropriate medication listed in Column II.

COLUMN I

51. _____ Tocolytic medication administered subcutaneously to suppress uterine
tachysystole.

52. _____ Classification of medications that can be used to ripen the cervix,
stimulate uterine contractions, or both.

53. _____ Cervical ripening agent in the form of a vaginal insert that is placed
in the posterior fornix of the vagina.

54. _____ Cervical ripening agent in the form of a gel that is inserted in the
cervical canal just below the internal os.

55. _____ Pituitary hormone used to stimulate uterine contractions in the
augmentation or induction of labor.

56. _____ Natural cervical dilator made from desiccated seaweed.

57. _____ Synthetic cervical dilator containing magnesium sulfate.

58. _____ Cervical ripening agent, used in the form of a tablet that is most commonly inserted intravaginally in the posterior fornix.

COLUMN II

A. oxytocin (Pitocin)
B. misoprostol (Cytotec)
C. dinoprostone (Cervidil)
D. dinoprostone (Prepidil)
E. terbutaline (Brethine)
F. prostaglandin
G. laminaria tent
H. Lamicel

59. DESCRIBE how each of the five factors of labor can cause labor to be long, difficult, or abnormal. EXPLAIN how
these factors interrelate.

60. EXPLAIN the treatment approach of therapeutic rest.

61. Angela (1-0-0-0-0) is experiencing hypertonic uterine dysfunction and Helena (3-1-0-1-1) is experiencing hypotonic uterine dysfunction. COMPARE and CONTRAST each woman's labor in terms of causes and precipitating factors, maternal-fetal effects, change in pattern of progress, and care management.
   A. Angela: hypertonic uterine dysfunction

   B. Helena: hypotonic uterine dysfunction

62. Identify four indications for oxytocin induction and four contraindications to the use of oxytocin to stimulate the onset of labor.
   Indications

   Contraindications

MULTIPLE CHOICE: Circle the correct option(s) and state the rationale for the option(s) chosen.

63. When assessing a pregnant woman, the nurse is alert for factors associated with preterm labor. Which factor, if exhibited by this woman, increases her risk for spontaneous preterm labor and birth? (Circle all that apply.)
   A. Caucasian race
   B. Obstetric history of 3-0-2-0-1
   C. History of bleeding at 20 weeks
   D. Currently being treated for second bladder infection in 2 months
   E. Employed as a nurse in a trauma intensive care unit (ICU)
   F. Body mass index (BMI) of 22 and height of 158 cm

64. A woman's labor is being suppressed using IV magnesium sulfate. Which measure should be implemented during the infusion?
   A. Limit intravenous fluid intake to 125 mL/hour.
   B. Discontinue infusion if maternal respirations are less than 14 breaths/minute.
   C. Ensure that indomethacin is available should toxicity occur.
   D. Assist woman to maintain a comfortable semirecumbent position.

65. A physician has ordered that dinoprostone (Cervidil) be administered to ripen a pregnant woman's cervix in preparation for an induced labor. In fulfilling this order, the nurse should:
    A. Insert the dinoprostone in the cervical canal just below the internal os
    B. Tell the woman to remain in bed for at least 15 minutes
    C. Observe the woman for signs of uterine tachysystole
    D. Remove the dinoprostone as soon as the woman begins to experience uterine contractions

66. A nulliparous woman experiencing a postterm pregnancy is admitted for labor induction. Assessment reveals a Bishop score of 9. The nurse should:
    A. Call the woman's primary health care provider to order a cervical ripening agent
    B. Mix 20 units of oxytocin (Pitocin) in 500 mL of 5% glucose in water
    C. Piggyback the oxytocin solution into the port nearest the drip chamber of the primary IV tubing
    D. Begin the infusion at a rate of 1 milliunit/minute as determined by the induction protocol

67. A woman's labor is being induced. The nurse assesses the woman's status and that of her fetus and the labor process just before an infusion increment of 2 milliunits/minute. The nurse discontinues the infusion and notifies the woman's primary health care provider if during this assessment she notes:
    A. Frequency of uterine contractions: every 1½ minutes
    B. Variability of fetal heart rate (FHR): present
    C. Deceleration patterns: early decelerations noted with several contractions
    D. Intensity of uterine contractions at their peaks: 80 to 85 mm Hg

68. A laboring woman's vaginal examination reveals the following: 3 cm, 50%, LSA, 0. The nurse caring for this woman should:
    A. Place the ultrasound transducer in the left lower quadrant of the woman's abdomen
    B. Recognize that passage of meconium would be a definitive sign of fetal distress
    C. Expect the progress of fetal descent to be slower than usual
    D. Assist the woman into a knee-chest position for each contraction

69. A nurse is caring for a pregnant woman at 30 weeks of gestation in preterm labor. The woman's physician orders betamethasone 12 mg IM for two doses, with the first dose to begin at 11 am. In implementing this order the nurse should:
    A. Consult the physician, because the dose is too high
    B. Explain to the woman that this medication will reduce her heart rate and help her to breathe easier
    C. Prepare to administer the medication intravenously between contractions
    D. Schedule the second dose for 11 am on the next day

70. A nurse caring for a pregnant woman suspected of being in preterm labor recognizes which sign as diagnostic of preterm labor?
    A. Cervical dilation of at least 2 cm
    B. Uterine contractions occurring every 15 minutes
    C. Spontaneous rupture of the membranes
    D. Presence of fetal fibronectin in cervical secretions

71. A woman at 27 weeks of gestation experiences some mild uterine cramping. Which actions should she take? (Circle all that apply.)
    A. Empty her bladder.
    B. Call her nurse-midwife immediately.
    C. Relax in a chair.
    D. Drink two to three glasses of water or juice.
    E. Palpate her uterus for 1 hour.
    F. Resume the activity she was doing if the cramping subsides.

72. A woman is in active labor. On spontaneous rupture of her membranes, the nurse caring for this woman notices variable deceleration patterns during evaluation of the monitor tracing. When preparing to perform a vaginal examination, the nurse observes a small section of the umbilical cord protruding from the vagina. What should the nurse do next?
   A. Increase the IV drip rate.
   B. Administer oxygen to the woman via mask at 8 to 10 L/minute.
   C. Place a sterile gloved hand into the vagina and hold the presenting part off the cord while calling for assistance.
   D. Wrap the cord loosely with a sterile towel saturated with warm normal saline.

III. THINKING CRITICALLY

1. Imagine that you are a nurse-midwife working at an inner-city women's health clinic. You are concerned about the rate of preterm labor and birth among the pregnant women who come to your clinic for care. OUTLINE a preterm labor and birth prevention program that you would implement at your clinic to reduce the rate of preterm labor and birth.

2. Sara, a primiparous client (2-0-1-0-1) at 22 weeks of gestation, comes to the clinic for her scheduled prenatal visit. She is anxious because her last labor began at 26 weeks and she is worried that this will happen again. "I had no warning the last time. Is there anything I can do this time to have my baby later or at least know that labor is starting so I can let you know?"
   A. IDENTIFY the signs of preterm labor that the nurse-midwife should teach Sara.

   B. EXPLAIN how the nurse-midwife could help Sara to implement a plan to reduce her risk for preterm labor.

   C. Three weeks later Sara calls the clinic and tells her nurse-midwife that she has been having uterine contractions about every 8 minutes or so for the last hour. She is admitted for possible tocolytic therapy. SPECIFY the criteria that Sara must meet before tocolysis can be safely initiated.

   D. Sara is started on a tocolysis regimen that involves IV administration of magnesium sulfate. OUTLINE the nursing care measures that must be implemented during the infusion to ensure the safety of Sara and her fetus.

   E. The nurse is preparing to give Sara a dose of betamethasone 12 mg as ordered by the physician.
      1. STATE the purpose of this medication.

2. EXPLAIN the protocol that the nurse should follow in fulfilling this order.

3. Debra has been experiencing signs of preterm labor. After a period of hospitalization, her labor was successfully suppressed and she was discharged to be cared for at home. Debra is receiving nifedipine (Procardia) 30 mg every 12 hours for 48 hours. She will palpate her uterine activity daily. Debra must also remain on bed rest for most of the day with time up to use the bathroom and for meals.

A. OUTLINE what the nurse should teach Debra regarding the self-administration of nifedipine.

B. IDENTIFY the side effects of nifedipine that the nurse should teach Debra before discharge.

C. DESCRIBE the instructions that Debra should be given regarding palpating her uterus for contractions.

D. Debra has two children who are 5 and 8 years old. SPECIFY the suggestions you would give to help Debra and her children cope with the bed rest requirement ordered by Debra's primary health care provider.

4. Denise, a primigravida, has reached the second stage of her labor with her fetus at zero station and positioned LOP. She is experiencing intense low back pain. Denise did not attend any childbirth classes and is having difficulty pushing effectively. Epidural analgesia is being used for pain control.

A. IDENTIFY the factors that can have a negative effect on the secondary powers of labor (bearing-down efforts). INDICATE those factors most likely implicated in Denise's situation.

B. DESCRIBE how you would help Denise to use her expulsive forces to facilitate the descent and birth of her baby.

C. SPECIFY the positions that would be recommended based on the position of the presenting part of Denise's fetus.

5. Anne, a primigravida, attended Lamaze classes with her husband, Mark. They were looking forward to working together during the labor and birth of their baby. Because of fetal distress, an emergency low-segment cesarean section with a transverse incision was performed after 18 hours of labor. Even though Anne and her son are in stable condition and she is glad that "everything turned out okay" for her son, she expresses a sense of failure, stating: "I could not manage to give birth to my son in the normal way and now I never will!"

    A. LIST the preoperative nursing measures that should have been implemented to prepare Anne physically and emotionally for the unexpected cesarean birth.

    B. SPECIFY the assessment measures that are critical when Anne is recovering following birth.

    C. STATE the postoperative nursing care measures that Anne requires.

    D. IDENTIFY the nursing diagnosis reflected in Anne's statement: "I could not manage to give birth to my baby in the normal way and now I never will." SPECIFY the support measures that the nurse could use to put the cesarean birth into perspective.

6. A vaginal examination reveals that Marie's fetus is RSA. SPECIFY the considerations that the nurse should keep in mind when providing care for Marie.

7. Angela (2-0-0-1-0) is at 42 weeks of gestation and has been admitted for induction of labor.

    A. Assessment of Angela at admission included determination of her Bishop score. STATE the purpose of the Bishop score and identify the factors that are evaluated.

    B. Angela's score was 5. INTERPRET this result in terms of the planned induction of her labor.

C. Angela's primary health care provider ordered that dinoprostone (Cervidil) be inserted. STATE the purpose of the dinoprostone, method of application, and its potential side effects.

D. Before induction of her labor, Angela's primary health provider performs an amniotomy.
   1. STATE the rationale for performing an amniotomy at this time.

   2. SPECIFY the nursing responsibilities before, during, and after this procedure.

E. INDICATE which of the following actions reflect appropriate collaborative care (A) for Angela during the induction of her labor with IV oxytocin. If the action is not appropriate (NA), state what the correct action would be.

   1. _____ Assist Angela into a lateral or upright position.

   2. _____ Apply an external electronic fetal monitor and obtain a 5-minute baseline strip of FHR and pattern.

   3. _____ Explain to Angela what to expect and techniques used.

   4. _____ Add 40 units of oxytocin (Pitocin) to 1000 mL of an isotonic electrolyte solution.

   5. _____ Piggyback the oxytocin solution into the port nearest the IV insertion site of the primary IV.

   6. _____ Begin infusion at 4 milliunits/minute.

   7. _____ Increase oxytocin by 1 to 2 milliunits/minute at 5- to 10-minute intervals after the initial dose until the desired pattern of contractions is achieved.

   8. _____ Stop increasing the dosage and maintain level of oxytocin when active labor is established and contractions occur every 2 to 3 minutes, last 80 to 90 seconds, and are estimated to be strong using palpation.

   9. _____ Monitor maternal blood pressure and pulse every 15 minutes and after every increment.

   10. _____ Monitor FHR and pattern and uterine activity every 15 minutes and before and after every increment; increase frequency to every 5 minutes during the active pushing phase of the second stage of labor.

   11. _____ Limit IV intake to 1500 mL in 8 hours.

F. STATE the reportable conditions associated with oxytocin (Pitocin) induction for which the nurse must be alert when managing Angela's labor.

G. The nurse notes a pattern of uterine tachysystole when evaluating Angela's monitor tracing. LIST the actions the nurse should take in order of priority.

8. Lora is a 37-year-old nulliparous client beginning her 42nd week of pregnancy. She and her primary health care provider have decided on a conservative "watchful waiting" approach because both she and her fetus are not experiencing distress.
   A. In helping Lora to make this decision, the risks that she and her fetus face as a result of a postterm pregnancy were explained. IDENTIFY the risks that Lora should have considered in making her decision.

   B. STATE the clinical manifestations that Lora is likely to experience as her pregnancy continues.

   C. OUTLINE the typical care management measures that should be implemented to ensure the safety of Lora and her fetus.

   D. SPECIFY the instructions that the nurse should give to Lora regarding her self-care as she awaits the onset of labor.

9. Suzanne is a 30-year-old primigravida who was just admitted in the latent phase of the first stage of labor. A major concern for her nurse will relate to Suzanne's BMI of 45, which indicates that she is obese. Additionally, Suzanne has been diagnosed with gestational hypertension and gestational diabetes.
   A. IDENTIFY the risk factors that this situation presents.

   B. DESCRIBE how the nurse will need to adjust care measures to ensure a safe environment and positive outcome for Suzanne and her baby.

33 Postpartum Complications

I. LEARNING KEY TERMS

FILL IN THE BLANKS: Insert the term that corresponds to each of the following descriptions of postpartum complications.

1. _____ Loss of 500 mL of blood or more after vaginal birth or of 1000 mL of blood or more after cesarean birth. Additional criteria that may be used are a 10% change in hematocrit between admission for labor and postpartum or the need for erythrocyte transfusion. It can be classified as _____ if it occurs within 24 hours of the birth or _____ if it occurs more than 24 hours but less than 6 weeks after the birth.

2. _____ Marked hypotonia of the uterus. It is the leading cause of early postpartum hemorrhage (PPH).

3. _____ Most common of all injuries in the low portion of the genital tract; they are classified as first, second, third, and fourth degree.

4. _____ Accumulation of blood in the connective tissue as a result of blood vessel damage. _____ are the most common type following birth.

5. _____ Term used to refer to slight penetration of the myometrium by placenta.

6. _____ Term used to refer to deep penetration of the myometrium by the placenta.

7. _____ Term used to refer to perforation of the uterus by the placenta.

8. _____ Turning of the uterus inside out after birth; it can be incomplete, complete, or prolapsed.

9. _____ Delayed return of the enlarged uterus to normal size and function following birth. Recognized causes of this delay include _____ and _____.

10. _____ Emergency situation in which profuse blood loss can result in severely compromised perfusion of body organs. Death may occur.

11. _____ Disorder in which coagulation is compromised, resulting in continuous bleeding.

12. _____ Abnormally low platelet level.

13. _____ Autoimmune disorder in which antiplatelet antibodies decrease the life span of the platelets.

14. _____ Type of hemophilia; it is probably the most common of all hereditary bleeding disorders.

15. _____ Formation of a blood clot or clots inside a blood vessel.

16. _____ Formation of a clot in a blood vessel as result of inflammation.

17. _____ Thromboembolic condition that involves the superficial saphenous venous system.

18. _____ Thromboembolic condition in which involvement varies but that occurs most often in the lower extremities; it can extend from the foot to the iliofemoral region.

19. _____ Complication of deep venous thrombosis (DVT) that occurs when part of a blood clot dislodges and is carried to the pulmonary artery, where it occludes the vessel and obstructs blood flow to the lungs.

20. _____ Any clinical infection of the genital canal that occurs within 28 days after miscarriage, induced abortion, or childbirth.

21. _____ Infection located in the lining of the uterus; it is the most common postpartum infection; it usually begins as a localized infection at the placental site but can spread to involve the entire lining.

22. _____ Infection of the breast soon after childbirth, most often affecting primiparous breastfeeding women.

II. REVIEWING KEY CONCEPTS

23. STATE the twofold focus of medical management of hemorrhagic shock.

24. STATE the standard of care for bleeding emergencies.

MULTIPLE CHOICE: Circle the correct option(s) and state the rationale for the option(s) chosen.

25. Methylergonovine (Methergine) 0.2 mg is ordered for a woman who gave birth vaginally 1 hour ago; it is to be administered intramuscularly to treat a profuse lochial flow with clots. Her fundus is boggy and does not respond well to massage. She is still being treated for preeclampsia with IV magnesium sulfate at 1 g/hour. Her blood pressure (BP), measured 5 minutes ago, was 155/98 mm Hg. In fulfilling this order, the nurse should:
    A. Measure the woman's blood pressure again 5 minutes after administering the medication
    B. Question the order, based on the woman's hypertensive status
    C. Administer the methylergonovine because it is the best choice to counteract the possible uterine relaxation effects of the magnesium sulfate infusion the woman is receiving
    D. Tell the woman that the medication will lead to uterine cramping

26. A postpartum woman in the fourth stage of labor received prostaglandin F$_2\alpha$ (Hemabate) 0.25 mg intramuscularly. The expected outcome of care for the administration of this medication is:
    A. Relief from the pain of uterine cramping
    B. Prevention of intrauterine infection
    C. Reduction in the blood's ability to clot
    D. Limitation of excessive blood loss that is occurring after birth

27. The nurse responsible for the care of postpartum women recognizes that the first sign of puerperal infection most likely is:
    A. Temperature elevation to 38°C or higher after the first 24 hours following birth
    B. Increased white blood cell count
    C. Foul-smelling profuse lochia
    D. Bradycardia

28. A breastfeeding woman's cesarean birth occurred 2 days ago. Investigation of the pain, tenderness, and swelling in her left leg led to a medical diagnosis of deep vein thrombosis (DVT). Care management for this woman during the acute stage of the DVT involves: (Circle all that apply.)
    A. Explaining that she will need to stop breastfeeding until anticoagulation therapy is completed
    B. Administering warfarin (Coumadin) orally
    C. Placing the woman on bed rest with her left leg elevated
    D. Fitting the woman with an elastic stocking so that she can exercise her legs
    E. Telling her to avoid changing her position for the first 24 hours
    F. Administering heparin intravenously for 3 to 5 days

III. THINKING CRITICALLY

1. Andrea is a multiparous client (6-5-1-0-7) who gave birth to full-term twins vaginally 1 hour ago. Oxytocin (Pitocin) was used to augment her labor when hypotonic uterine contractions protracted the active stage of her labor. Special forceps were used to assist the birth of the second twin. Currently her vital signs are stable; her fundus is at the umbilicus, midline and firm; and her lochial flow is moderate to heavy without clots.
    A. Early postpartum hemorrhage is a major concern. STATE the factors that have increased Andrea's risk for hemorrhage at this time.

    B. IDENTIFY the priority nursing diagnosis at this time.

    C. During the second hour after birth, the nurse notes that Andrea's perineal pad became saturated in 15 minutes and that a large amount of blood had accumulated on the bed under her buttocks. DESCRIBE the nurse's initial response to this finding. STATE the rationale for the action you described.

    D. The nurse prepares to administer 10 units of oxytocin intravenously as ordered by Andrea's physician. EXPLAIN the guidelines the nurse should follow in fulfilling this order.

    E. During the assessment of Andrea, the nurse must be alert for signs of developing hemorrhagic shock. CITE the signs the nurse would be watching for.

F. DESCRIBE the measures that the nurse should use to care for Andrea's physiologic needs and to support her and her family and attempt to reduce their anxiety.

2. Nurses working on a postpartum unit must be constantly alert for signs and symptoms of puerperal infection in their clients. You have been assigned to present a nursing in-service presentation titled "Postpartum Uterine Infection—An Update." PREPARE a teaching plan that includes each of the following components.
   A. Factors that can increase a postpartum woman's risk for puerperal infection.

   B. Infection prevention measures that nurses should be using when caring for postpartum women.

   C. Typical clinical manifestations of endometritis for which nurses should be alert when assessing postpartum women.

   D. Two nursing diagnoses that are appropriate for women diagnosed with endometritis.

   E. Critical nursing measures that are essential in care management related to the prevention and early detection of puerperal infection.

3. Sara, a primiparous breastfeeding mother at 2 weeks postpartum, calls her nurse-midwife to tell her that her right breast is painful and she is "not feeling well."
   A. EXPLAIN the assessment findings the nurse-midwife would be alert for to determine whether Sara is experiencing mastitis.

B. A medical diagnosis of mastitis of Sara's right breast is made. STATE two nursing diagnoses appropriate for this situation.

C. DESCRIBE the treatment measures and health teaching that Sara, who wishes to continue to breastfeed, needs regarding her infection and breastfeeding.

D. IDENTIFY several measures that Sara should learn and implement to prevent recurrence of mastitis.

4. Susan is a 36-year-old obese multiparous client (4-3-0-1-3) who experienced a cesarean birth 2 days ago. She has no previous history of pregnancy-related complications. When asked, she admits to smoking but has been trying to cut down from her usual half-pack every 1 to 2 days. A major complication of the postpartum period for Susan is the development of thromboembolic disease.
A. STATE the risk factors for this complication that Susan presents.

B. When assessing Susan on the afternoon of her second postpartum day, the nurse notes signs indicative of deep vein thrombosis (DVT). LIST the signs the nurse most likely observed.

C. A medical diagnosis of DVT is confirmed. STATE one nursing diagnosis appropriate for this situation.

D. OUTLINE the expected care management for Susan during the acute phase of DVT.

E. On discharge, Susan will be taking warfarin for at least 3 months. SPECIFY the discharge instructions that Susan and her family should receive.

34 Nursing Care of the High Risk Newborn and Family

I. LEARNING KEY TERMS

FILL IN THE BLANKS: Insert the term that corresponds to each of the following descriptions related to gestational age and intrauterine growth.

1. _____ Infant whose birth weight is less than 2500 g, regardless of gestational age.

2. _____ Infant whose birth weight is less than 1500 g.

3. _____ Infant whose birth weight is less than 1000 g.

4. _____ or _____ Infant born before completion of 37 weeks of gestation, regardless of birth weigh. These infants are at risk because their organ systems are immature and they lack adequate physiologic reserves to function in an extrauterine environment.

5. _____ Infant born between 34 $^5/_7$ and 36 $^6/_7$ weeks of gestation, regardless of birth weight; by nature of their limited gestation, these infants remain at risk for problems related to thermoregulation, hypoglycemia, hyperbilirubinemia, sepsis, and respiratory function.

6. _____ Infant born between the beginning of 38 weeks and the completion of 42 weeks of gestation, regardless of birth weight.

7. _____ or _____ An infant born after 42 weeks of gestation, regardless of birth weight.

8. _____ Infant whose birth weight falls above the 90th percentile on intrauterine growth curves and charts.

9. _____ Infant whose birth weight falls between the 10th and the 90th percentiles on intrauterine growth curves and charts.

10. _____ Infant whose rate of intrauterine growth was restricted and whose birth weight falls below the 10th percentile on intrauterine growth curves and charts.

11. _____ Rate of fetal growth that does not meet expected growth patterns.

12. _____ Type of inhibited fetal growth in which the weight, length, and head circumference are all affected.

13. _____ Type of inhibited fetal growth in which the head circumference remains within normal parameters while the birth weight falls below the 10th percentile.

14. _____ Birth in which the neonate manifests any heartbeat, breathes, or displays voluntary movement, regardless of gestational age.

15. _____ Death of a fetus after 20 weeks of gestation and before birth, with absence of any signs of life after birth.

247

16. _____ Death that occurs in the first 27 days of life; it is described as early if it occurs in the first week of life and as late if it occurs at 7 to 27 days.

17. _____ Total number of fetal and early neonatal deaths per 1000 live births.

18. _____ Respiratory pattern commonly seen in preterm infants; such infants exhibit 5- to 10-second respiratory pauses followed by 10 to 15 seconds of compensatory rapid respirations.

19. _____ Cessation of respirations for 20 seconds or more or a shorter pause accompanied by bradycardia, cyanosis, or hypotonia.

20. _____ Noninvasive, effective means for detecting alterations in systemic blood pressure (hypotension or hypertension) and for identifying the need to implement appropriate therapy to maintain cardiovascular function.

21. _____ The environmental temperature at which oxygen consumption is minimal but adequate to maintain the body temperature.

22. _____ Surface-active phospholipid secreted by the alveolar epithelium; it reduces the surface tension of fluids that line the alveoli and respiratory passages, resulting in uniform expansion and maintenance of lung expansion at low intraalveolar pressure.

23. _____ Evaporative loss that occurs largely through the skin (70%) and respiratory tract (30%); it is increased in preterm infants.

24. _____ Method of providing breast milk or formula through a nasogastric tube or orogastric tube; feeding can be accomplished either with a tube inserted at each feeding (bolus) or continuously through an indwelling catheter.

25. _____ Nutritional method used to stimulate or prime the gastrointestinal tract to achieve better absorption of nutrients when bolus or regular intermittent gavage feedings can be given.

26. _____ Method of feeding that involves the surgical placement of a tube through the skin of the abdomen into the stomach.

27. _____ Supplemental parenteral fluids administered to infants who are unable to obtain sufficient fluids or calories by enteral feedings.

28. _____ Sucking on a pacifier during tube or parenteral feeding or between oral feedings to improve oxygenation and facilitate earlier transition to nipple feeding; this type of sucking may lead to decreased energy expenditure with less restlessness and to positive weight gain and better sucking skills.

29. _____ Method that can be used to provide maternal or paternal skin-to-skin contact with their newborn, to reduce stress in the infant and to create a positive healing effect for the mother who had a high-risk pregnancy.

30. _____ Form of grieving experienced by parents as they prepare themselves for the possibility of their infant's death while still clinging to the hope that the infant will survive.

II. REVIEWING KEY CONCEPTS

31. The preterm infant is vulnerable to a number of complications related to immaturity of physiologic functions. IDENTIFY the potential problems and their physiologic basis for each of the areas listed below.
   - Respiratory function

- Cardiovascular function

- Body temperature

- Central nervous system function

- Adequate nutrition

- Renal function

- Hematologic status

- Infection

- Growth and development potential

MATCHING: Match the description in Column I with the appropriate complication associated with the high-risk newborn in Column II.

COLUMN I

32. _____ Complex, multicausal disorder that affects the developing blood vessels in the eyes of preterm infants; it is often associated with oxygen tensions that are too high for the level of retinal maturity, initially resulting in vasoconstriction and continuing problems after the oxygen is discontinued. Scar tissue formation and consequent visual impairment may be mild or severe.

33. _____ Acute inflammatory disease of the gastrointestinal mucosa commonly complicated by bowel necrosis and perforation; intestinal ischemia, colonization by pathogenic bacteria, and enteral feeding all play an important role in its development.

34. _____ Occurs when the fetal shunt connecting the left pulmonary artery and the dorsal aorta fails to close after birth or reopens after constriction has occurred.

35. _____ Chronic lung disease with a multifactorial etiology that includes pulmonary immaturity, surfactant deficiency, lung injury and stretch, barotrauma, inflammation caused by oxygen exposure, fluid overload, ligation of a patent ductus arteriosus (PDA), and familial predisposition. Incidence has decreased with prenatal use of maternal steroids when preterm birth is expected coupled with the use of exogenous surfactant; it occurs most commonly in preterm infants requiring mechanical ventilation.

36. _____ Lung disorder, usually affecting preterm infants, caused by a lack of pulmonary surfactant, which leads to progressive atelectasis, loss of functional residual capacity, and ventilation-perfusion imbalance with an uneven distribution of ventilation.

37. _____ Combined findings of pulmonary hypertension, right-to-left shunting, and a structurally normal heart; it is also called persistent fetal circulation because the syndrome includes reversion to fetal pathways for blood flow.

38. _____ One of the most common types of brain injuries encountered in the neonatal period and among the most severe in both short- and long-term outcomes; incidence is decreasing related to prenatal use of corticosteroids and postnatal use of surfactant.

COLUMN II

A. Bronchopulmonary dysplasia (BPD)
B. Retinopathy of prematurity (ROP)
C. Patent ductus arteriosus (PDA)
D. Persistent pulmonary hypertension of the newborn (PPHN)
E. Germinal matrix hemorrhage–intraventricular hemorrhage (GMH-IVH)
F. Necrotizing enterocolitis (NEC)
G. Respiratory distress syndrome (RDS)

39. Joshua was born at 35 weeks of gestation and James was born at 41 weeks of gestation. COMPARE the care management needs of Joshua and James based on needs and risks associated with their gestational ages.

MULTIPLE CHOICE: Circle the correct option(s) and state the rationale for the option(s) chosen.

40. Preterm infants are at increased risk for developing respiratory distress. The nurse should assess for signs that would indicate that the newborn is having difficulty breathing. Signs of respiratory distress are: (Circle all that apply.)
    A. Use of abdominal muscles to breathe
    B. Expiratory grunting
    C. Periodic breathing pattern
    D. Suprasternal retraction
    E. Nasal flaring
    F. Acrocyanosis

Chapter **34** **Nursing Care of the High Risk Newborn and Family**

41. When caring for a preterm infant at 30 weeks of gestation, the nurse should recognize that the newborn's primary nursing diagnosis is:
    A. Risk for infection related to decreased immune response
    B. Ineffective breathing pattern related to surfactant deficiency and weak respiratory muscle effort
    C. Ineffective thermoregulation related to immature thermoregulation center
    D. Imbalanced nutrition: less than body requirements related to ineffective suck and swallow

42. A nurse is preparing to insert a gavage tube and feed a preterm newborn. As part of the protocol for this procedure the nurse should: (Circle all that apply.)
    A. Determine the length of tubing to be inserted by measuring from tip of nose to lobe of ear to midpoint between xiphoid process and umbilicus
    B. Lubricate the tip of the gavage tube with sterile water to ease passage
    C. Insert the tube through the nose as the preferred route for most infants
    D. Check placement of the tube by injecting 2 to 3 mL of sterile water into the tube and listening for gurgling with a stethoscope
    E. Assess residual gastric aspirate every 2 to 4 hours when continuous feedings are administered
    F. Provide nonnutritive sucking during gavage feedings

43. Evaluating blood gas values provides essential information about the effectiveness of the preterm newborn's respiratory effort and oxygen administration measures. Which arterial blood gas values indicate adequate gas exchange? (Circle all that apply.)
    A. pH 7.40
    B. PaO_2 75 mm Hg
    C. $PaCO_2$ 48 mm Hg
    D. HCO_3 28 mEq/L
    E. Base excess –6
    F. Oxygen saturation 93%

44. Preterm newborns are at increased risk for infection. The most important measure to prevent iatrogenic infections in the preterm newborn is to:
    A. Monitor vital signs for instability
    B. Teach parents infection control measures
    C. Cleanse the newborn's skin with plain warm water
    D. Perform hand hygiene

45. Preterm infants are at risk for cold stress. Which signs should alert the nurse that the preterm infant he or she is caring for may be hypothermic? (Circle all that apply.)
    A. Acrocyanosis
    B. Hypoglycemia
    C. Irritability
    D. Periodic breathing pattern
    E. Bradycardia
    F. Abdominal distention

III. THINKING CRITICALLY

1. Baby girl Jane was born 12 hours ago at 28 weeks of gestation. Oxygen therapy is a vital component of her care because she has been experiencing respiratory distress since birth.
    A. IDENTIFY the criteria that were used to determine that baby Jane needed supplemental oxygen.

Chapter **34** Nursing Care of the High Risk Newborn and Family

B. CREATE a set of general guidelines that reflects the recommended principles for safe and effective administration of oxygen to a compromised newborn.

C. Baby girl Jane's respiratory status is improving and her health care providers are preparing to begin the process of weaning her from the oxygen. DESCRIBE signs that indicate that Jane is ready to be weaned from oxygen therapy.

D. OUTLINE the guidelines that should be followed when weaning Jane from oxygen therapy.

2. Anne, a 3 lb, 12 oz (1705 g) preterm newborn at 32 weeks of gestation, is admitted to the neonatal intensive care unit (NICU) after her birth for observation and supportive care. Anne's nutritional needs are a critical concern in her care. Oral feedings of maternal colostrum and breast milk are attempted first.
A. STATE the assessment data that the nurse should document after each of Anne's feedings to indicate feeding method effectiveness.

B. The nurse determines that Anne's suck is weak and she becomes too fatigued during oral feedings to obtain sufficient nutrients and fluid. The nurse confers with the neonatologist and a decision is made to provide intermittent gavage feedings with occasional oral feedings. DESCRIBE the guidelines the nurse should follow when inserting the gavage tube.

C. STATE the priority nursing diagnosis for Anne.

D. DISCUSS the principles the nurse should follow before, during, and after a gavage feeding to ensure safety and maximum effectiveness.

E. OUTLINE the protocol that should be followed when advancing Anne back to full oral feeding.

3. The NICU is a stressful environment for preterm infants and their families.
    A. IDENTIFY the common sources of stress facing infants and their families in an intensive care environment.
        Infant stressors

        Family stressors

    B. Nurses working in the NICU and parents must be aware of infant behavioral cues and adjust stimuli accordingly. LIST infant behavioral cues that indicate readiness for interaction and stimulation and behavioral cues that signal a need for a time-out.
        Approach behaviors (cues to a relaxed state)

        Avoidance behaviors (cues to overstimulation)

    C. IDENTIFY specific measures that can be used to protect infants from overstimulation and yet provide appropriate stimulation to meet the developmental and emotional needs of infants.

    D. SPECIFY the guidelines that should be followed regarding infant positioning.

4. Marion is beginning her 43rd week of pregnancy.
    A. SUPPORT this statement: Perinatal mortality is significantly higher in the postmature fetus and neonate.

B. STATE the assessment findings that are typical of a postmature infant.

C. DISCUSS the two major complications that can be experienced by a postmature infant.

5. Janet, a pregnant client at term, is in labor. On the basis of serial ultrasound findings, her fetus is estimated to be smaller than it should be as a consequence of Janet's heavy smoking during pregnancy and her high-risk status related to preeclampsia.
   A. IDENTIFY three major complications facing Janet's baby during labor, birth, and the postpartum period.

   B. DESCRIBE the physiologic basis for each potential complication and the signs and symptoms indicative of its presence.

6. Marion is at 24 weeks of gestation and is in preterm labor. Her primary health care provider determines that preterm birth is inevitable and has elected to transport Marion to a tertiary center before she gives birth, to maximize the survival potential of her unborn infant.
   A. EXPLAIN the advantages of transport before birth.

   B. Marion gives birth before she can be transported. Her baby will be transported to the tertiary center once stable. INDICATE the needs of this preterm baby that must be stabilized before transport.

   C. IDENTIFY the measures that the nurse should use to support Marion and her family as her newborn is transported to the tertiary center.

7. Anita and Juan are the parents of a 2-day-old preterm newborn boy. Their baby, who is 27 weeks' gestation and weighs 1 kg, is in the NICU and will be in the hospital for several weeks or longer. The nurse caring for this baby recognizes that he must also provide supportive care for Anita and Juan.

   A. As parents of a preterm infant, Anita and Juan must accomplish several tasks as they develop a relationship with their baby boy and prepare to care for him. IDENTIFY these tasks and a nursing care measure that can be used to help Anita and Juan successfully accomplish each task.

   B. STATE the behaviors the nurse should assess as he observes Anita and Juan with their baby. CATEGORIZE these behaviors in terms of behaviors that indicate effective coping and those that indicate ineffective coping and maladaptation.

8. IMAGINE that you are a nurse working in an NICU caring for an infant at 26 weeks of gestation born 2 hours ago. He is exhibiting signs of increasing dyspnea. The neonatologist orders that surfactant be administered. The baby's parents become very upset and tell you, "Our baby is already having a hard time breathing. What can this surfactant stuff do except make it worse for him?"

   A. DESCRIBE what you would tell these parents regarding the purpose of exogenous surfactant administration to the preterm newborn.

   B. EXPLAIN how you would inform the parents about how the surfactant is administered.

9. The nurse manager of an NICU attended a national nursing conference on NICU innovations in care. She was very impressed by the presentation on kangaroo care and decides to institute it at the NICU she manages. DESCRIBE the approach that she should take to inform her nurses about the change she wishes to make and encourage their full participation in its implementation.

10. Imagine that you are a nurse working in an NICU. You have been assigned to care for Tim, a 1-day-old infant born at 30 weeks of gestation. As you begin his care you take note of all of the lines and tubes attached to him and realize that you must consider the pain Tim is experiencing as part of your plan of care.

    A. EXPLAIN how you would distinguish common newborn responses from those that could indicate that Tim is experiencing discomfort and pain.

B. Reports indicate that newborns have memory of the pain they experience. DESCRIBE behaviors that you would look for that could indicate that Tim is forming a memory of painful experiences.

C. DESCRIBE what could happen to Tim if you neglected to recognize his pain experience and incorporate pain relief measures in your plan of care.

D. DISCUSS how you would use each of the following strategies to manage the pain Tim is experiencing:
   - Nonpharmacologic measures

   - Pharmacologic measures

35 Acquired Problems of the Newborn

I. LEARNING KEY TERMS

FILL IN THE BLANKS: Insert the term that corresponds to each of the following descriptions.

1. _____ Physical injury sustained by a neonate during labor and birth.

2. _____ Rupture of the capillaries within the eye caused by increased intracranial pressure during birth. They usually clear within 5 days after birth and present no problems.

3. _____ Bruises; may appear on the face as the result of a face presentation or on the buttocks and genitalia with a breech presentation.

4. _____ Pinpoint hemorrhagic areas.

5. _____ The bone most frequently fractured during birth.

6. _____ or _____ Brachial paralysis of the upper portion of the arm; it is the most common type of paralysis associated with a difficult birth.

7. _____ Failure of the kidney to develop.

8. _____ Sacral agenesis with weakness or deformities of the lower extremities, malformation and fixation of the hip joints, and shortening or deformity of the femurs.

9. _____ Excessive fetal growth resulting in a large for gestational age (LGA) newborn; often associated with women who have pregestational or gestational diabetes.

10. _____ Blood glucose levels less than 40 mg/dL in term infants.

11. _____ Disease affecting the structure and function of the heart.

12. _____ Increased number of red blood cells; results in increased viscosity of the blood.

_____ Results when the excessive red blood cells are hemolyzed.

13. _____ Presence of microorganisms or their toxins in blood or other tissues; it is one of the most significant causes of neonatal morbidity and mortality.

14. _____ Generalized infection in the bloodstream.

15. _____ Disorder that results from toxins released into the bloodstream by microorganisms. The most common sign is hypotension. The infant will appear gray or mottled and will have cool extremities and rapid, irregular respirations and pulse.

16. _____ Administration of an antibiotic ointment (e.g., erythromycin) into the eyes of the newborn within 1 hour of birth to prevent ophthalmia neonatorum.

17. _____ Elevated wartlike lesions characteristic of congenital syphilis.

18. _____ Copious clear mucous discharge from the nose characteristic of congenital syphilis.

19. _____ Circumoral radiating scars that form as mucocutaneous lesions of the lips heal; occurs with congenital syphilis.

20. _____ Combination antiviral drug treatment used during antepartum, intrapartum, and neonatal periods that has almost completely eliminated mother-to-child human immunodeficiency virus (HIV) transmission in developed countries; it is also used to treat HIV-positive children.

21. _____ Infections caused by an organism that usually does not cause illness; it is an outcome of HIV infection related to the suppression of immunologic activity. These infections include candidiasis and *Pneumocystis jiroveci* pneumonia (PCP).

22. _____ Infection known as fifth disease or "slapped cheek illness" in older children.

23. _____ Microorganism that is a leading cause of neonatal morbidity and mortality in the United States. Women who are positive for this microorganism are given prophylactic antibiotics when in labor.

24. _____ Primarily a food-borne infection causing maternal and neonatal illness; it is one of the three major causes of neonatal meningitis globally.

25. _____ Oral candidiasis; it is characterized by adherent white plaques on the oral mucosa, gums, and tongue.

26. _____ Acute and long-term outcome of alcohol ingestion during pregnancy; it is characterized by prenatal and postnatal growth restriction, central nervous system (CNS) malfunctions (e.g., cognitive impairment), and distinctive craniofacial features (e.g., microcephaly, small eyes).

27. _____ Term given to the group of signs and symptoms associated with drug withdrawal in the neonate.

II. REVIEWING KEY CONCEPTS

28. IDENTIFY the most common congenital anomalies experienced by infants with diabetic mothers in terms of each of the following:
Cardiac

Central nervous system

Musculoskeletal

Renal

29. STATE the infections(s) represented by each letter in the acronym TORCH.

T

O

R

C

H

30. Sepsis is one of the most significant causes of neonatal morbidity and mortality.
    A. INDICATE the primary modes of infection transmission for each of the periods listed below.
    - Prenatal

    - Perinatal

    - Postnatal

    B. IDENTIFY the major risk factors that, if present, should alert the nurse to an increased potential for infection in the neonate.

C. LIST the signs a neonate might exhibit that would indicate that sepsis is present.

D. DESCRIBE two effective nursing measures for each of the following categories:
- Preventive measures

- Curative measures

MULTIPLE CHOICE: Circle the correct option(s) and state the rationale for the option(s) chosen.

31. When assessing a newborn after birth, the nurse notes the following: limited movement of left arm with crepitus at the shoulder and absence of Moro reflex on left side. The nurse suspects:
    A. Brachial plexus injury
    B. Fracture of the clavicle
    C. Phrenic nerve injury
    D. Intracranial hemorrhage on the right side of the brain

32. A nurse is caring for a male newborn whose mother had gestational diabetes during pregnancy. His estimated gestational age is 41 weeks and his weight indicates that he is macrosomic. When assessing this newborn, the nurse should be alert for which findings associated with macrosomia? (Circle all that apply.)
    A. Fracture of the femur
    B. Hypocalcemia
    C. Blood glucose level of 38 mg/dL
    D. Signs of a congenital heart defect
    E. Pale complexion
    F. Round "cherubic" face

33. A woman who developed hepatitis B during pregnancy gives birth vaginally to a healthy baby boy. Her baby is receiving hepatitis B immunoglobulin (HBIg) 0.5 mg IM 2 hours after birth. When should he receive his first dose of the hepatitis B vaccine?
    A. At the same time as the HBIg but in a different site
    B. One month after birth
    C. Six months after birth
    D. One year after birth

34. A woman was discovered to be HIV positive as part of routine screening during pregnancy. She was immediately treated with HAART. She just gave birth to a baby girl. Care management of this newborn includes:
    A. Encouraging the mother to breastfeed to protect her infant from infection
    B. Teaching the mother about the importance of taking her infant for routine immunizations
    C. Isolating the newborn in a special nursery
    D. Initiating HAART treatment as soon as the newborn is diagnosed as HIV positive

35. A woman in labor admits that she used heroin during her pregnancy. After the birth of her baby boy, the nurse caring for him must be alert for which signs that indicate neonatal abstinence syndrome? (Circle all that apply.)
    A. Sleepiness
    B. Poor feeding
    C. Bradypnea
    D. Below normal body temperature
    E. Diarrhea
    F. Frequent yawning

III. THINKING CRITICALLY

1. Birth trauma, although decreasing in incidence, is still an important source of neonatal morbidity. Nurses caring for women in labor should be aware of the factors that predispose infants to injury during the process of birth.
    A. IDENTIFY the factors that increase fetal vulnerability to injury and trauma at birth.

    B. DESCRIBE an approach to labor and birth care that can reduce the incidence of birth injuries.

    C. Baby boy Timothy's right clavicle was fractured during birth as a result of shoulder dystocia. DESCRIBE the signs that Timothy most likely exhibited that alerted the nurse that his clavicle was fractured.

    D. EXPLAIN to Timothy's parents the most likely care approach related to his fracture.

2. Baby boy Robert, weighing 11 lb, 4 oz, was born 1 hour ago. His mother, a primipara, had gestational diabetes mellitus.
    A. Robert's mother is thrilled at his size, stating: "He looks so healthy and well nourished, not like the skinny babies in the nursery." EXPLAIN what the nurse caring for Robert should tell his parents about the reason for his large size.

    B. DESCRIBE the typical characteristics exhibited by a macrosomic infant such as Robert.

C. Robert, as a macrosomic infant, is at increased risk for the development of hypoglycemia. DESCRIBE the physiologic basis for his increased risk for hypoglycemia.

D. IDENTIFY the signs that Robert would exhibit if he developed hypoglycemia.

3. Baby girl Susan was born 2 hours ago. Her mother tested positive for HBsAg antibodies as a result of infection with hepatitis B virus (HBV).
   A. DESCRIBE the protocol that should be followed in providing care for Susan.

   B. Susan's mother asks the nurse if she can breastfeed her baby daughter. DISCUSS the nurse's response to the mother.

4. Baby boy Andrew is a full-term newborn who was just now born by spontaneous vaginal delivery. Genital herpes recurred in his mother and her membranes ruptured before the onset of labor.
   A. IDENTIFY the four modes of transmission for herpes simplex virus (HSV) to the newborn. INDICATE the mode most likely to have transmitted the infection to Andrew.

   B. LIST the clinical signs that Andrew would exhibit as evidence of a disseminated infection, CNS involvement, and localized HSV infection.

   C. DESCRIBE the recommended nursing measures related to each of the following:
   Management after birth, prior to discharge

   Administration of vidarabine and acyclovir

5. Baby girl Mary is 1 day old. Her mother is HIV positive but received no treatment during pregnancy.
   A. DISCUSS Mary's potential for HIV infection.

   B. IDENTIFY four strategies that can be used to prevent the transmission of HIV to newborns.

   C. OUTLINE the protocol that most likely will be followed to determine if Mary is HIV positive.

   D. Name the opportunistic infections, if contracted by Mary, that would strongly suggest that she is infected with HIV.

   E. DESCRIBE the care measures recommended for Mary.

   F. Mary's mother wishes to breastfeed Mary because she has read that it can prevent infection. DISCUSS the nurse's response to this mother.

6. Thomas, a healthy 2-day-old newborn, has developed thrush.
   A. DESCRIBE the signs most likely exhibited by Thomas that led to this diagnosis.

   B. NAME the modes of transmission for this infection.

   C. DISCUSS the care management required by Thomas as a result of his yeastlike fungal infection.

7. Jane, a newborn, has been diagnosed with fetal alcohol syndrome (FAS) as a result of moderate to sometimes heavy binge drinking by her mother throughout pregnancy.

    A. DESCRIBE the characteristics Jane most likely exhibited to establish the diagnosis of FAS.

    B. STATE three long-term effects Jane could experience as she gets older.

    C. DESCRIBE two nursing measures that could be effective in promoting Jane's growth and development.

8. Maternal substance abuse can be harmful to fetal and newborn health status as well as to growth and development. Susan has just been born. Her mother used cocaine during pregnancy.

    A. IDENTIFY the effects that Susan may exhibit as a result of exposure to cocaine while in utero.

    B. Outline the care measures appropriate for both Susan and her mother during hospitalization and after discharge.

9. Tony is a 2-hour-old newborn. It is suspected that his mother abused drugs during pregnancy.

    A. LIST the signs associated with neonatal abstinence syndrome that the nurse should observe for when assessing Tony.

    B. Tony begins to exhibit signs that confirm that his mother used heroin during pregnancy. CITE two nursing diagnoses that would be appropriate for Tony.

    C. OUTLINE the care management that Tony and his mother will require as Tony progresses through withdrawal.

36 Hemolytic Disorders and Congenital Anomalies

I. LEARNING KEY TERMS

FILL IN THE BLANKS: Insert the hematologic disorder or congenital anomaly represented by each of the following descriptions.

1. _____ Condition in which the total serum bilirubin level in the blood is increased.

2. _____ Yellow discoloration of the skin, mucous membranes, sclera, and various organs associated with elevated bilirubin levels in the blood. It is termed _____ when it occurs more than 24 hours after birth and _____ when it is evident beginning in the first 24 hours after birth.

3. _____ Condition that occurs when an Rh-negative mother has an Rh-positive fetus who inherits the dominant Rh-positive gene from the father.

4. _____ Term used to refer to an Rh-negative mother's formation of antibodies capable of destroying the red blood cells of an Rh-positive fetus; this occurs with exposure of the mother to Rh-positive blood during pregnancy, birth, abortion, amniocentesis, or trauma.

5. _____ Complication of Rh incompatibility in which erythrocytes are destroyed by maternal Rh-positive antibodies; this can result in an increase in fetal bilirubin levels.

6. _____ Complication of Rh incompatibility that results in fetal compensation for red blood cell destruction by producing large numbers of immature erythrocytes to replace those that are hemolyzed.

7. _____ The most severe form of Rh incompatibility; it is characterized by marked anemia, cardiac decompensation, cardiomegaly, hepatosplenomegaly, hypoxia, and fluid leakage out of the intravascular space, resulting in generalized edema and fluid effusion into the peritoneal, pericardial, and pleural spaces.

8. _____ Disorder caused by deposition of bilirubin in the brain, resulting in acute central nervous system manifestations during the first weeks after birth.

9. _____ Term used to refer to the chronic and permanent results of bilirubin toxicity.

10. _____ Maternal blood test, used to determine whether the mother has antibodies to the Rh antigen.

11. _____ Test performed on cord blood to determine whether there are maternal antibodies to the Rh antigen in the fetal blood.

12. _____ Defect present at birth that is caused by genetic or environmental factors, or both.

13. _____ A biochemical autosomal recessive genetic disorder that causes a blockage in a critical metabolic pathway; examples include phenylketonuria and galactosemia.

14. _____ A small head circumference restricting brain growth and leading to cognitive impairment.

15. _____ Urinary meatus opens below the glans penis or anywhere along the ventral surface of the penis, scrotum, or peritoneum.

16. _____ Urinary meatus opens on the dorsal surface of the penis.

17. _____ Abnormal development of the bladder, abdominal wall, and pubic symphysis that causes the bladder, urethra, and ureteral orifices to be exposed.

18. _____ Excess cerebrospinal fluid (CSF) in the ventricles of the brain as a result of overproduction, decrease in reabsorption, or aqueductal flow obstruction of CSF; it is characterized by bulging fontanels, widening of sutures, an abnormal increase in the circumference of the head, and increasing CSF pressure.

19. _____ Term used to refer to the group of anatomic abnormalities of the heart that are present at birth and are the most common of all congenital malformations; ventricular septal defects and tetralogy of Fallot are two common forms of this type of congenital disorder.

20. _____ The most common form of clubfoot. The foot points downward and inward, the ankle is inverted, and the Achilles tendon is shortened, all making the foot appear C shaped.

21. _____ The most common congenital anomaly of the nose consisting of a unilateral or bilateral bony or soft tissue septum obstructing the posterior nares.

22. _____ The most common defect of the central nervous system (CNS) resulting from failure of the neural tube to close at some point during fetal development.

23. _____ Type of neural tube defect in which the posterior portion of the laminae fail to close but the spinal cord or meninges do not herniate or protrude through the defect and there is no abnormality of the spinal cord, nerve roots, or meninges; often a birthmark or hairy patch is present above the defect.

24. _____ Type of neural tube defect in which an external sac containing the meninges and cerebrospinal fluid protrudes through a defect in the vertebral column and is typically covered in skin.

25. _____ Covered (with a peritoneal sac) defect of the umbilical ring into which varying amounts of the abdominal organs may herniate.

26. _____ Herniation of the bowel through a defect in the abdominal wall to the right of the umbilical cord. No membrane covers the intestines.

27. _____ Congenital anomaly in which the passageway from the mouth to the stomach ends in a blind pouch, thus failing to form a continuous passageway to the stomach.

28. _____ Congenital anomaly characterized by an abnormal connection between the esophagus and the trachea.

29. _____ Term used to describe absence of an anal opening; commonly it is accompanied by a fistula from the rectum to the perineum or to the genitourinary system.

30. _____ Term used to describe a spectrum of disorders related to the abnormal development of one or all of the components of the hip joint that may develop at any time during fetal life, infancy, or childhood.

31. _____ Herniation of the brain and meninges through a skull defect, usually in the occipital area.

32. _____ Congenital disorder characterized by the absence of both cerebral hemispheres and the overlying skull. It is incompatible with life.

33. _____ Disorder characterized by displacement of the abdominal organs into the thoracic cavity through a defect in the formation of the diaphragm.

34. _____ Type of neural tube defect in which an external sac containing the meninges, cerebrospinal fluid (CSF), and spinal cord protrudes through a defect in the vertebral column; the sac can tear, allowing CSF to leak out and pathogens to enter.

35. _____ Commonly occurring congenital midline fissure, or opening, in the lip or palate resulting from failure of the primary palate to fuse; one or both deformities may occur and nasal deformity may also be present.

36. _____ Defect in which there are extra digits on the hands or feet.

37. _____ Erroneous or abnormal sexual differentiation.

38. _____ An excessive amount of amniotic fluid.

39. _____ An insufficient amount of amniotic fluid.

40. _____ Studies involving the analysis of chromosomes and molecular DNA; they are done to confirm or rule out a suspected genetic disorder.

II. REVIEWING KEY CONCEPTS

41. EXPLAIN the pathogenesis of ABO incompatibility.

42. Congenital anomalies affect the health and well-being of infants. SPECIFY the assessment techniques and considerations that guide prenatal diagnosis of congenital anomalies.

43. Congenital heart defects (CHDs) are a major cause of death in the first year of life.
    A. LIST several maternal factors associated with a higher incidence of CHDs.

    B. IDENTIFY the four physiologic classifications of CHDs, and GIVE one example for each classification.

    C. Nurses caring for newborns after birth need to include assessment for CHDs in a thorough and ongoing assessment of their health status. DESCRIBE the signs that may be exhibited at birth by an infant with a CHD.

MULTIPLE CHOICE: Circle the correct option(s) and state the rationale for the option(s) chosen.

44. A nurse is caring for a full-term newborn who is Rh positive. His mother (3-2-0-1-2), who is Rh negative, was never treated to prevent sensitization with her previous pregnancies. When assessing the newborn, the nurse must be alert for signs indicative of pathologic jaundice. Which sign alerts the nurse to this disorder?
    A. Jaundice in face, including sclera, beginning at 36 hours after birth
    B. Serum bilirubin level of 16 mg/dL on the second day of life
    C. Serum bilirubin concentration of 2 mg/dL in cord blood
    D. Total serum bilirubin level increase of 3 mg/dL in 24 hours

45. An Rh-negative woman (2-2-0-0-2) just gave birth to an Rh-positive baby boy. The direct and indirect Coombs test results are negative. Based on these data, the nurse anticipates:
    A. Preparing to administer RhoGAM to the newborn within 24 hours of his birth
    B. Observing the newborn closely for signs of pathologic jaundice
    C. Telling the woman that she will not need to receive RhoGAM after this birth because both Coombs test results are negative
    D. Administering Rh$_o$(D) immunoglobulin (RhoGAM) intramuscularly to the woman within 72 hours of her baby's birth

46. A newborn female has been diagnosed with myelomeningocele. An important nursing measure to protect the newborn from injury and further complications during the preoperative period is:
    A. Maintain the newborn in a lateral position
    B. Measure the frontal-occipital circumference to assess for hydrocephalus
    C. Cover the sac with Vaseline gauze to protect it from drying out
    D. Change the diaper frequently to prevent contamination of the sac with meconium

III. THINKING CRITICALLY

1. Pathologic jaundice is a serious health problem with the potential for severe complications that can permanently affect the life and health of the infant.
    A. CONTRAST physiologic and pathologic jaundice in terms of time of onset, time of resolution, and expected serum levels of unconjugated bilirubin.

    B. EXPLAIN the underlying physiologic process that leads to hyperbilirubinemia in the newborn.

    C. LIST the potential causes for pathologic jaundice.

    D. IDENTIFY the measures found to be effective in preventing hyperbilirubinemia.

2. Angela, who is Rh negative, had a spontaneous abortion at 13 weeks of gestation, which resulted in what she said was just a heavier than usual menstrual period. Six months later she became pregnant again.

   A. DESCRIBE the physiologic basis for Rh incompatibility and the occurrence of sensitization.

   B. An indirect Coombs test is positive. STATE the meaning of this finding.

   C. INDICATE if Angela is or is not a candidate for RhoGAM. SUPPORT your answer.

   D. DESCRIBE RhoGAM (Rh immunoglobulin) and its use.

   E. Angela's fetus is at risk for erythroblastosis fetalis and hydrops fetalis. EXPLAIN each of these conditions—what they are and the implications of their occurrence for the health status of Angela's baby.
      - Erythroblastosis fetalis

      - Hydrops fetalis

   F. DESCRIBE the treatment approaches that can be used to prevent intrauterine fetal death and early neonatal death for Angela's baby.

3. Baby girl Jennifer was born with spina bifida cystica with myelomeningocele. DESCRIBE the measures the nurse should use to manage Jennifer's care and help her parents to cope with this congenital anomaly.

4. Baby boy Thomas was just born. He is exhibiting signs that the nurse-midwife and the neonatologist believe are consistent with a diaphragmatic hernia.
   A. IDENTIFY the clinical manifestations that Thomas most likely exhibited to cause his health care providers to suspect diaphragmatic hernia.

   B. STATE the priority nursing diagnosis for Thomas.

   C. OUTLINE the essential care measures during the immediate postbirth period.

5. Baby girl Denise was born with a cleft lip and palate.
   A. STATE three nursing diagnoses faced by Denise and her parents. DISCUSS the rationale for each nursing diagnosis stated.

   B. OUTLINE several nursing measures that will need to be implemented to ensure Denise's well-being until surgical repair can be accomplished.

37 Perinatal Loss, Bereavement, and Grief

I. LEARNING KEY TERMS

FILL-IN-THE-BLANKS: Insert the term that corresponds to each of the following descriptions related to perinatal loss and grief.

1. _____ Experiences in which a valued person or object can no longer be seen, touched, heard, known, or otherwise experienced.

2. _____ State of being without a valued other, especially by death. It is characterized by the emotional state of _____, the profound sadness and despair that accompany a loss.

3. _____ The immediate reaction to news of perinatal loss or infant death; it is characterized by a state of shock and numbness, a sense of unreality, loss of innocence, powerlessness, disbelief, and denial.

4. _____ Phase of the grief response that encompasses many difficult emotions as the parents work through their pain and adjust to life without the wished-for child; it is characterized by feelings of loneliness, emptiness, and yearning that occur in the early months after the loss.

5. _____ Phase of the grief response characterized by behavioral changes such as difficulty in getting things done, an inability to concentrate, restlessness, confused thought processes, difficulty solving problems, and poor decision making.

6. _____ Phase of the grief response when parents attempt to understand "why" and search for meaning; they are better able to function at home and at work, experience a return of self-esteem and confidence, can cope with new challenges, and have placed the loss in perspective.

7. _____ The grief response that occurs with reminders of the loss; it typically happens at special anniversary dates related to the loss and during subsequent pregnancies and after birth.

8. _____ Model developed by Swanson that conceptualizes intervention with women and families experiencing perinatal loss. It involves five components, namely, _____, _____, _____, _____, and _____.

9. _____ Extremely intense grief reaction that lasts for a very long time.

10. _____ Formalized end-of-life (EOL) interdisciplinary care model specifically aimed at intervening when pregnancy is expected to end in stillbirth or neonatal death.

11. _____ The culturally mandated traditions and rituals in the time after a death; these rituals are intertwined with cultural norms and expectations and can vary greatly across families, religions, nationalities, and ethnicities.

12. _____ Type of loss in which the object of grief, such as a fetus that has never been physically seen or held by his or her parents and is unknown to others, is missing.

13. _____ Losses surrounding pregnancy that are not openly acknowledged and mourned publicly, thereby limiting social support and leading to a sense of isolation in bereaved persons.

14. Mary, a pregnant client at 24 weeks of gestation, has been admitted to the labor unit following a prenatal visit at her health care provider's office. Fetal death is suspected and eventually confirmed. IDENTIFY the phase of grief response represented by each of the following comments made by Mary as she reacts to her loss. DESCRIBE each phase in terms of expected duration, behaviors typically exhibited, and emotions experienced.

    A. "The doctor says he cannot find my baby's heartbeat or feel my baby move. He thinks my baby has died. I know you will hear my baby's heartbeat because you have a monitor here. My baby is okay—I just know it!"

    B. "I know this never would have happened if I had quit my job as a legal secretary. My mom told me that pregnant women should take it easy. If I had listened I would have my baby in my arms right now!"

    C. "Since my baby died I just cannot seem to concentrate on even the simplest things at home and at work. I always seem to feel tired and out of sorts."

    D. "It is going to be hard. I will always remember my little baby boy and the day he was supposed to be born. But I know that my husband and I have to go on with our lives."

15. EXPLAIN how a father's grief response may differ from that of his partner, the mother.

16. EXPLAIN how you would use each of the five components of the caring theory to support grieving parents and families.

17. DESCRIBE how you, as a nurse, would help parents and other family members to actualize the loss of their newborn.

18. Nurses working with families who are experiencing loss must be able to distinguish normal grieving behaviors from those that indicate complicated bereavement.
   A. IDENTIFY those behaviors that characterize complicated bereavement.

   B. DESCRIBE the approach a nurse should take if signs of complicated bereavement are noted.

MULTIPLE CHOICE: Circle the correct option(s) and state the rationale for the option(s) chosen.

19. A woman gave birth to twin girls, one of whom was stillborn. Which nursing action would be *least* helpful in supporting the woman as she copes with her loss?
   A. Remind her that she should be happy that one daughter survived and is healthy.
   B. Assist the woman to take pictures of both babies.
   C. Encourage the woman to hold the deceased twin in her arms to say goodbye.
   D. Offer her the opportunity for counseling to help her with her grief and the grief of the surviving twin as she gets older.

20. During the acute distress phase of the grief response parents are most likely to experience:
   A. Fear and anxiety about future pregnancies
   B. Difficulty with cognitive processing
   C. Search for meaning
   D. Shock and numbness

21. A 17-year-old woman experiences a miscarriage at 12 weeks of gestation. When she is informed about the miscarriage she begins to cry, stating that she was upset about her pregnancy at first and now is being punished for not wanting her baby. The nurse's best response is:
   A. "You are still so young, you probably were not ready for a baby right now."
   B. "This must be so hard for you—I am here if you want to talk."
   C. "At least this happened early in your pregnancy before you felt your baby move."
   D. "God must have a good reason for letting this happen."

III. THINKING CRITICALLY

1. Jane (2-1-0-0-1) is a 21-year-old admitted with vaginal bleeding at 13 weeks of gestation. She experiences a miscarriage. Jane is accompanied by her husband, Tom. Her 5-year-old daughter is at home with Jane's mother.
   A. DESCRIBE the approach you would take to develop a plan of individualized support measures for Jane as she and her family cope with their loss.

   B. CITE questions and observations you would use to gather the information required to create an individualized plan of care.

C. IDENTIFY the therapeutic communication techniques you should use to help Jane and Tom acknowledge and express their feelings and emotions about their loss.

D. At discharge, Jane is crying. She tells you, "I know it must have been something I did wrong this time, since my first pregnancy was okay. We wanted to give our daughter a baby brother or sister." INDICATE whether the following responses would be therapeutic (T) or nontherapeutic (N). SPECIFY how you would change the responses determined to be nontherapeutic.

_____ 1. "You are still young. As soon as your body heals, you will be able to try to have another baby."

_____ 2. "What can I do that would help you and Tom to cope with what happened?"

_____ 3. "Do not worry. I am sure you did everything you could to have a healthy pregnancy."

_____ 4. "It was probably for the best. Fetal loss at this time is usually the result of defective development."

_____ 5. "You sound like you are blaming yourself for what happened. Let's talk about it."

_____ 6. "This must be difficult for you and your family."

_____ 7. "If it had to happen, it is best that it happened this early in the pregnancy before you and your family became attached to the fetus."

_____ 8. "You really should concentrate on your daughter rather than thinking so much about the baby you lost."

_____ 9. "I feel sad about the loss that you and Tom are experiencing."

_____ 10. "Would you and Tom like to speak to our hospital's grief counselor before you are discharged?"

2. Angela gave birth vaginally to a stillborn fetus at 38 weeks of gestation. In addition to emotional support, her physical needs must be recognized and met. IDENTIFY these physical needs and how you would meet them.

3. Anita gave birth to a baby boy who died shortly thereafter as a result of multiple congenital anomalies, including anencephaly. She and her husband, Bill, are provided with the opportunity to see their baby.
A. DISCUSS how the nurse can help Anita and Bill to make a decision that is right for them about seeing their baby.

B. Anita and Bill decide to see their baby. SPECIFY the measures the nurse can use to make the time that Anita and Bill spend with their baby as easy as possible and to provide them with an experience that will facilitate the grieving process.

4. Tara is at 16 weeks of gestation. A sonogram reveals that her fetus has anencephaly. Her primary health care provider recommends a therapeutic abortion. DISCUSS the role of the nurse in supporting Tara as she makes her decision about the abortion and copes with her grief.

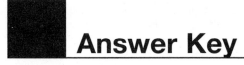

Answer Key

CHAPTER 1: 21ST CENTURY MATERNITY AND WOMEN'S HEALTH NURSING

I. Learning Key Terms

1. C, 2. H, 3. D, 4. I, 5. F, 6. A, 7. G, 8. B, 9. E, 10. J
11. Maternity nursing
12. Women's health care
13. *Healthy People 2020*
14. Millennium Developmental Goals (MDGs)
15. Interprofessional education
16. Affordable Care Act 2010
17. Human trafficking
18. Female genital mutilation, infibulation, circumcision
19. Doulas
20. Health literacy
21. Nursing Interventions Classification (NIC)
22. Evidence-based practice
23. Cochrane Pregnancy and Childbirth Database
24. Outcomes of care
25. Standards of practice
26. Standard of care
27. Risk management
28. Sentinel event
29. Failure to rescue
30. QSEN
31. SBAR
32. TeamSTEPPS

II. Reviewing Key Concepts

33. Four major objectives of *Healthy People 2020*: see *Healthy People 2020* section and Box 1-2.
34. Factors contributing to infant mortality: see Infant Mortality section, which identifies several physical and psychosocial factors.
35. Problems of the U.S. health care system: see sections related to each of the problems listed to help you with your answer.
36. Increase in high-risk pregnancies: see Problems with U.S. Health Care System section for a discussion of physical, psychosocial, and economic factors that have led to the increase in incidence.
37. Factors and conditions affecting health of women: see Health of Women section; discuss such factors as race, violence, aging, adolescent pregnancy, cancer, poverty, and access to health care.
38. Choice B is correct; while choices A, C, and D are major mortality risks for women, the leading cause of death is heart disease.

39. Choice C is correct; although the other options are important, inability to pay, which relates to inadequate or lack of health care insurance, is the most significant barrier.
40. Choice D is correct.
41. Choices A, B, and D are correct; African-American women have a maternal mortality rate that is three times higher than Caucasian women whereas the rate for Hispanic women is the lowest; the leading cause of neonatal death is congenital anomalies.
42. Choice B is correct; smoking is not associated with anomalies; because smoking adversely affects circulation and thus placental perfusion, choices A, C, and D are all possible complications of smoking.
43. Choice D is correct; both diabetes and hypertension associated with pregnancy are the risk factors most commonly reported with obesity.

III. Thinking Critically

1. Nursing director of inner-city prenatal clinic: answer should incorporate application of each of the following:
   - Biostatistics and contributing factors
   - Factors associated with high-risk pregnancy and measures to reduce them
   - Benefits of prenatal care; effect of and reasons for inadequate prenatal care
   - Importance of self-management and consumer involvement; devise ways to enhance health literacy and to encourage participation in prenatal care by overcoming barriers
2. High technology will not reduce the rate of preterm and LBW infants: discuss the following topics when formulating an answer:
   - Factors associated with LBW and IMR
   - Factors that escalate rate of high-risk pregnancy
   - High-tech care: what it can and cannot do; answer should reflect factors associated with IMR, the high cost of care management for high-risk pregnancies and compromised infants compared with the cost and effectiveness of early, ongoing, and comprehensive prenatal care.
3. Three proposed changes with rationales: changes proposed should reflect efforts toward improving access to care, using evidence-based approaches and standards to guide care, and creating health care services that address the factors associated with poor pregnancy outcomes and medical errors.
4. Barriers to prenatal care: see Limited Access to Care section; address solutions to such barriers as inability

to pay, lack of transportation, dependent child care, minority status, cultural beliefs, young maternal age, and single status. Be creative and innovative in the approaches that you propose.

5. Involving consumers and promoting self-management: care measures proposed should include health teaching, self-assessment measures, guiding decision making by providing information regarding the pros and cons of care choices available, communication and counseling techniques, substance abuse counseling, and referral to support groups.

6. Facilitating health literacy: see Health Literacy section; include therapeutic communication techniques, culturally sensitive approaches, and preparation of bilingual written materials in your answer.

7. Process to use to prevent medical errors: see Reducing Medical Errors section and access the Patient Fact Sheet identified when formulating your answer.

8. Value of evidence-based practice: see Introduction to Evidence-Based Practice, Cochrane Pregnancy and Childbirth Database, and Joanna Briggs Institute sections for ideas for your answer.

9. Using social media to enhance the efficacy of health care: see Social Media section.

10. Two international concerns affecting health and safety of women and their children: see International Concerns section to discuss human trafficking and female genital mutilation.

CHAPTER 2: COMMUNITY CARE: THE FAMILY AND CULTURE

I. Learning Key Terms

1. B, 2. E, 3. D, 4. G, 5. C, 6. F, 7. A, 8. B, 9. E, 10. C, 11. D, 12. A
13. Culture
14. Subculture
15. Cultural relativism
16. Acculturation
17. Assimilation
18. Ethnocentrism
19. Cultural competence
20. Future orientation
21. Past orientation
22. Present orientation
23. Personal space
24. Family
25. Nuclear
26. Extended
27. Cohabitating parent
28. Single parent
29. Married blended
30. Homosexual
31. No-parent family
32. Multigenerational
33. Married parent
34. Family systems theory
35. Family life cycle theory

36. Family stress theory
37. McGill model of nursing
38. Health belief model
39. Human developmental ecology
40. Genogram
41. Ecomap
42. Walking survey (community walkthrough)
43. Vulnerable populations
44. Health disparities
45. Primary prevention
46. Secondary prevention
47. Tertiary prevention

II. Reviewing Key Concepts

48. Discuss purpose of incorporating "products of culture" when providing care: see Childbearing Beliefs and Practices section for a discussion of communication, personal space, time orientation, and family roles, including how the nurse should consider each area when communicating with and caring for clients in a culturally sensitive manner.

49. Components of culturally competent care: see Developing Cultural Competency section, which identifies the key components of this approach.

50. Rationale for increasing emphasis on home- and community-based health care: see Home Care in the Community and Guidelines for Nursing Practice sections to formulate your answer. Consider changes in length of hospital stays, portability of technology, influence of insurance reimbursement, and the need to reduce health care costs in your answer; describe the need for nurses to broaden their scope of practice.

51. Community-based health promotion activities for childbearing families: see Community Health Promotion and Levels of Preventive Care sections to formulate an answer.

52. Cite problems faced by several vulnerable populations: see separate sections for each of the identified vulnerable populations listed to formulate an answer.

53. Ways in which nurses can use technology to provide health services: see Communication and Technology Applications section; include the Internet, warm lines, advice lines, and telephonic nursing assessment, consultation, and education.

54. Choice A is correct; choices B, C, and D reflect the characteristics of families with closed boundaries; they are more prone to crises because they have a narrow network to help them in times of stress.

55. Choice B is correct; providing explanations, especially when performing tasks that require close contact, can help to avoid misunderstandings; touching the client, putting the client in proximity to others, overuse of eye contact, and taking away the right to make decisions can be interpreted by clients in some cultures as invading their personal space and thereby increase the level of anxiety and stress experienced.

56. Choice D is correct; choices A, B, and C are incorrect interpretations based on the woman's culture and

customs; Native Americans may use cradleboards and avoid handling their newborn often; newborns should not be fed colostrum.

57. Choices A, C, E, and F are correct; prenatal care should begin late in pregnancy and chamomile tea is thought to ensure effective labor.

58. Choices A, B, D, and E are correct; birthing in an institutional setting is valued and breastfeeding should start as soon as possible after birth.

59. Choice C is correct; the student should be looking at the woman while speaking and asking questions through the interpreter; a normal tone of voice should be used.

60. Choices B, C, and F are correct; choices A and D are secondary levels of prevention and choice E is a tertiary level of prevention.

61. Choice C is correct because it represents the primary level of prevention.

62. Choice D is correct; although choices A and B are appropriate, they are not the most important; gloves are not needed unless the possibility of contacting body substances is present.

III. Thinking Critically

1. Process for providing culturally competent care: see Developing Cultural Competence section and Box 2-3; incorporate the components of culturally competent care in your answer; use questions in Cultural Considerations box to assess a client's cultural expectations regarding childbearing.

2. Imagine that you are a nurse working in a multicultural prenatal clinic: use Table 2-2 to formulate your answer; consider components of communication, personal space, time orientation, and family roles; identify the degree to which each woman and family adheres to their cultures, beliefs, and practices; do not stereotype.

3. Pamela, a Native-American pregnant woman.
   A. Questions to ask: see questions listed in the Cultural Considerations box.
   B. Communication approach to use: see Childbearing Beliefs and Practices section; include concepts of communication patterns, space, time, and family roles when formulating your answer.
   C. Identify Native-American beliefs and practices: see Table 2-2 to formulate your answer; remember to determine her individual beliefs and practices to avoid stereotyping.

4. Hispanic family—recent birth of twin girls: describe cultural beliefs and practices; Table 2-2 outlines newborn care guidelines for several ethnic groups, including those that Hispanic families are likely to follow.

5. Sunni refugee couple from Iraq seeking prenatal care: see Communication: Use of an Interpreter section, Box 2-2, and Cultural Considerations box.
   - Consider the process of working with a translator; show respect for this couple by addressing questions and comments to them and not to the translator; recognize that the husband may wish to be present and a female interpreter would be required.
   - Box 2-2 outlines the preparation measures, interaction during the interview, and consultation with translator before, during, and after the interview; learn about the culture and prepare questions.
   - Consider the stressors faced by refugees and immigrants and the health care needs they present.
   - Research Iraq and become familiar with Sunni cultural and religious beliefs and practices and the current political and religious turmoil that led to this couple coming to the United States.

6. Home care nurse must become familiar with neighborhoods and their resources: see Assessing the Community and Data Collection and Sources of Community Health Data sections.
   A. Community walkthrough (walking survey): a walking survey involves use of observation skills during a trip through a community.
   B. Components of a community walkthrough are outlined in Box 2-4.
   C. Use of findings: discuss each of the survey's components; describe how each of these components can reflect a community's strengths and problems; strengths can be used to provide clients with needed support; nurse can mobilize community leaders to solve identified problems; try using the survey to assess your community and the community in which your college is located.

7. Marie, a single parent of two children, is homeless: see Homeless Women and Implications for Nursing sections.
   A. Basis for health problems (cite what these problems may be) to which she and her children are most vulnerable: lack of preventive care and resources, limited to no access to primary care resulting in the use of emergency departments for health care.
   B. Marie's vulnerability for pregnancy: victimization, economic survival, lack of access to health care and birth control measures, need for closeness and intimacy, doubt fertility.
   C. Principles to guide nurse when providing care: treat with respect and dignity, case management to coordinate care to meet multiple needs, flexible appointment times providing service when they come in, make each interaction count, be purposeful, keep Marie empowered, help her to reconnect with her support system if possible and appropriate.

8. Consuelo, pregnant wife of a migrant worker and mother of two: see Immigrant, Refugee, and Migrant Women section.
   - Begin by confirming that she is pregnant.
   - Consider pregnancy risks she faces; evaluate exposure to teratogens.

- Concerns to address include limited access to and use of contraceptives, increased rate of STIs, and poor nutrition.
- Lack of trust and fear of deportation may be barriers to seeking and continuing with prenatal care.

9. List questions for a postpartum follow-up telephone call: see Communication and Technology Applications section; include questions guided by expected postpartum physical and emotional changes; ask her how she is feeling and managing, condition of her newborn (eating, sleeping, eliminating), response of other family members to newborn, sources of happiness and stress, adequacy of help and support being received, and need for additional support or referrals.

10. Home visit to a postpartum woman at 36 hours after birth: see Boxes 2-5 and 2-6 and Care Management—Preparing for a Home Visit section to answer each component of this exercise, including the approach you would take to prepare, your actions during the visit, the safety precautions and infection control measures you would follow, how you would end the visit, and the interventions you would follow after the visit, including documentation of assessments, actions, and responses.

11. Angela, a pregnant woman with hyperemesis gravidarum: see Home Care in the Community—Perinatal Services and Client Selection and Referral sections for parts A and B and Care Management section for part C.
   A. Criteria for discharge readiness: include criteria related to Angela's health status and that of her fetus, availability of qualified home care professionals, family resources, and cost effectiveness of discharging her to home care.
   B. Information needed to institute high-tech care in the home: medical diagnosis and prognosis, treatment required, medication history, drug dosing information, and type of infusion access device that will be used.
   C. Home environment criteria: safe place to store medications and infusion supplies; do a walk-through inspection to determine temperature of the home, general cleanliness, and adequacy of area to prepare and administer prescribed treatment.

12. Importance and cost effectiveness of home health care services for postpartum women and their families: see Perinatal Services section; include the following in your answer:
   - Ability to observe firsthand the home environment and family dynamics; adequacy of resources; safety.
   - Teaching can be tailored to the woman, her family, and her home.
   - Services are less expensive than hospital.
   - Prevention, early detection, and treatment measures can be offered.
   - Services may lead to long-term positive effects on parenting and child health.

- Use research findings and recommendations of professional organizations to validate proposal.
- Investigate insurance reimbursement for home care.

CHAPTER 3: NURSING AND GENOMICS

I. Learning Key Terms

1. S, 2. Q, 3. J, 4. D, 5. G, 6. U, 7. I, 8. T, 9. E, 10. R, 11. A, 12. C, 13. O, 14. L, 15. V, 16. P, 17. H, 18. B, 19. K, 20. M, 21. F, 22. N
23. Genetics
24. Genomics
25. Genetic testing
26. Direct (molecular) testing
27. Linkage analysis
28. Biochemical testing
29. Cytogenic testing
30. Carrier screening tests
31. Predictive testing; presymptomatic; predispositional
32. Pharmacogenomics
33. Gene therapy
34. Multifactorial inheritance
35. Unifactorial inheritance
36. Autosomal dominant inheritance
37. Autosomal recessive inheritance
38. Inborn error of metabolism
39. X-linked dominant inheritance
40. X-linked recessive inheritance

II. Reviewing Key Concepts

41. Identify five main genetics-related nursing activities: see Nursing Expertise in Genetics and Genomics section.
42. Explain the difference between occurrence and recurrence risk: see Genetic Counseling—Estimation of Risk section.
43. Ethical issues related to Human Genome Project: see Human Genome Project—Ethical, Legal, and Social Implications section; consider effect of being able to determine vulnerability to certain disorders and the effect this can have on an individual physically, socially, economically, and emotionally; consider possibility of altered relationships engendered by the information and the potential for discrimination and stigmatization.
44. Choice A is correct; autosomal dominant inheritance is unrelated to exposure to teratogens; each pregnancy has the same potential for expression of the disorder; there is no reduction if one child is already affected; if the gene is inherited, the disorder is always expressed.
45. Choice D is correct; there is a 25% chance that females will be carriers; if males inherit the X chromosome with the defective gene, the disorder will be expressed and they can transmit the gene to female offspring; females are affected if they receive the defective gene from both parents.

46. Choice D is correct; cystic fibrosis, as an inborn error of metabolism, follows an autosomal recessive pattern of inheritance; two defective genes (one from each parent) are required for the disorder to be expressed; the woman does not have the disorder and the father does not have the defective gene; therefore none of their children will have the disorder but there will be a 50% chance they will be carriers of the defective gene.
47. Choice C is correct; factor V Leiden (FVL) affects the body's clotting mechanism by increasing the woman's risk for deep vein thrombosis (DVT) and pulmonary embolism (PE).

III. Thinking Critically

1. Factors influencing decision regarding genetic testing: see Factors Influencing the Decision to Undergo Genetic Testing section. Factors can include family pressures, responsibility to others, access to testing, and cultural and ethical beliefs.
2. Support of statement that nurses should have basic understanding of genetics: see Nursing Expertise in Genetics and Genomics section. Your answer should reflect the rapid advance in genetic-based treatment and the ability to diagnose genetic disorders; emphasize the nurse's role as teacher, counselor, and advocate.
3. Questions to determine if risk factors for inheritable disorders are present: ask questions that would elicit information regarding health status of family members, abnormal reproductive outcomes, history of maternal disorders, drug exposures, illnesses, advanced maternal and paternal age, and ethnic origin.
4. Couple facing a genetic disorder.
   A. Nurse's role in determining genetic risk: Tay-Sachs is an autosomal recessive disorder that follows a unifactorial pattern of inheritance; Joshua needs to be tested because he must also be a carrier, which would produce a child with the disorder; emphasize the nurse's role in terms of emotional support, facilitation of the decision-making process, and interpretation of diagnostic test results and how they can influence future childbearing decisions. Consider factors that can influence the decision to participate or not participate in testing.
   B. Inheritance possibility when both parents carry the defective recessive gene: there is a 25% chance the child will be normal, a 25% chance that the child will express the disorder, and a 50% chance that the child will be a carrier; this pattern is the same for every pregnancy; there is no reduction in risk from one pregnancy to another.
   C. Education and emotional support: discuss the nature of this disorder, extent of risk, and consequences if the child inherits the disorder; discuss options available, including amniocentesis and continuing or not continuing the pregnancy if the child is affected; discuss use of reproductive technology or adoption; be sensitive to cultural and religious beliefs; encourage expression of feelings; refer the couple for further counseling or support groups as appropriate.

ANSWER KEY UNIT II

CHAPTER 4: ASSESSMENT AND HEALTH PROMOTION

I. Learning Key Terms

1. Mons pubis
2. Labia majora
3. Labia minora
4. Prepuce
5. Frenulum
6. Fourchette
7. Clitoris
8. Vestibule
9. Urethra (urinary meatus)
10. Perineum
11. Vagina; rugae; Skene; Bartholin
12. Fornices
13. Uterus; cul-de-sac of Douglas
14. Corpus
15. Isthmus
16. Fundus
17. Endometrium
18. Myometrium
19. Cervix
20. Endocervical canal; internal os; external os
21. Squamocolumnar junction; Papanicolaou (Pap)
22. Uterine (fallopian) tubes
23. Ovaries; ovulation; estrogen; progesterone; androgen
24. Bony pelvis
25. Breasts
26. Tail of Spence
27. Nipple
28. Areola
29. Montgomery glands (tubercles)
30. Acini
31. Myoepithelium
32. E, 33. K, 34. N, 35. S, 36. P, 37. A, 38. T, 39. M, 40. I, 41. R, 42. B, 43. L, 44. G, 45. C, 46. O, 47. F, 48. Q, 49. H, 50. J, 51. D

II. Reviewing Key Concepts

52. Guidelines for performing a Pap test: guidelines for each component of the procedure are outlined in Box 4-11, Papanicolaou Smear/Test.
53. Characteristics of a palpated lump: location, size, mobility, consistency, tenderness, and types of borders.
54. Choices A and D are correct; a woman should perform BSE every month at the end of menstruation when the breasts are the least tender; she should use the fingerpads of her three middle fingers for palpation.
55. Choice D is correct; clean gloves are required only if open lesions are present and when compressing the

nipple if discharge is anticipated; fingers should not be lifted; two hands are used for women with large, pendulous breasts.

56. Choice C is correct; self-examination should not be used for self-diagnosis but rather to detect early changes, which would call for the guidance of a health care provider.

57. Choice B is correct; do not ask questions during the examination because it may distract the client, interfering with relaxation measures she may be using; offer explanations only as needed during the examination.

58. Choice A is correct; all women should be screened because abuse can happen to any woman; abuse can begin or escalate during pregnancy; the most commonly injured sites are head, neck, chest, abdomen, breasts, and upper extremities. If abuse is suspected, the nurse needs to assess further to encourage disclosure and then assist the woman to take action and formulate a safety plan. Nurses should follow the laws of their state with regard to reporting instances of abuse.

59. Choice B is correct; bone mineral density testing should be initiated at 65 years of age or older unless risk factors are present; endometrial biopsies are not recommended on a routine basis for most women but women at risk for endometrial cancer should have one done at menopause; mammograms should be done annually for women 50 years of age and older.

60. Choice A is correct; all women—not just specific groups—should participate in preconception care approximately 1 year before planning to become pregnant.

61. Choice C is correct; women should not use vaginal medications or douche for 24 to 48 hours before the test; oral contraceptives can continue; the best time for the test is midcycle.

III. Thinking Critically

1. Importance of preconception care: see Preconception Counseling and Care section and Box 4-2; this nurse should:
   - Define preconception counseling and what it entails and stress the importance of both partners' participation.
   - Identify the effect that a woman's health status and lifestyle habits have on the developing fetus during the first trimester.
   - Describe how preconception counseling can assist a couple to choose the best time to begin a pregnancy.

2. Establishing a woman's health clinic.
   A. Services to be offered: see the Reasons for Entering the Health Care System section, in which several services are discussed, including those related to pregnancy, health promotion and screening, fertility, sexuality, menstruation, and menopause.

   B. Barriers: see the Barriers to Seeking Health Care section. Discuss financial, cultural, and gender issues as barriers; use barriers to create strategies, including advocating for universal health insurance, providing culturally sensitive services, and improving access, including transportation and child care provisions and longer clinic hours; innovative incentives.

   C. Services for health promotion and prevention: see Health Risks to Women section, Box 4-5, and Table 4-3.
      - Consider common risk factors for health problems, leading causes of death among women, and behaviors that increase risk for health problems.
      - Create programs that address age-specific issues; for example, puberty, teen pregnancies, and menopause.
      - Address the appropriate focus areas for women in Healthy People 2020.
      - Follow recommended health screening guidelines in Table 4-4.

3. State how age, disabilities, and abuse can influence health assessment of women: see specific sections for each factor in the health assessment.

4. Woman requesting advice regarding diet and exercise to lose weight: see Nutrition, Obesity, and Exercise sections.
   - BMI falls in the obese range.
   - Review risks for health disorders associated with being overweight.
   - Start with 24-hour to 3-day nutritional recall; based on analysis of woman's current nutritional habits, suggest use of the MyPlate system; emphasize complex carbohydrates and foods high in iron and calcium; recommend reduced fat intake; ensure adequate fluid intake, avoiding those high in sugar, alcohol, or caffeine; use weight changes and activity patterns to determine adequacy of caloric intake.
   - Aerobic exercise: discuss weight-bearing vs. non–weight-bearing exercises as well as frequency and duration of exercise sessions for maximum benefit; associate exercise with weight loss and the maintenance of appropriate weight.

5. Woman experiencing stress.
   A. Physical and emotional signs of stress: see Stress section and Box 4-7 for a listing of typical physical, behavioral, and psychologic signs of stress.

   B. Stress management: see Stress and Stress Management sections.
      - Help Alice to formulate her goals in life and set priorities; work on time management to allow for relaxation time.
      - Discuss her interests and hobbies, to be incorporated into a stress management program designed for her; develop alternatives to alcohol and smoking for relaxation, such as biofeedback, guided imagery, and yoga.
      - Refer to a support group for stress management.

- Suggest literature and Internet sites that may be beneficial.
  C. Smoking cessation: see Smoking and Substance Use Cessation sections and Box 4-12.
  - Use the four As formula.
  - Have Alice describe her smoking.
  - Discuss how she stopped before.
  - Suggest a variety of strategies for smoking cessation; encourage her to choose a method that is right for her.
6. Woman's concern regarding violence against women: see Violence Against Women, Abused Women, Health Risk Prevention, and Health Protection sections and Fig. 4-10.
   - Discuss the woman's current circumstances and what she does now to protect herself.
   - Discuss how she changed her behavior based on the experiences of her friends; how she helped or did not help her friends; her evaluation of how the legal and health care system met the needs of her friends; what could have and should have been done to help her friends.
   - Discuss protective and legal services, including hotlines and emergency centers; facilitate access to services to promote assertiveness, self-defense techniques, and self-help groups.
7. Nurses' responses to concerns and questions of women.
   A. How to prepare for first gynecologic examination: explain what will occur and each guideline to follow for preparation and why each is important for the accuracy of the test.
   B. Signs indicating ovulation: see Ovarian Cycle and Other Cyclic Changes sections, in which signs of ovulation are described.
   C. Breast characteristics across the life span: see Table 4-2, which outlines characteristics of the breasts of adolescent, adult, and postmenopausal women.
   D. Douching: see Internal Structures section; describe how vaginal secretions protect the reproductive tract and how douching could alter this function and also injure the mucosa, thereby increasing the risk for infection; describe how she should cleanse her genitalia.
8. Woman anxious about first gynecologic examination: see Pelvic Examination section and Box 4-10, Assisting with Pelvic Examination.
   - Teach her about the examination.
   - Encourage her to ask questions and verbalize concerns.
   - Describe simple relaxation measures.
   - Ensure privacy and be sensitive to her modesty.

9. Health history of a new client at a women's health clinic.
   A. Components: see Health Assessment-Interview section and Box 4-9 for a list and description of components.

   B. Writing questions: use components of the health history as a guide; write questions that are open-ended, clear, and concise; address only one issue; progress from the general to the specific.
   C. Therapeutic communication techniques with examples: see Interview, Cultural Considerations, and Women with Special Needs sections for a description of communication techniques to use.
   - How to be sensitive and nonjudgmental in your approach; use a relaxed, confident, and professional manner.
   - Consider the culture of the client and any special needs, including those related to sensory deficit.
   - Adjust the environment and provide privacy.
   - Ensure confidentiality.
10. Teaching self-examination techniques: each teaching plan should include cognitive, psychomotor, and affective teaching-learning techniques; describe a variety of methodologies, including discussion, exploration of feelings, and provision of literature; demonstrate and have client redemonstrate using practice models and then the clients themselves as appropriate.
    - Breast self-examination: see Teaching for Self-Management—BSE box.
    - Vulvar (genital) self-examination: see Vulvar Self-Examination section.
11. Culturally sensitive approach to women's health care: review the Cultural Competence section in Chapter 2 and take note of the 4 Cs of cultural competence to determine how to:
    - Approach the woman in a respectful and calm manner.
    - Consider modifications in the examination to maintain the woman's modesty.
    - Incorporate communication variations such as conversational style, pacing, spacing, eye contact, touch, and time orientation.
    - Take time to learn about the woman's cultural beliefs and practices regarding well-woman assessment and care.
12. Screening for abuse when providing well-woman care.
    A. Adjusting the environment: provide for comfort and privacy; assess the woman alone, without her partner or adult children present.
    B. Abuse indicators: see the Abused Women section for identification of several indicators of possible abuse and areas of the body most commonly injured, including during pregnancy; specific somatic complaints; and inadvisable behaviors, including a pattern of canceling health care appointments.
    C. Questions to ask: see Fig. 4-10, which lists questions that all women should be asked in a very direct manner.

D. Use the following approach if abuse is confirmed:
- Acknowledge the abuse and affirm that it is unacceptable and common; tell her that you are concerned and that she does not deserve the abuse; know the requirements in your state regarding reporting abuse.
- Communicate that abuse can recur; cite the cycle of violence (see Chapter 5); tell her that help is available; empower her to use this help.
- Help her to formulate an escape plan.

13. Describe events in each cycle composing the menstrual cycle: see Hypothalamic-Pituitary Cycle, Ovarian Cycle, and Endometrial Cycle sections and Fig. 4-7 for a full description of the events and changes characteristic of each cycle; include teaching methodologies you would use to enhance the effectiveness of presentation. Encourage the young women to discuss their concerns regarding these changes.

14. Assisting with a pelvic examination: see Boxes 4-10 and 4-11 and Pelvic Examination section to formulate your answer; information is included regarding client preparation and assisting the health care provider.

15. Adolescent client at women's health clinic who exhibits signs of a possible eating disorder: based on her BMI of 16 this woman is underweight; see Nutritional Deficiencies section.
A. Use the SCOFF questions (Box 4-6) to screen for an eating disorder and what it could be; complete a nutritional assessment including what she eats, how much she eats, when, and where; discuss her exercise patterns; ask her about how she should look and how much she should weigh; discuss the connection between her BMI and nutritional patterns and her lack of menses and breast development.
B. See sections for each of the eating disorders listed and compare them.

CHAPTER 5: VIOLENCE AGAINST WOMEN

I. Learning Key Terms

1. Intimate partner violence (IPV)
2. Cycle of violence model; tension building; battering; "honeymoon"
3. Feminist perspective
4. Ecological model; individual woman; microsystem; mesosystem, exosystem; macrosystem; chronosystem (see Fig. 5-2)
5. Sexual violence
6. Sexual harassment
7. Sexual assault
8. Rape
9. Statutory rape
10. Molestation
11. Rape-trauma syndrome; acute (disorganization); outward adjustment; long-term process (reorganization)
12. Sexual assault nurse examiner (SANE)

II. Reviewing Key Concepts

13. Sociologic factors associated with violence: see Sociologic Perspective section for several significant factors, including expectation of male aggression, patriarchal viewpoints, and multigenerational transmission of violence.

14. Cultural influence on violence against women: see Cultural Considerations section. Answer should reflect:
- Factors true for all cultures, such as role and expected behavior of men and women, importance of family, and roles within the family; to whom you go when experiencing problems; approach to health care; definition of what violence and abuse means; effect of environmental stressors; and availability of resources.
- Examples from a variety of cultures should be given for each factor.

15. Characteristics of women in abusive relationships and men who are abusers.
A. Characteristics of women in abusive relationships contrasted with those who are not: see Women Experiencing IPV section for the identification of several characteristics of women in violent and nonviolent relationships.
B. Characteristics of women who seek help: see Care Management section; beaten severely and frequently, never experienced or witnessed abuse in their own families, and have alternatives in terms of jobs or careers.
C. Barriers to seeking help: see Care Management section; avoid stigma and involvement of police and fear that they will not be believed or of reprisal from abuser.
D. Characteristics of persons who are likely to abuse: see Box 5-1 for a list of many characteristics of a potential male batterer.

16. Forms of abuse: forms of abuse are discussed in IPV section.

17. The use of the ABCDEs tool when caring for an abused woman: see Nursing Interventions section for a full description of this tool and how it is used.

18. Strategies to prevent cycle of violence: see Prevention section of Plan of Care and Interventions, which describes many prevention strategies across the life span.

19. Factors that deter women from reporting rape: see Sexual Violence section, which discusses several deterrents to reporting rape.

20. Choices A and D are correct; characteristics of a potential batterer include deficits in assertiveness, low tolerance for frustration, inadequate verbal skills especially with regard to expressing feelings, and an unusual amount of jealousy leading to often expecting his partner to spend all of her time with him (see Box 5-1).

21. Choice D is correct; battered women are often isolated as a result of fear, the stigma that society places

on them because of the false belief that they must enjoy being abused, and restrictions on their activities by their partner; typical feminine characteristics are more apparent in women in abusive relationships whereas assertiveness, independence, and willingness to take a stand are more characteristic of women who are in nonviolent relationships.

22. Choices B, C, and E are correct; anxiety and depression can lead to use of alcohol, tobacco, and drugs as a means of coping; inadequate diet results in low maternal weight gain, increasing the risk for anemia and giving birth to an LBW newborn; the rate of preterm birth and LBW is increased; abused women are more likely to experience STIs, pelvic pain, and bleeding.

23. Choice A is correct; women who experience repeated and severe abuse, have never witnessed or experienced abuse in their own families, and have alternatives such as a job or career are more likely to seek assistance.

24. Choices C, D, and E are correct; there is no recall after taking a drink laced with the drug; severe headache is not characteristic of having been drugged but feeling fuzzy when waking up is characteristic.

III. Thinking Critically

1. Disproving myths regarding violence against women: use the Introduction section for statistical information regarding the incidence and demographics of violence against women, Table 5-2, and Perspectives on Violence and IPV sections to disprove myths A, B, C, and D; use IPV during Pregnancy section to disprove myth E; in addition to your text, you can use the Internet to gather information to dispel the myths.

2. Ecological framework: see Ecological Model section and Fig. 5-2 to create your outline.

3. Cues indicative of physical abuse.
    A. Identify cues: see Care Management—Assessment section, including the following in your answer:
        ■ Typical injuries
        ■ Psychosocial findings
        ■ Behaviors related to health care
    B. Suspicion that pregnant woman is being abused: see Care Management and IPV during Pregnancy sections.
        ■ Use appropriate communication techniques, including direct questions (see Fig. 5-3).
        ■ Perform interview and examination in a private setting; a female health care provider might be helpful.
        ■ If injuries are noted, tell her that these are common in women who are abused; tell her that she is not responsible for another person's abusive behavior.
        ■ Consider legal implications.
    C. Abuse is confirmed: see Nursing Interventions section; describe how you would use the

ABCDEs of caring as a framework for helping Carol.
    D. Why pregnancy leads to violence: see IPV during Pregnancy section; discuss such factors as stress of pregnancy, jealousy of fetus, anger, and attempt to end the pregnancy.
    E. Approaches to avoid: avoid being judgmental, such as evaluating Carol's actions and responses to violence in terms of how the nurse would act in the same situation, or rushing her; Carol needs to be helped at her own pace, but formulating an escape plan is critical.
    F. Use Fig. 5-3 to evaluate the degree of danger.
    G. Adverse effects of violence on pregnancy: many adverse effects are identified in IPV during Pregnancy section.
    H. Indicators for readiness to leave abusive relationship:
        ■ Exhibits capability to plan for and invest in herself
        ■ Recognizes that abuse is part of a continuing pattern
        ■ Expresses desire to leave; needs to leave when no abuse is occurring with reassurance of available economic and social support to make it on her own
    I. Legal responsibilities of the nurse: see Mandatory Reporting of Domestic Violence section.
        ■ Full documentation of the abuse should be done (see Box 5-2 for guidelines to follow).
        ■ Know your state's requirement regarding the reporting of abuse/battering.

4. For a woman who has been raped, see Sexual Violence section.
    A. Sexual assault nurse examiner: see Care Management section; this nurse is fully prepared to care for rape victims and collect essential evidence.
    B. Nurse's responsibility to assess and collect and preserve evidence of the rape: see Sexual Examination section and Legal Tips for adult sexual assault protocol to follow; ensure that your answer includes data that must be collected, how to care for evidence, and legal requirements.
    C. Nurse's actions to meet emotional needs: emotional support measures can be found throughout the Care Management section, including the section on psychologic first aid; consider how you would help her before, during, and after the examination as well as the importance of follow-up care after discharge.
    D. Phases of rape-trauma syndrome: behaviors and emotions and counselor support required (see Rape-Trauma section for a discussion of each phase).
    E. Discharge interventions: see Discharge and After Discharge sections; describe each of the following in your answer: medications, instructions, resources, getting home, and follow-up.

CHAPTER 6: REPRODUCTIVE SYSTEM CONCERNS

I. Learning Key Terms

1. Amenorrhea
2. Hypogonadotropic amenorrhea
3. Female athlete triad
4. Cyclic perimenstrual pain and discomfort (CPPD); dysmenorrhea; premenstrual syndrome (PMS); premenstrual dysphoric disorder (PMDD)
5. Dysmenorrhea
6. Primary dysmenorrhea
7. Secondary dysmenorrhea
8. Premenstrual syndrome (PMS)
9. Premenstrual dysphoric disorder (PMDD)
10. Endometriosis
11. Oligomenorrhea
12. Hypomenorrhea
13. Metrorrhagia; intermenstrual bleeding
14. Mittlestaining
15. Breakthrough bleeding
16. Menorrhagia; hypermenorrhea
17. Abnormal uterine bleeding (AUB)
18. Dysfunctional uterine bleeding (DUB)
19. Menarche
20. Menopause
21. Perimenopause; climacteric
22. Surgical menopause
23. Postmenopause
24. Dyspareunia
25. Hot flush
26. Hot flash
27. Night sweats
28. Osteoporosis
29. Phytoestrogens; isoflavones

II. Reviewing Key Concepts

30. Describe changes associated with perimenopause: use separate section for each expected change in the Menopause section to complete this activity.
31. Choice B is correct; the 14-year-old reflects several of the risk factors associated with this menstrual disorder, namely participating in a sport that is stressful, is subjectively scored, and requires contour-revealing clothing and in which success is favored by a prepubertal body shape.
32. Choice C is correct; choices A, B, and D all interfere with prostaglandin synthesis whereas acetaminophen has no antiprostaglandin properties; prostaglandins are a recognized factor in the etiology of primary dysmenorrhea.
33. Choice A is correct; decreasing the ingestion of salty foods and refined sugars 7 to 10 days before menses decreases fluid retention; asparagus and cranberry juice have a natural diuretic effect that can reduce edema and related discomforts; valerian is an herb that reduces menstrual cramping.
34. Choices B, C, and E are correct; alcohol as well as tobacco and caffeine can worsen symptoms whereas

exercise, especially during the luteal phase, relieves symptoms, as can fruits, especially peaches and watermelon, and whole grains; sodium intake should be less than 3 g daily; bugleweed and evening primrose oil can reduce breast discomfort.

35. Choices C, D, and F are correct; women taking danazol often experience reversible masculinizing changes; it is taken orally; ovulation may not be fully suppressed, so birth control is essential because the medication is teratogenic; amenorrhea, not increased bleeding, occurs.
36. Choice A is correct; oligomenorrhea is infrequent menses; menorrhagia is excessive bleeding during menses; hypomenorrhea is scanty bleeding at normal intervals.
37. Choice C is correct; DUB is most commonly associated with anovulatory cycles in women at the extremes of their reproductive years (puberty, perimenopause); it can also occur when women secrete low levels of progesterone; it is associated with obesity; increased prostaglandins are associated with dysmenorrhea.
38. Choice A is correct; dysmenorrhea is painful menstruation; dysuria is painful urination; dyspnea is difficulty breathing.
39. Choice D is correct; alendronate sodium (Fosamax) should be taken on an empty stomach with a glass of water to enhance absorption; remaining upright will help to decrease gastrointestinal (GI) symptoms.
40. Choice B is correct; see Table 6-2 for an explanation of each herb.

III. Thinking Critically

1. Woman with hypogonadotropic amenorrhea: see Hypogonadotropic Amenorrhea section.
   A. Risk factors exhibited: athletic competition that is subjectively scored, endurance sport favoring low body weight, inappropriate body composition, nutritional deficits related to need to maintain body size, stress and vigorous exercise, need to wear body-revealing clothing, prepubertal body shape or weight categories favor success or ability to participate.
   B. Nursing diagnosis: disturbed body image related to delayed onset of menstruation and development of secondary sexual characteristics; anxiety can also be a nursing diagnosis.
   C. Expected outcomes: Maria will:
      ■ Describe the basis for delayed onset of pubertal changes accurately
      ■ Participate in a therapeutic regimen that will favor age-appropriate physical development
   D. Care management: see Management section for several nursing interventions.
   E. See Hypogonadotropic Amenorrhea section for a list of sports of concern and the rationale for the concern; measures should include education, one-on-one counseling, and screening in terms of BMI and nutrition; involve coaches and families in the program.

2. Woman with primary dysmenorrhea: see Primary Dysmenorrhea section.
   A. Questions regarding pain: gather data related to timing of the pain, its characteristics, its severity, and relief measures she has tried and their level of effectiveness; what makes the pain worse or better; woman's knowledge level regarding reason for the pain; effect of pain on daily activities and relationships.
   B. Nursing diagnoses: consider the areas of acute pain and ineffective role performance as the focus for nursing management of this woman's primary dysmenorrhea; use assessment data to determine which nursing diagnosis will take precedence.
   C. Physiologic basis of the pain: dysmenorrhea, in this case, is a physiologic process rather than a pathologic process associated with ovulatory cycles and the secretion of estrogen and progesterone, leading to the release of prostaglandins, which cause the uterus to contract and vasospasm to occur, resulting in uterine ischemia and pain.
   D. Relief measures: see Management section and Tables 6-1 and 6-2 for several measures; be sure to discuss basis of the problem, how each measure suggested works to provide relief, and how and when they should be used; assist woman to choose measures that are best for her.
3. Woman experiencing PMS: see PMS and PMDD sections.
   A. Signs and symptoms of PMS: see PMS section for a full description of signs and symptoms; include physical and psychologic signs and symptoms; clinical manifestations are usually related to effects of fluid retention, behavioral and emotional changes, cravings, headache, fatigue and energy levels, and backache.
   B. Nursing diagnosis: nursing diagnoses could include acute pain, activity intolerance, disturbed sleep pattern, and ineffective role performance; use assessment findings to determine those that apply to a particular client, including those that are priority.
   C. Nursing approach: see Management section, Tables 6-1 and 6-2, and Nursing Care Plan for several pharmacologic and nonpharmacologic measures; include how you would work with the woman to explain the basis of the pain and choose the measures to include in an individualized plan of care.
   D. Symptoms of premenstrual dysphoric disorder: see PMDD section for a full description of this disorder.
4. Woman with endometriosis: see Endometriosis section.
   A. Clinical manifestations: dysmenorrhea (secondary), pelvic pain and heaviness, thigh pain, GI symptoms, diarrhea, constipation, dyspareunia, abnormal bleeding, metrorrhagia, menorrhagia, and infertility.
   B. Pathophysiology of the disorder: growth of endometrial tissue outside uterus, mainly in the pelvis; implants respond to cyclic changes in hormones; bleeding of implants leads to inflammatory response, formation of scar tissue and adhesions, fibrosis, and anemia; impaired fertility can occur.
   C. Pharmacologic management: each medication is discussed in the Management section.
   D. Support measures: see Management section and Nursing Care Plan for several measures such as education regarding the disease process; discuss treatment options; refer to support groups and counseling as appropriate; work with couple together and separately to allow for expression of feelings and concerns; review options for pregnancy since infertility can be an outcome.
5. Woman at risk for osteoporosis: see Osteoporosis section.
   A. Risk factors exhibited: Caucasian, age, perimenopausal, slender or thin, family history of osteoporosis, smokes, sedentary lifestyle indoors, dietary risks related to inadequate calcium and vitamin D coupled with excess intake of fast food, caffeine, and soft drinks.
   B. Prevention measures: see Box 6-2; specifically address risk factors presented by the woman, in this case including nutrition, smoking, and exercise and activity patterns; encourage bone density testing.
   C. Signs of osteoporosis: see Fig. 6-2; decrease in height, back pain (especially lower back), dowager's hump (kyphosis), and fractures.
6. Woman experiencing perimenopausal changes: see Menopause section.
   A. Relief measures: see specific subsection for each change, Teaching for Self-Management—Comfort Measures box, and Alternative Therapies, Sexual Counseling, and Midlife Support Groups sections; discuss each change, why it occurs, and several relief options; encourage the woman and her partner to be involved in the process of coping with the changes of the perimenopausal period and the decisions that must be made.
   B. Decision making regarding MHT: see Menopausal Hormonal Therapy section and Table 6-4; answer should include benefits, risks, side effects, preparations and administration, duration of treatment, and alternatives.
   C. Instructions for use of transdermal patch: see Treatment Guidelines section; apply to trunk and upper arms, not on breasts; check site for irritation; alternate sites; apply at recommended frequency to hairless, clean, dry, intact site; emphasize importance of regular and ongoing health care to monitor effects of hormone use.
   D. Heart disease concerns: see Coronary Heart Disease section and sections related to nutrition and exercise for the information needed to tell this client why there is risk for heart disease and what she can do about it; with a BMI indicating obesity, weight loss will decrease the risk for not only heart disease but also hypertension and type 2 diabetes.

E. Use of Internet: provide Heidi with a list of appropriate websites with which to start; give her guidelines regarding how to find sites and how to evaluate sites she finds, including sponsor, currency, and accuracy; caution her to seek advice of health care provider before beginning a recommended treatment or to seek information if she has questions.

CHAPTER 7: SEXUALLY TRANSMITTED AND OTHER INFECTIONS

I. Learning Key Terms

1. Sexually transmitted infections (STIs) or sexually transmitted diseases (STDs); chlamydia; HPV; gonorrhea; HSV-2; syphilis; HIV
2. Risk-reduction measures
3. Condom (male, female)
4. Chlamydia
5. Gonorrhea
6. Syphilis; chancre; condylomata lata
7. Pelvic inflammatory disease (PID)
8. Human papillomavirus (HPV); condylomata acuminata; Gardisil; Cervarix
9. Genital herpes simplex virus (HSV)
10. Hepatitis A virus (HAV)
11. Hepatitis B virus (HBV)
12. Hepatitis C virus (HCV)
13. Human immunodeficiency virus (HIV); cellular immune; acquired immunodeficiency syndrome (AIDS)
14. Group B streptococci (GBS)
15. Bacterial vaginosis (BV)
16. Vulvovaginal candidiasis
17. Trichomoniasis
18. TORCH
19. Toxoplasmosis
20. Rubella
21. Cytomegalovirus (CMV)
22. Standard Precautions

II. Reviewing Key Concepts

23. Common risk behaviors for STIs: Box 7-2 cites many common risk behaviors according to the 5 Ps.
24. Infection control principles and practices: see Box 7-3 for a full explanation of standard precautions.
25. Outline common reproductive infections: see Tables 7-2 and 7-5 and each infection's section for information related to typical clinical manifestations and management guidelines.
26. Meaning of TORCH: see TORCH Infections section and Table 7-7 for the infections represented by each letter.
27. Choice A is correct; because these infections are often asymptomatic, they can go undetected and untreated, causing more severe damage, including ascent of the pathogen into uterus and pelvis, resulting in PID and infertility; many effective treatment measures are available, including treatment for chlamydia.

28. Choice B is correct; choice A is indicative of candidiasis; choice C is indicative of genital HSV; choice D is indicative of trichomoniasis.
29. Choice B is correct; metronidazole is used to treat bacterial vaginosis and trichomoniasis; benzathine penicillin G is used to treat syphilis; acyclovir is used to treat genital herpes.
30. Choice C is correct; cesarean section or isolation is not required; there are no lesions with this bacterial infection; antiviral medication is not appropriate.
31. Choices A, D, and E are correct; recurrent infections commonly involve only local symptoms that are less severe; stress reduction, healthy lifestyle practices, cleansing lesions, and acyclovir can reduce recurrence rate and prevent secondary infection; viral shedding can occur before lesions appear during the prodromal stage; acyclovir cannot cure herpes but can keep it in control.
32. Choice B is correct; although choices A, C, and D are measures that should be followed, knowing her partner—including the partner's sexual history and presence of any manifestations of infection—is essential.
33. Choice B is correct; several HPV serotypes are thought to have oncogenic potential and are therefore the primary cause of cervical cancer.
34. Choice C is correct; the vaccine is given in three doses over a 6-month period.

III. Thinking Critically

1. Woman attending first visit at a women's health clinic.
   A. Determining risk for STIs: see Box 7-2 to determine areas of risk; discuss the development of a therapeutic relationship, including use of therapeutic communication techniques in order to facilitate trust and full disclosure; consider importance of vulvar self-examination and examination of partner for early detection.
   B. Major points to emphasize for STI prevention: see Prevention and Risk-Reduction Measures sections and Table 7-1.
      - Know partner.
      - Avoid many partners or partners who have had many previous partners.
      - Insist on barrier method; be prepared.
      - Do not make decisions based on appearances and unfounded assumptions.
      - Carefully examine partner.
      - Know low-risk sexual practices and those that are unsafe or risky.
   C. Measures to help client develop assertiveness and communication skills related to safer sexual practices.
      - Begin by stressing the seriousness of the infections and the risk for transmission she faces by not using prevention measures; emphasize importance of discussing prevention measures, including condom use, with partner at a time removed from sexual activity.

- Role-play using possible partner responses for woman to react to; rehearse how she will handle various situations so she can sort out her feelings and fears ahead of time.
  - Reassure her that her reluctance is not unusual.
  D. HPV vaccine: see Risk-Reduction Measures and HPV sections; emphasize that although she is still within the age range of 13 to 26 to receive a catch-up vaccine, it is less effective when given after the woman is sexually active; it is also not effective for all forms of HPV or other infections, so regular Pap tests and clinical examinations are still very important.
2. Pregnant woman diagnosed as HIV positive at 4 weeks of gestation.
  A. Heterosexual transmission of HIV to women: see HIV section; consider exchange of body fluids (semen, blood, vaginal secretions); intravenous (IV) drug use by herself or her partner; history of multiple STIs.
  B. Clinical manifestations during seroconversion: viremic, influenza-type responses along with abnormal CBC results.
  C. Management: see Management section for a discussion of measures for nonpregnant and pregnant women, including education, transmission prevention infection control measures to maintain resistance to infection, and contraception; signs of disease progress; multidisciplinary care with a holistic focus; use of antiviral prophylaxis; referrals as needed.
  D. Measures to reduce transmission to baby: see HIV—Counseling for HIV Testing and HIV and Pregnancy sections; discuss several measures, including use of ART or HAART, scheduled cesarean at 38 weeks, avoiding breastfeeding, and lifestyle.
3. Woman with severe PID: see Pelvic Inflammatory Disease section.
  A. Risk factors: several factors are listed, including those related to menstrual history, age, contraceptive method used, recent reproductive tract problem or procedure, sexual behavior, and genital hygiene, including douching.
  B. Diagnostic criteria: include such findings as oral temperature of 38.3°C or higher, discharge, elevated erythrocyte sedimentation rate, bilateral adnexal tenderness, cervical motion tenderness, elevated C-reactive protein, and lower abdominal tenderness.
  C. Nursing diagnoses during acute phase: nursing diagnoses most likely will include acute pain, anxiety (effect on sexuality and future fertility), impaired physical mobility, constipation or diarrhea, and impaired urinary elimination.
  D. Management guidelines: see Management section; management outline should include measures for each of the following areas:
    - Position and activity or rest

- Comfort measures; nutrition and fluid balance
- Emotional support measures
- Health education: for now and with discharge
  E. Self-management during recovery phase: see Management section and Teaching for Self-Management—Sexually Transmitted Infections and Prevention of Genital Tract Infections boxes for several suggestions and prevention of genital tract infection for the future; emphasize activity restrictions, importance of rest, good nutrition, taking medications completely, and follow-up.
  F. Reproductive risks: tubal obstructions and adhesions leading to ectopic pregnancy or infertility, chronic pelvic pain, dyspareunia, and abscesses.
4. Woman diagnosed with gonorrhea: see Gonorrhea section and Nursing Care Plan.
  A. Essential assessment areas during health history: Box 7-2 outlines points to emphasize during assessment; be sure to discuss with her measures she has been using to reduce the risk of STIs; determine why she may or may not be using these measures.
  B. Nursing diagnosis: anxiety related to potential effect of STI on future sexual function or ineffective sexuality pattern related to recent diagnosis of STI is indicated.
  C. Self-management
    - Educate about STIs.
    - Discuss self-care measures: see Teaching for Self-Management—Sexually Transmitted Infections and Prevention of Genital Tract Infections boxes.
    - Discuss risk-reduction practices (see Table 7-1) and practice assertiveness with partners.
    - Review genital self-examination: see technique in Chapter 4.
5. Reducing pain of condylomata associated with HPV infection: see HPV—Management section for several suggestions related to cleansing, reducing moisture, what to wear, and measures to enhance healing.
6. Woman diagnosed with herpes simplex virus 2: see HSV—Management section.
  A. Measures to relieve pain and prevent secondary infection: see HSV—Management section for several measures to include in the answer.
    - Correct use of antiviral medications (Table 7-2)
    - Care of lesions
    - Use of alternative treatments
    - What to wear
    - Comfort measures, including use of analgesics
    - Diet and lifestyle to enhance healing
  B. Preventing or reducing recurrence.
    - Educate regarding HSV.
    - Keep diary.
    - Educate regarding stress-reduction measures and how to prevent transmission.

7. Measures to prevent transmission of hepatitis B virus: see HBV—Management section; use immunoprophylaxis for household members and sexual contacts,

maintain high levels of personal hygiene, carefully dispose of items contaminated with blood or body fluids including saliva, and use risk-reduction practices (Table 7-1).

8. Woman concerned about exposure to HIV: see HIV section.
   A. Risky behaviors: see Box 7-2 and Table 7-1; exposure to contaminated body fluids, including semen and blood; discuss sexual practices and partners as well as possible IV drug use.
   B. Testing procedure: see Screening and Diagnosis section and Legal Tip—HIV Testing for full description of types of tests and testing protocol, counseling required, and legal implications; nurse should witness an informed consent, tell the woman how long it will take for the results to be available, consider ethical issues of confidentiality and privacy, and use a nonjudgmental and empathic approach.
   C. Counseling protocol: see Counseling for HIV Testing section; counseling should occur before and after testing, by the same person, in a private area with no interruptions; all assessments, actions, and responses should be documented; describe pretest and posttest counseling and teaching.
   D. Instructions following a negative test result: use Sonya's risky behaviors as a basis for discussing prevention measures, including safer sex practices; discuss effect HIV could have on Sonya's health and on the health of her fetus when she is pregnant.

CHAPTER 8: CONTRACEPTION AND ABORTION

I. Learning Key Terms

1. Contraception
2. Birth control
3. Family planning
4. Contraceptive failure rate
5. Coitus interruptus
6. Fertility awareness–based methods, natural family planning (NFP), and periodic abstinence
7. Calendar rhythm method
8. Two-day method
9. Cervical mucus ovulation method
10. Spinnbarkeit
11. Basal body temperature (BBT) method
12. Thermal shift
13. Symptothermal
14. Biologic marker methods
15. Spermicide
16. Condom
17. Diaphragm
18. FemCap (cervical cap)
19. Contraceptive sponge
20. Monophasic pill
21. Multiphasic pill (biphasic, triphasic)
22. Withdrawal bleeding
23. Transdermal contraceptive system
24. Vaginal contraceptive ring
25. Minipill
26. Depo-Provera (DMPA, depot medroxyprogesterone acetate)
27. Implanon; Jadelle
28. Intrauterine device (IUD)
29. Sterilization; oviducts (uterine/fallopian tubes); sperm ducts (vas deferens); vasectomy
30. Tubal reconstruction
31. Lactation amenorrhea method (LAM)
32. Induced abortion; elective abortion; therapeutic abortion
33. Aspiration (vacuum or suction curettage)
34. Medical abortion; methotrexate; misoprostol; mifepristone
35. Dilation and evacuation

II. Reviewing Key Concepts

36. Couple making decision regarding contraceptive method to use.
    A. Factors influencing effectiveness: see full list in Box 8-1.
    B. Informed consent: see Legal Tip—Informed Consent in Care Management section; use BRAIDED format.
37. Purpose for self-assessment of cervical mucus: see Ovulation Method section and Teaching for Self-Management—Cervical Mucus Characteristics box for a description of the rationale for checking cervical mucus.
38. Fertility awareness (natural family planning) methods for contraception.
    A. ovulation; exercising restraint; irregular menstrual cycles
    B. 5; 22
    C. decrease; 0.5; progesterone; increase; 0.2 to 0.5; 2 to 4
    D. cervical mucus; amount; consistency
    E. basal body temperature (BBT); cervical mucus
    F. luteinizing hormone (LH); 12 to 24
39. Use of nonprescription barrier methods.
    A. I
    B. C
    C. C
    D. I
    E. C
    F. I
    G. I
40. Choice A is correct; oral contraception provides no protection from STIs; therefore a condom and spermicide are still recommended to prevent transmission; choices B, C, and D reflect appropriate actions and recognition of the effects of oral contraceptive pills (OCPs).
41. Choice B is correct; benefits of low dose pills are decreased menstrual blood loss and iron deficiency

anemia; cervical mucus is thickened, thereby inhibiting sperm penetration; ovulation and the development of the endometrium are also inhibited; there is no protection from STIs; the overall effectiveness rate is nearly 100% if used correctly.

42. Choice A is correct; women often complain of the irregular bleeding that occurs with progestin-only contraceptives.

43. Choice A is correct; the injection is repeated every 11 to 13 weeks (four times per year); choices B, C, and D are accurate.

44. Choice A is correct; the string should be checked after menses, before intercourse, at the time of ovulation, and if expulsion is suspected; a missing string or one that becomes longer or shorter should be checked by a health care professional.

45. Choice D is correct; spermicide should be inserted no longer than 1 hour prior to intercourse; douching or rinsing should not occur for at least 6 hours after the last act of coitus; frequent use of N-9, especially for anal intercourse, may disrupt mucosa, increasing rather than decreasing the risk of HIV transmission.

46. Choice B is correct; spermicide should be applied inside the cap but not around the rim because a seal will not form to keep the cap in place; use during menses increases the risk for toxic shock syndrome (TSS); checking the cap's position is all that is required before each subsequent act of coitus.

47. Choices A, C, and D are correct; spermicide should be spread on both surfaces of the diaphragm; it should not be removed for at least 6 hours after intercourse nor should it be used during menses because of the risk for TSS.

48. Choices A, B, and D are correct; BBT rises during the luteal phase and libido increases.

49. Choices C and D are correct; there is no hormone in this IUD; copper serves as a spermicide and it inflames the endometrium, preventing fertilization; NSAIDs are recommended to decrease cramping.

50. Choices A and D are correct; condoms are still needed to reduce risk for STIs and to prevent pregnancy until two consecutive sperm counts are at zero; he may become sexually active when desired but needs to use a condom since sperm may still be in the ejaculate.

III. Thinking Critically

1. Toxic shock syndrome: see Diaphragms section.
   A. Prevention measures when using diaphragm or cervical cap: removal 6 to 8 hours after intercourse as recommended; avoid use during menses; awareness of danger signs of TSS.
   B. Clinical manifestations: see Safety Alert for several signs.

2. Woman seeking assistance with making choice regarding birth control method: see Care Management—Assessment section and Nursing Care Plan.
   A. Nursing diagnosis: deficient knowledge related to methods of contraception *or* anxiety related to lack of knowledge regarding contraception.

B. Approach for nurse to use to assist with decision making: include the following areas in answer:
   ■ Assess level of knowledge and health status.
   ■ Describe methods; determine preferences for or objections to methods; involve partner as appropriate.
   ■ Determine level of contraceptive involvement desired.

3. Woman choosing to use combination estrogen-progestin oral contraceptive: see Hormonal Methods section.
   A. Mode of action: see Oral Contraceptive section for a description of how method works.
   B. Advantages: see Advantages section for several benefits of COC pills.
   C. Contraindications: see Disadvantages and Side Effects section, which lists several reasons for not using COC pills.
   D. Specify side effects related to changing levels of estrogen and progesterone: see Disadvantages and Side Effects section.
   E. Signs and symptoms requiring woman to stop taking the pill and notify her health care provider: see Signs of Potential Complications—Oral Contraceptives box for full explanation of ACHES.
   F. Instructions for the client: include a description of each of the following in your answer: directions on package, importance of using own pills and taking at same time every day, side effects and adverse reactions, interactions with other medications, need for STI protection, backup method, and what to do when missing a pill or pills.

4. Woman using a cervical cap: see FemCap (Cervical Cap) section and Teaching for Self-Management—Insertion and Removal of Cervical Cap box.
   A. Factors making client a poor candidate for using cap: several factors are identified in this section.
   B. Client instructions for safe and effective use: include a discussion of each of the following:
      ■ Know when and how to insert and remove, check placement before each act of coitus, use spermicide.
      ■ Avoid using during menses or for at least 6 weeks postpartum.
      ■ Check fit annually and after gynecologic surgery, birth, or major weight changes.

5. Instructions following IUD insertion: see IUD section.
   ■ See Signs of Complications—IUDs box, which defines the acronym PAINS to identify signs of problems.
   ■ Teach how and when to check string.
   ■ Stress importance of appropriate genital hygiene and risk-reduction measures.
   ■ Inform when IUD needs to be replaced.

6. Couple contemplating sterilization: see Sterilization section.
   A. Decision-making approach: nurse acts as facilitator to help couple explore the pros and cons of sterilization itself and the options available for male and female.
   B. Preoperative and postoperative care measures and instructions for vasectomy: fully discuss each of these areas in your answer:
      ■ Preoperative: health assessment; witness an informed consent.
      ■ Postoperative: prevention and early detection of bleeding and infection; self-management measures.
      ■ Caution that sterility is not immediate and what to do.
      ■ STI protection.
7. Woman contemplating elective abortion: see Induced Abortion section and Box 8-4.
   A. Nursing diagnosis: decisional conflict related to unplanned pregnancy and need to complete education.
   B. Describe approach: use therapeutic communication techniques to establish trusting relationship; discuss alternatives available to her and the consequences of each; nurse facilitates decision-making process and the client makes the decision; make appropriate referrals to help her with the decision.
   C. Procedure for vacuum aspiration: see Aspiration section for full description of procedure.
   D. Nursing diagnoses: consider fear and anxiety, anticipatory grieving, risk for deficient fluid volume (blood loss), risk for infection, and acute pain.
   E. Nursing measures for care and support: answer should reflect assessment and physical care and emotional support.
   F. Discharge instructions: answer should include observation for signs of complications (see Safety Alert), infection prevention, activity restrictions, resumption of sexual relations, use of birth control and risk-reduction measures, follow-up appointment, and importance of stress reduction.
8. Drugs used for medical abortions and how they work: see Medical Abortion section; describe methotrexate, misoprostol (Cytotec), and mifepristone.
9. Woman seeking assistance following unprotected intercourse: see Emergency Contraception section.
   A. Nursing approach:
      ■ Explore possibility of pregnancy and options related to continuing pregnancy if it occurs (keeping baby, adoption).
      ■ Explore options for emergency contraception to prevent pregnancy: methods available, how each works, timing, side effects, how administered.

   ■ Emphasize importance of follow-up to check for effectiveness of method used and occurrence of infection.
   ■ Discuss methods of contraception and safer sex measures to prevent recurrence of this situation.
   B. Using Plan B One Step: see Emergency Contraception section, Medication Alert, and Table 8-2 for the information to complete this exercise.
   C. Nurse must emphasize that while risk for pregnancy is significantly reduced it is still possible; therefore follow-up is essential.

CHAPTER 9: INFERTILITY

I. Learning Key Terms

1. E, 2. F, 3. C, 4. G, 5. D, 6. B, 7. A
8. Infertility
9. Sterility
10. Assisted reproductive technology (ART)
11. In vitro fertilization and embryo transfer (IVF & ET)
12. Intracytoplasmic sperm injection
13. Gamete intrafallopian transfer (GIFT)
14. Zygote intrafallopian transfer (ZIFT)
15. Therapeutic donor insemination
16. Gestational carrier (embryo host)
17. Surrogate motherhood
18. Assisted hatching
19. Donor embryo (embryo adoption)
20. Preimplantation genetic diagnosis
21. Cryopreservation of human embryos
22. Intrauterine insemination

II. Reviewing Key Concepts

23. Medications used in the treatment of infertility: use Medication Guide—Infertility Medications and Medical section to describe the mode of action and purpose of each medication listed.
24. Choice B is correct; spinnbarkeit refers to stretchiness of cervical mucus at ovulation to facilitate passage of sperm; there is an LH surge prior to ovulation; BBT rises in response to increased progesterone after ovulation; cervical mucus becomes thinner and more abundant with ovulation.
25. Choice A is correct; both male and female obesity can adversely affect fertility; water-soluble lubricants can be safely used; daily hot tubs or saunas may increase scrotal temperature enough to interfere with spermatogenesis; although excessive alcohol use can cause erectile dysfunction, abstention from alcohol is not necessary.
26. Choice C is correct; this medication provides LH and FSH, causing a powerful ovulation stimulation that can result in multiple pregnancy; therefore regular ovarian ultrasound and monitoring of estradiol levels are required to prevent hyperstimulation. It is administered intramuscularly and is used when clomiphene fails to induce ovulation; it is followed by

administration of human chorionic gonadotropin (hCG).

27. Choice A is correct; Clomid is used to increase FSH and LH secretion by stimulating the pituitary gland.

28. Choice D is correct; with passage of radiopaque dye, this test could straighten or unblock the uterine tube if that is the cause of the infertility but it is not a guarantee she will conceive; it is performed 4 to 5 days after menstruation (proliferative phase); uterine cramping and referred pain to the shoulder are expected findings and are treated with mild analgesics and position changes.

II. Thinking Critically

1. Couple receiving care for infertility: see Factors Associated with Infertility section, Nursing Care Plan for Infertility, and Boxes 9-1 and 9-2.
   A. Identify and describe components for normal fertility: components required for conception and pregnancy are identified and described in this section.
   B. Support statement that assessment for infertility must involve both partners: Box 9-4 identifies findings favorable for fertility and indicates male and female factors; cite statistics related to male and female factors associated with infertility.

2. Couple undergoing testing for infertility.
   A. Nursing support measures: see Psychosocial section of Interventions, Box 9-5, and Table 9-2; nurses must feel comfortable with their own sexuality and recognize common responses to infertility; help couple to:
      ▪ Express feelings and openly discuss sexuality issues
      ▪ Grieve the loss of fertility and the inability to have biologic children if that is the outcome
      ▪ Find support groups and adoption agencies as appropriate
   B. Female and male assessment components: see appropriate text sections and Boxes 9-1 and 9-2 for a full explanation of the components for each assessment.
   C. Procedure for semen analysis: see Semen Analysis section for essential guidelines to ensure test result accuracy.
   D. Effect of lifestyle practices on male fertility: see Male Infertility section and Box 9-2; smoking can result in abnormal sperm, decreased number of sperm, and chromosomal damage; include in your answer the potential effect of secondhand smoke on the smoker's partner and on the fetus, should pregnancy occur; alcohol use can result in erectile dysfunction depending on the amount of alcohol used; exposure of the scrotum and testes to increased temperatures can alter sperm production and obesity can decrease sperm quality.

3. Concerns engendered by assisted reproductive technologies: see Assisted Reproductive Therapies section and Boxes 9-3 and 9-5; in your answer, discuss who should pay; who are the biologic parents; marital status; ownership of ovum, sperm, and embryos; seeking the "perfect" child; risk for multiple gestation; and reduction abortions.

4. Woman scheduled for a diagnostic laparoscopy: see Laparoscopy section, Fig. 9-4, and Table 9-1.
   A. Timing: early in menstrual cycle to avoid disturbing a possible fertilized ovum.
   B. Preprocedure care measures: nothing by mouth (NPO) for 8 hours, void before procedure, bowel preparation may be required.
   C. Purpose and process of the procedure: describe diagnostic and therapeutic purposes and process (what will happen).
   D. Postprocedure care measures: discuss assessment of status; physical care and emotional support measures; timing of discharge—criteria, discharge instructions, and prevention of complications.

5. Couple experiencing problems with fertility.
   A. Typical responses and nursing actions: see Table 9-2 for descriptions of reactions and several recommended nursing actions.
   B. Guiding the decision-making process: see Box 9-5.
      ▪ Discuss meaning of fertility and having biologic children for this couple and for their family.
      ▪ Fully inform couple of diagnostic tests and treatment options so that informed decision can be made.
      ▪ Review financial considerations, including what insurance will cover.
      ▪ Encourage couple to define what they are willing to endure physically, emotionally, and financially to have a biologic child; discuss alternatives to biologic children.
      ▪ Refer to support groups.
   C. Religious and cultural beliefs and practices that can influence decision making regarding treatment of infertility: see Box 9-3.

CHAPTER 10: PROBLEMS OF THE BREAST

I. Learning Key Terms

1. B, 2. E, 3. G, 4. A, 5. F, 6. H, 7. D, 8. C

II. Reviewing Key Concepts

9. Definitions of treatment approaches: see section for each method and Table 10-4 for a full description of each treatment approach.

10. Choices B and C are correct; breast cancer is more common among Caucasian women but the mortality rate is higher among African-American women; it is most prevalent among women between 45 and 66 years of age and approximately 80% of women with breast cancer do not have a family history.

11. Choice D is correct; tamoxifen reduces growth and inhibits recurrence of estrogen-sensitive breast

cancer; usual dose is 20 mg, by mouth, once a day; because it is an antiestrogen medication, signs of estrogen deficit such as hot flashes and menstrual irregularities can occur.

12. Choice B is correct; the right arm should be used as much as possible to maintain mobility and prevent lymphedema; tingling and numbness are expected findings for as long as a few months after surgery; deodorant may be used but not a strong one.

13. Choice A is correct; acute pain is a common finding; it usually begins a week before the onset of menses; leakage from nipples is not associated with this disorder; surgery is unlikely; cancer risk is not high because fibrocystic changes are part of the normal involutional patterns of the breast.

14. Choice D is correct; fibroadenomas are generally small, unilateral, firm, nontender, movable lumps; borders are discrete and well defined; discharge is not associated with this breast disorder.

15. Choices B, D, and E are correct; the woman should continue to take her calcium supplement because the medication will also treat her osteoporosis; the medication is taken daily with or without food.

III. Thinking Critically

1. Educating women about breast cancer: see Malignant Conditions of the Breast section.
   A. Information regarding risk factors: see Incidence and Etiologies section and Box 10-1 to determine risk factors to teach women; identify factors and degree of risk they represent alone and in combination; include research findings; discuss how risk factors can influence health care, including suggestions for assessment methods and frequency, lifestyle changes, and prevention methods for very-high-risk women.
   B. Breast screening recommendations: see Table 10-3 and Screening section for recommendations for women ages 20 to 39 years and 40 years and older.
   C. Factors inhibiting women from participating in breast screening and strategies to encourage compliance: see Clinical Manifestations and Diagnosis section and Cultural Considerations—Breast Screening Practices box.
      - Inhibiting factors: culture, lack of knowledge and time, fear, finances and insurance coverage, age, and access
      - Strategies: reminder postcards, buddy system, insurance coverage, teaching days and programs for women and health care providers, advertisements in the media, mobile clinics to bring health screening to neighborhoods, flexible clinic hours, free screening and walk-in self-referrals; present several and get their feedback; encourage them to offer other suggestions.
   D. Manifestations suggestive of breast cancer: see Clinical Manifestations and Diagnosis section for a full explanation of the manifestations.

   E. Diagnostic tests if a lump is found: describe each test and its importance in the diagnostic process—mammography, ultrasound, MRI, biopsy of tumor tissue or fluid.
   F. Genetic basis for breast cancer: see Etiology and Genetic Considerations sections; discuss pros and cons of genetic testing and the risks for genetically transmitted breast cancer.

2. Woman's concern regarding the genetic risk for breast cancer: see Malignant Conditions of the Breast—Etiology and Genetic Considerations section and Box 10-1.
   - Tell her most cancers are not related to genetic factors; 80% to 85% of women with breast cancer do not have a family history.
   - Obtain a full family history regarding breast and other cancers, focusing on other family members diagnosed with breast cancer.
   - Discuss *BRCA* gene testing and its meaning; discuss the Genetic Information Nondiscrimination Act (GINA).
   - Help her to explore what she would do if results are positive.
   - Encourage her participation in appropriate screening measures such as clinical breast examinations, mammograms, and MRIs; BSE should also be discussed.

3. Woman with fibrocystic breast change: see Fibrocystic Changes section.
   A. Assessment process to diagnose fibrocystic change: include a description of each component.
      - History, physical assessment, clinical breast examination
      - Diagnostic testing: ultrasonography, fluid aspirated if necessary, fine-needle aspiration
   B. Clinical manifestations: describe the bilateral changes that occur in size and tenderness with the menstrual cycle.
   C. Nursing diagnosis: based on assessment findings and time in menstrual cycle; can include acute pain and anxiety.
   D. Relief measures: try several approaches to find the combination that works the best; keep a diary: include such measures as analgesics, support, dietary changes, vitamins E and B_6, diuretics, and avoiding caffeine.
   E. Risk for cancer: very low and depends on type of cellular change; risk is primarily related to atypical hyperplasia.

4. Woman with lump in left breast: see Malignant Conditions of the Breast section and Nursing Care Plan.
   A. Diagnostic protocol: describe each component (see Clinical Manifestations and Diagnosis section).
      - History and physical examination, including clinical breast examination; document characteristics of the lump and associated findings
      - Mammography, ultrasound, biopsy, MRI
      - Laboratory testing

B. Emotional effect of cancer diagnosis: see Care Management—Emotional Support after Diagnosis section; answer should include:
- Description of emotional reactions, such as shock, denial, and fear
- Disruption caused by diagnosis: role changes, finances, body image, and sexual function
- Review of decision-making questions she and her family should ask; see Box 10-3

C. Nursing diagnoses and care management:
- Preoperative period
  - Nursing diagnoses: see Preoperative Care section; could include fear and anxiety, anticipatory grieving; risk for ineffective family and individual coping are likely to be priority diagnoses.
  - Preoperative teaching and typical surgical care measures: Reach for Recovery volunteer may be asked to speak to the woman and her family.
- Immediate postoperative period: see Immediate Postoperative Care section and Nursing Care Plan.
  - Nursing diagnoses: acute pain, risk for infection, impaired skin integrity, and risk for deficient fluid volume.
  - Typical postoperative care along with elevation of arm: avoid using arm for BP, IV, blood draws, and medications; follow protocol for movement and use of affected arm; check for bleeding; assist with position changes; leg exercises; coughing and deep breathing.
  - Emotional support throughout

D. Preparing Molly for self-management at home: see Box 10-4 and Teaching for Self-Management—After a Mastectomy box; instructions should address pain control; signs of expected changes and complications; infection prevention; wound, dressing, and drainage care; BSE; arm exercises and use of arm for activities of daily living; and time for follow-up appointment.

E. Support measures.
- Help woman and partner to deal with change in appearance and treatment regimen.
- Refer to community resources and support groups.
- Discuss follow-up treatments, the process of reconstruction, and use of prostheses; provide emotional support with first view of incision.

5. Tamoxifen therapy: see Tamoxifen section of Adjuvant Therapy and the Medication Guide for Tamoxifen.
- Oral antiestrogen medication; be prepared for menopause-like symptoms, such as hot flashes.
- Plan should include action and purpose, dosage, and how to take effectively as well as adverse reactions to watch for and what to do if they occur.

6. Woman with breast cancer beginning chemotherapy: see Chemotherapy and Teaching Needs for the Client and Family Undergoing Adjuvant Therapy sections.

A. Teaching plan:
- Name of medication, route of administration, treatment schedule, timing, length of time for administration
- Payment, insurance coverage
- Side effects and how to manage them, including use of alternative therapies
- Teratogenic potential
- Required follow-up care
- Expected effect of treatment on her daily life; adjustments that will need to be made

B. Nursing diagnoses: use assessment findings to determine which diagnoses would apply and their priority for this client.
- Imbalanced nutrition: less than body requirements
- Risk for infection
- Disturbed body image
- Interrupted family processes
- Ineffective role performance
- Fear/anxiety

Nursing interventions: see Nursing Interventions section and Nursing Care Plan.

CHAPTER 11: STRUCTURAL DISORDERS AND NEOPLASMS OF THE REPRODUCTIVE SYSTEM

I. Learning Key Terms

1. C, 2. F, 3. L, 4. J, 5. G, 6. H, 7. M, 8. A, 9. B, 10. O, 11. N, 12. I, 13. D, 14. E, 15. K
16. Pessary
17. Anterior repair (colporrhaphy)
18. Posterior repair (colporrhaphy)
19. Myomectomy
20. Uterine artery embolization (UAE)
21. Laser surgery
22. Hysteroscopic uterine ablation
23. Hysterectomy
24. Bilateral salpingo-oophorectomy (BSO)
25. Colposcopy
26. Conization
27. Cryosurgery
28. Loop electrosurgical excision procedure (LEEP)
29. Radical hysterectomy
30. Pelvic exenteration
31. Simple vulvectomy
32. Complete radical vulvectomy

II. Reviewing Key Concepts

33. Ovarian cancer, a "silent" cancer: see Cancer of Ovary—Incidence and Etiology and Clinical Manifestations sections for full explanation.
34. Choices B and E are correct; a knee-chest position is appropriate for a retroverted uterus; anterior colporrhaphy is performed to repair a cystocele; vaginal or abdominal hysterectomy would be performed

if needed; estrogen may be used to improve tissue tone.

35. Choices C and E are correct; fibroids are dependent on estrogen for growth; therefore they will increase in size during pregnancy and shrink with menopause; abnormal uterine bleeding is the most common clinical manifestation and can lead to anemia if severe; constipation, low dull abdominal pain and pressure, dysmenorrhea, and backache are other common signs and symptoms as the tumors enlarge.

36. Choice B is correct; reducing fluid intake can be dangerous because fluids are required to prevent urinary tract infection; choices A, C, and D are all effective in reducing urinary incontinence.

37. Choice B is correct; only the uterus was removed; therefore HRT will not be needed; turning, coughing, and deep breathing should be performed at least every 2 hours for the first 24 hours; no douching is required and it should be avoided.

38. Choice C is correct; CIS is noninvasive and therefore cervical conization with follow-up is the appropriate treatment choice; the LEEP procedure can be used for the conization; UAE is used in the treatment of fibroid tumors and radiation for invasive forms of cancer.

III. Thinking Critically

1. Reproductive tract cancers.
   A. Risk factors: see Incidence and Etiology section for each of the cancers listed for identification of risk factors.
   B. Use of risk factors: encourage early detection; teaching measures such as more frequent, earlier examination for those at high risk; use the risk factors to identify specific measures for each type of cancer (e.g., infection prevention measures for cervical cancer).

2. Woman diagnosed with moderate uterine prolapse along with cystocele and rectocele: see Uterine Displacement and Prolapse and Cystocele and Rectocele sections.
   A. Clinical manifestations: see Clinical Manifestations section; several manifestations are described for each disorder.
   B. Two priority nursing diagnoses with expected outcomes:
      ■ Constipation related to altered position of uterus, rectum, and bladder; woman will experience regular, soft-formed bowel elimination.
      ■ Ineffective sexuality patterns related to vaginal change associated with uterine prolapse, cystocele, and rectocele; woman will openly discuss measures to enhance sexual function.
   C. Management of uterine prolapse, cystocele, and rectocele: see Medical and Surgical Management and Nursing Interventions sections; answer should include use of Kegel exercises, diet changes, stool softeners, mild laxatives, and pessary.

D. Using a pessary:
   1. Nursing diagnosis: risk for infection related to altered tissue integrity associated with insertion of pessary.
   2. Instructions for use: tailor instructions for the type of pessary used; include how to insert and remove, how to care for and cleanse, genital hygiene measures, and signs indicative of infection; use discussion, demonstrations, and anatomic models and illustrations to enhance learning.
E. Postoperative care following vaginal hysterectomy and colporrhaphy: see Postoperative Nursing Interventions section, Box 11-3, and Teaching for Self-Management—Care after Myomectomy and Hysterectomy box; discuss each of the following measures:
   ■ Ensure cleanliness; prevention of postoperative complications.
   ■ Keep bowel and bladder empty; discuss activity and rest requirements; maintain venous return with leg exercises.
   ■ Check for pain, bleeding, and infection.

3. Woman with fibroids: see Benign Neoplasms—Leiomyomas section.
   A. Clinical manifestations: see Clinical Manifestations and Diagnosis section for several manifestations.
   B. Compare treatment approaches and factors considered for choice: see Medical Management and Surgical Management sections; discuss medications used to shrink the tumor and medications used to treat symptoms, uterine artery embolization, myomectomy, laser surgery, electrocautery, and hysterectomy.
   C. Care management after UAE: see UAE section and Teaching for Self-Management—Home Care after UAE box for several measures that should be implemented.

4. Woman with endometrial cancer.
   A. Nursing diagnosis for preoperative and postoperative periods: see Endometrial Cancer section and Nursing Care Plan.
      ■ Preoperative: fear related to diagnosis of uterine cancer and anticipated surgery; woman will openly discuss fears and concerns with health care provider and family.
      ■ Postoperative: acute pain, risk for deficient fluid volume, and risk for infection; eventually disturbed body image and ineffective sexuality patterns; an expected outcome for pain would be that woman will experience reduction in pain when relief measures are implemented.
   B. Nursing care and support:
      ■ Preoperative: see Preoperative Care section and Box 11-2; preoperative teaching; typical physical measures for major abdominal surgery; consider issue of informed consent; see Box 11-1.

- Postoperative: see Postoperative Care section and Box 11-3; measures included in plan should be assessment of physical and emotional status, fluid intake, measures to prevent postoperative complications, wound care, perineal care, pain relief and comfort measures, recommended position changes.
  C. Discharge instructions: see Discharge Planning and Teaching section and Teaching for Self-Management—Woman Who Has Had a Myomectomy or Hysterectomy box for a full explanation of teaching topics.
  D. Cultural issues: see Cultural Considerations—Meaning of Cancer box; body image; meaning of uterus and fertility in her culture; meaning of death; responses to pain.
  E. Nursing diagnosis related to diagnosis and treatment: Anxiety *or* disturbed body image related to effects of surgery and possibility of ongoing treatment for cancer; also consider ineffective sexuality patterns that could interfere with her emotional health and recovery.
  F. Support measures during recovery:
   - Provide time to discuss fears, ask questions, explore feelings regarding self as woman and sexuality.
   - Involve significant others.
   - Teach about effects of surgery and other treatment measures that may be used; discuss the use of alternative therapies.
   - Refer to support groups.
5. Woman with invasive cancer of the cervix: see Cancer of Cervix section.
  A. Nursing diagnoses with expected outcomes: see Box 11-6, Woman Having Radiation Therapy.
   - Fear related to concerns about cancer and effects of radiation treatments; woman will openly express fears regarding diagnosis and treatment with health care provider and family.
   - Impaired skin integrity related to effects of radiation on tissue; will use appropriate measures to reduce skin breakdown and enhance healing; see Box 11-4 related to the importance of nutrition.
  B. Outline the care and support required for external radiation and internal radiation: see sections for each type of radiation therapy, the Teaching for Self-Management boxes related to radiation therapy, and Box 11-4 for points to highlight when completing the outline; be sure to include emotional support measures along with the physical care measures.
  C. Self-protection measures: see Internal Radiation Therapy section and Safety Alert for precautions to follow; emphasize wearing of film badge, use of careful isolation techniques, and planning nursing care to reduce exposure; distance, time, and shielding are three ways to control exposure.

6. Woman recovering from a radical vulvectomy: see Cancer of the Vulva section.
  A. and B. Nursing measures to prevent infection and maintain sexual functioning: see Nursing Interventions section of Cancer of the Vulva for a full list of nursing care measures for each expected outcome of care.
  C. Discharge instructions: see Teaching for Self-Management—Care After Radical Vulvectomy box to determine critical discharge instructions that should be given to this woman to enhance healing and prevent complications.
7. Cancer during pregnancy: see Cancer and Pregnancy section; answer should include:
   - Issues and emotions regarding the mother, fetus, and impact of treatment
   - Potential for termination of pregnancy
   - Review of options for treatment, with their potential effect on the maternal-fetal unit
   - Ethical considerations for treatment and its effect on fetal well-being—a critical component of decision making
8. Woman receiving chemotherapy for treatment of advanced ovarian cancer: see Cancer of Ovary section.
  A. Measures to relieve selected chemotherapy-related problems: see Box 11-4; be sure to include an explanation of why the problems occur and why suggested relief measures are safe and effective.
  B. Support measures: see Nursing Interventions section and Legal Tip—Advance Directives; consider discussion of such issues as stages of grief, advance directives, services of hospice, Internet resources, and alternative and complementary therapies.

ANSWER KEY UNIT III

CHAPTER 12: CONCEPTION AND FETAL DEVELOPMENT

I. Learning Key Terms

1. Conception
2. Gametes; sperm; ovum (egg)
3. Mitosis
4. Meiosis
5. Haploid
6. Diploid
7. Gametogenesis; spermatogenesis; oogenesis
8. Fertilization
9. Zygote
10. Morula
11. Blastocyst; trophoblast
12. Implantation
13. Chorionic villi
14. Decidua
15. Embryo
16. Fetus

17. Amniotic membranes; chorion; amnion
18. Amniotic fluid; oligohydramnios; hydramnios
19. Umbilical cord; arteries; vein; Wharton jelly; nuchal cord
20. Placenta; human chorionic gonadotropin (hCG)
21. Viability
22. Ductus arteriosus
23. Ductus venosus
24. Foramen ovale
25. Hematopoiesis
26. Pulmonary surfactants; lecithin-sphingomyelin (L/S)
27. Quickening
28. Meconium
29. Dizygotic; fraternal
30. Monozygotic; identical; conjoined
31. Congenital disorders
32. Teratogens

II. Reviewing Key Concepts

33. Describe the functions of yolk sac, amniotic fluid and membranes, umbilical cord, and placenta: see individual sections for each of these structures in Development of the Embryo.
34. Name the primary germ layers and identify tissues and organs developed from each layer: see Primary Germ Layers section to complete this activity.
35. Choices B, E, and F are correct; feeling of movement is called quickening; the sex of a baby is determined at conception; the heart begins to pump blood by the end of the 3rd week and a heartbeat can be heard with ultrasound by the 8th week of gestation.
36. Choice B is correct; the L/S ratio is a test to determine the presence of the surfactants lecithin and sphingomyelin; it becomes 2:1, indicating lung maturity, at approximately 35 weeks of gestation; an elevated alpha-fetoprotein level is an indicator for an open neural tube defect; renal disorders usually are indicated by a decreased amount of amniotic fluid.
37. Choice C is correct; the healthy newborn of a well-nourished mother will not need iron sources until about 5 months of age; iron-fortified cereal is usually introduced at this time.
38. Choice A is correct; if a woman's diabetes is uncontrolled, maternal hyperglycemia will produce fetal hyperglycemia and stimulate hyperinsulinemia, resulting in increased fetal growth (macrosomia or large for gestational age); lung maturation is inhibited and neonatal hypoglycemia can occur; strict control of maternal glucose levels before and during pregnancy will reduce the risk.

III. Thinking Critically

1. A. Progress of development at 2 months, 5 months, and 7 months: see Table 12-1 to formulate your answer; use of illustrations and life-sized models will facilitate learning.
   B. Survival after 35 weeks of gestation: discuss how the respiratory system develops, including the critical factor, surfactant production; describe how surfactant helps the newborn to breathe.
   C. Quickening: explain that this is the woman's perception of fetal movement that occurs at about 16 to 20 weeks of gestation; describe how the fetus moves; it will not hurt but can be uncomfortable and interfere with sleep toward the end of pregnancy; fetus will develop its own sleep-wake cycle.
   D. Fetal sensory perception: discuss sensory capability of the fetus using the Sensory Awareness section in Fetal Maturation; fetus can hear sounds such as parents' voices and respond to light and touch; encourage Susan to interact with her fetus.
   E. Sex determination: discuss functions of X and Y chromosomes; sex of her fetus will become recognizable around 12 weeks of gestation.
   F. Multiple gestation—twins: see section for each type of twinning to formulate your answer; discuss monozygotic (identical) and dizygotic (fraternal) twinning and how each occurs; emphasize that fraternal twinning tends to occur in families.
   G. Influence of activity and position on fetal growth and development: see Placental Functions section; discuss differences in circulation through placenta in various positions, including supine, lateral, sitting, and standing; discuss the effect of excessive exercise on placental circulation; emphasize that efficient circulation through the placenta is important to ensure an adequate supply of oxygen and nutrients for growth and development.

CHAPTER 13: ANATOMY AND PHYSIOLOGY OF PREGNANCY

I. Learning Key Terms

1. C, 2. P, 3. K, 4. T, 5. S, 6. U, 7. J, 8. N, 9. V, 10. B, 11. G, 12. A, 13. O, 14. I, 15. X, 16. E, 17. M, 18. W, 19. F, 20. H, 21. D, 22. R, 23. L, 24. Q
25. Gravidity
26. Parity
27. Gravida
28. Nulligravida
29. Nullipara
30. Primigravida
31. Primipara
32. Multigravida
33. Multipara
34. Viability
35. Preterm
36. Term
37. Postdate, postterm
38. Human chorionic gonadotropin (hCG)
39. Presumptive changes
40. Probable changes
41. Positive signs
42. Braxton Hicks contractions

43. Uterine soufflé/bruit
44. Funic soufflé
45. Quickening
46. Supine hypotensive syndrome (vena caval syndrome)
47. Pruritus gravidarum; pruritic urticarial papules and plaques of pregnancy (PUPPP)
48. Pica
49. Ptyalism

II. Reviewing Key Concepts

50. Obstetric history using 2-digit and 5-digit systems: see Gravidity and Parity section and Table 13-1: Nancy (3-2; 3-1-1-0-1); Marsha (4-2; 4-2-0-1-2); Linda (4-2; 4-1-1-1-3).
51. Changes in vital signs as pregnancy progresses.
    - Blood pressure and heart rate patterns: see Table 13-4 and Cardiovascular System section; blood pressure decreases and returns to prepregnant levels by term; blood pressure is affected by several factors, including maternal position and level of anxiety; pulse increases by 10 to 15 beats/minute; murmurs, dysrhythmias, and palpitations can occur.
    - Respiratory patterns: see Table 13-5 and Respiratory System section; breathing becomes more thoracic in nature and volume is deeper with a slight increase in rate; some shortness of breath may be experienced in the second trimester as the diaphragm is pushed upward by the enlarging uterus; continues until lightening occurs.
    - Temperature: baseline temperature rises slightly as a result of the increase in basal metabolic rate (BMR) and the progesterone effect; women may complain of heat intolerance.
52. Mean arterial pressure (MAP) calculation: see Box 12-2; use the following formula:

$$\frac{Systolic + 2(Diastolic)}{3}$$

    Answers are: 91, 81, 90, 110.
53. Specify value changes for selected laboratory tests during pregnancy.
    - CBC: see Tables 13-3 and 13-4 and Blood Volume and Composition section.
    - Clotting activity: see Circulation and Coagulation Times section and Table 13-3.
    - Acid-base balance: see Acid-Base section and Table 13-3.
    - Urinalysis: see Fluid and Electrolyte Balance section and Table 13-3.
54. Changes in endocrine function and secretions of hormones: see Table 13-6 for a description of each hormone and how and why hormonal levels change with pregnancy.
55. Choices A, E, and F are correct; hCG indicates a positive pregnancy test and is a probable sign along with ballottement and Hegar sign; breast tenderness and morning sickness are presumptive signs; fetal heart sounds are a positive sign of pregnancy.
56. Choice D is correct; use 5-digit system GTPAL: **g**ravida (total number of pregnancies, including the present one, is 5), para (**t**erm birth of daughter at 39 weeks = 1, **p**reterm stillbirth at 32 weeks and triplets at 30 weeks = 2, spontaneous **a**bortion at 8 weeks = 1, total number of **l**iving children = 4).
57. Choice C is correct; although little change occurs in respiratory rate, breathing becomes more thoracic in nature with the upward displacement of the diaphragm; women normally experience a greater awareness of breathing and may even complain of dyspnea and an increased awareness to breathe at rest as pregnancy progresses; supine hypotension syndrome occurs as a result of vena cava and aorta compression by the uterus when the woman is in a supine position; baseline pulse rate increases by 10 to 15 beats/minute; systolic and diastolic pressure decreases slightly (or may stay the same; it should not increase) beginning in the second trimester, returning to prepregnancy levels in the third trimester.
58. Choice D is correct; recording cycle information assists with accuracy of diagnosis; choice C reflects the most common error of performing this test too soon and she will need to repeat the test in 1 week if the result is negative; first-voided morning specimens should be used because they are the most concentrated and are apt to have the largest amount of hCG; anticonvulsants, tranquilizers, diuretics, and promethazine can result in inaccurate results.
59. Choice B is correct; friability refers to cervical fragility resulting in slight bleeding when the cervix is scraped or touched; Chadwick sign refers to a deep bluish cervix and vagina as a result of increased circulation; Hegar sign refers to softening and compressibility of the lower uterine segment.

III. Thinking Critically

1. Responses to client concerns and questions.
    A. Spotting after intercourse: discuss cervical and vaginal friability and increased vascularity; makes the vagina and cervix softer and more delicate, so spotting after intercourse is expected; caution that any bleeding should be reported so it can be evaluated.
    B. Use of home pregnancy test: see Teaching for Self-Management—Home Pregnancy Testing box; emphasize the importance of following directions because each brand of test is slightly different; use first-voided morning specimen for the most concentrated urine and notify health care provider regardless of the test result.
    C. Bladder and vaginal infections: discuss the effect of increased vaginal secretions and of changes in urinary elimination, including stasis of urine that contains nutrients and has a higher pH; review prevention measures at this time.

D. Breast changes with pregnancy: discuss changes in beasts, such as enlargement of Montgomery glands and tubercles and development of lactation structures, resulting in larger breasts that are tender during the first trimester; changes in consistency and presence of lumpiness during BSE and leakage of fluid; changes are bilateral.

E. Effects of pregnant woman's position: discuss supine hypotensive syndrome and importance of the lateral position when at rest.

F. Nosebleeds: discuss effect of estrogen-stimulated increase in upper airway vascularity.

G. Ankle edema: explain the effect of the enlarging uterus and the dependent position of her legs on circulation; discuss measures to reduce edema; caution her to never take someone else's medications or to self-medicate.

H. Posture and low back pain: explain why lordosis occurs and what she can do to relieve low back pain.

I. Braxton Hicks contractions: the woman is describing false labor contractions because they diminish with activity; these contractions facilitate blood flow and promote oxygen delivery to the fetus; compare these contractions with true labor contractions.

J. Shortness of breath: explain that what she is experiencing is a result of increased sensitivity of her respiratory center to carbon dioxide, compensation for mild respiratory alkalosis, and the elevation of her diaphragm by the enlarging uterus; assess the woman for signs of pulmonary edema to ensure that the shortness of breath is physiologic rather than pathologic.

K. Changes in bowel function: explain changes in elimination patterns, why they occur, and what she can safely do to prevent constipation and enhance bowel elimination.

2. Blood pressure protocol: see Blood Pressure section and Box 13-1; consider the effects of maternal age, activity and stress level, health status, arm, and position; protocol should emphasize consistency in arm and position used, size of cuff, time provided for relaxation prior to measurement; repeat if finding is inconsistent with woman's baseline or is abnormal.

CHAPTER 14: NURSING CARE OF THE FAMILY DURING PREGNANCY

I. Learning Key Terms

1. Presumptive
2. Probable
3. Positive
4. Nägele's; 3 calendar months; 7 days; 1 year; 7 days; 9 calendar months
5. Trimester
6. Supine hypotension; vena cava; aorta
7. Fundal height

8. Pinch
9. Accepting the pregnancy; identifying with role of parent; reordering personal relationships; establishing relationship with the fetus; preparing for childbirth
10. Emotional lability (mood swings and changes)
11. Ambivalence
12. Biologic fact of pregnancy; "I am pregnant"; growing fetus as distinct from herself; "I am going to have a baby"; birth; parenting of the child; "I am going to be a mother"
13. Couvade syndrome
14. Announcement phase; biologic fact of pregnancy; moratorium; accept the pregnancy; focusing; labor; parenthood
15. Prescriptions
16. Proscriptions; taboos
17. Sequential Integrated Screening (SIS)
18. Noninvasive prenatal testing
19. Doula
20. Birth plan

II. Reviewing Key Concepts

21. Calculate expected date of birth: use Nägele's rule: subtract 3 months and add 7 days and 1 year (if appropriate) to the first day of the last normal menstrual period.
    A. February 12, 2015
    B. October 21, 2014
    C. June 11, 2015
22. Cultural beliefs and practices: see Variations in Prenatal Care—Cultural Influences section.
    A. Describe how cultural beliefs affect participation in prenatal care: consider beliefs regarding pregnancy and health care during pregnancy, finances, transportation, communication difficulties, and concerns regarding modesty.
    B. Prescriptions and proscriptions: see specific sections for emotional response, clothing, physical activity and rest, sexual activity, and diet.
23. Outline components of initial and follow-up visits: see Initial Visit and Follow-up Visits sections to complete the outline.
24. Components of fetal assessment: see Follow-up Visits section, which describes several assessment measures of the mother and fetus directly; include what a mother can do to assess her fetus, such as daily fetal movement counts beginning at approximately 27 weeks of gestation.
25. Warning signs of potential complications during pregnancy.
    A. List signs of complications: see Signs of Potential Complications box, which lists signs according to the first, second, and third trimesters.
    B. Nursing approach when discussing signs of complications with pregnant woman and her family: see Recognizing Potential Complications section.
    ■ Discuss the signs, possible causes, and when and to whom to report.

- Present the signs verbally and in written form.
- Provide time to answer questions and discuss concerns; make follow-up phone calls.
- Gather full information of signs that are reported; use information as a basis for action.
- Document all assessments, actions, and responses, including the date(s) that information regarding these signs was given, the methodology used, and the woman's reaction to the information.

26. Creating a protocol for fundal measurement: see Measurement of Fundal Height section and Fig. 14-8; consider woman's position, type of measuring device used, measurement method, and conditions of the examination, such as an empty bladder and relaxed or contracted uterus. Document any variations from the protocol when recording a measurement.

27. Factors used to estimate gestational age: see Fetal Assessment—Gestational Age section for a discussion of these factors.

28. Prevention of injury.
    A. Principles of body mechanics: see Fig. 14-12 and Teaching for Self-Management—Posture and Body Mechanics box.
    B. Safety guidelines: see Teaching for Self-Management—Safety During Pregnancy box and the safety measures identified in Education for Self-Management section.

29. Feeding method decision making: see Preparation for Breastfeeding section, which identifies several reasons why breastfeeding may not be chosen; discuss how a nurse can help a pregnant woman/couple to overcome doubts they may have about breastfeeding.

30. Choices A, B, and E are correct; choices C and F are probable signs and choice D is a positive sign, diagnostic of pregnancy.

31. Choice C is correct; use Nägele's rule by subtracting 3 calendar months and adding 7 days and 1 year (if appropriate) to the first day of the last normal menstrual period, which in this case is November 9, 2014.

32. Choice D is correct; supine hypotension related to compression of the aorta and vena cava is being experienced; the first action is to remove the cause of the problem by turning the woman onto her side; this should alleviate the symptoms being experienced, including nausea; assessment of vital signs can occur after the woman's position is changed.

33. Choices A and D are correct; during this normal quiet period a woman focuses on her fantasy child as the attachment process is occurring; sexual desire is decreased during the first and third trimesters and increased in the second; ambivalence and mood swings are common responses when preparing for a new role and reacting to hormonal changes; safe passage and birth preparation are primary concerns during the third trimester; a woman's partner is usually the most important person.

34. Choices A, D, and E are correct; intake of at least 2 to 3 L per day is recommended; she does not have to reduce frequency of intercourse but rather void before and after intercourse and then drink a large glass of water; the effectiveness of cranberry juice has not been proven; additional methods of preventing UTIs include frequent, regular urination; good genital hygiene; and avoiding wearing tight-fitting jeans for long periods.

35. Choice D is correct; continuous support is critical and involves praise, encouragement, reassurance, comfort measures, physical contact, and explanations; the doula does not get involved in clinical tasks; she is not a substitute for the father but rather encourages his participation as a partner in supporting the laboring woman.

III. Thinking Critically

1. Health history interview: see Initial Visit and Follow-up Visits sections.
   A. Purpose of the health history interview:
      - Establish therapeutic relationship.
      - Planned time for purposeful communication to gather baseline data related to the woman's subjective appraisal of her health status and to gather objective information based on observation of the woman's affect, posture, body language, skin color, and other physical and emotional signs.
      - Update information and compare with baseline information during follow-up interviews.
   B. Write two questions for each component of initial health history interview: ensure that questions reflect principles of effective questioning; consider the need to ask follow-up questions to clarify and gather further information when a problem is identified.
   C. Write four questions for the follow-up health history interviews: focus on updating baseline information and asking questions related to anticipated events and expected changes for the woman's gestational age at the time of the visit.

2. Care of woman at initial visit who is anxious and unsure about prenatal care: answer should emphasize:
   - Establishing a therapeutic, trusting relationship so woman will feel comfortable continuing with prenatal care.
   - Teaching the woman about the importance of prenatal care for her health and that of her baby; determine if barriers are present that may limit participation in prenatal care.
   - Involving her boyfriend in the care process so he will encourage her participation in prenatal care; consider that the father of the baby is often considered to be the most significant support person.
   - Following guidelines for health history interview, physical examination, and laboratory testing; ensure privacy and comfort during the examination and teach her about how her body is changing and will continue to change with pregnancy.

- Evaluating the desire for this pregnancy and the need for community agency support.
3. Couple during first trimester—concerns and questions.
   A. Accuracy of EDB: reliability depends on the accuracy of date used and the regularity of woman's menstrual cycles; most women give birth within 1 week before or 1 week after the expected date of birth.
   B. Kegel exercises: use pelvic muscle exercises to maintain muscle tone and ability to support pelvic organs; see Kegel Exercises section of Education for Self-Care; see Chapter 5: Teaching for Self-Management—Kegel Exercises box.
   C. Effect of pregnancy on sexuality: see Sexual Counseling section, Teaching for Self-Management—Sexuality in Pregnancy box, and Fig. 14-18; emphasize that intercourse is safe as long as pregnancy is progressing normally and it is comfortable for the woman; sexual expression should be in tune with the woman's changing needs and emotions; inform that spotting can normally occur related to the fragility of the vaginal mucosa and cervix and that changes in positions and activities may be helpful as pregnancy progresses.
   D. Morning sickness: see Table 14-2 (first trimester section), Nursing Care Plan, and Box 14-6; fully assess what she is experiencing, then discuss why it happens, how long it will likely last, and relief measures that are safe and effective, including complementary and alternative approaches; also see Nutritional Discomforts section in Chapter 15.
4. Physical activity and exercise during pregnancy: see Physical Activity section of Education for Self-Management and Teaching for Self-Management—Exercise Tips for Pregnant Women box; assess her usual pattern of exercise and activity and consider their safety during pregnancy; discuss precautions and guidelines for safe, effective exercise; emphasize that moderate physical activity benefits her and her baby and will prepare her for the work of labor and birth; caution her to take note of the effects of exercise in terms of her temperature, heart rate, and feeling of well-being.
5. Nursing diagnoses, expected outcomes, and nursing measures for women in various situations during pregnancy.
   A. Risk for urinary tract infection related to lack of knowledge regarding changes of the renal system during pregnancy.
      - Woman will drink at least 2 to 3 L of fluids per day; will empty bladder at first urge.
      - Explain changes that occur in the renal system during pregnancy; increase fluid intake; use acid-ash–forming fluids; void frequently, including before going to bed to keep bladder empty; void before and after intercourse, then drink a full glass of water; perform good perineal hygiene and wear appropriate clothing; use lateral position to enhance renal perfusion and urine formation.
   B. Acute pain in lower back related to neuromuscular changes associated with pregnancy at 23 weeks of gestation.
      - Woman will experience lessening of lower back pain following implementation of suggested relief measures.
      - Explain basis for lower back pain and relief measures, including back massage, pelvic rock, and posture changes (see Teaching for Self-Management—Posture and Body Mechanics box, Table 14-2, and Fig. 14-12); encourage woman to change her footwear for better stability and safety.
   C. Anxiety related to lack of knowledge concerning the process of labor and birth and appropriate measures to cope with the pain and discomfort.
      - Couple will enroll in a childbirth education program in the seventh month of pregnancy.
      - Explain the childbirth process and describe the many nonpharmacologic and pharmacologic measures to relieve pain; discuss role of coach and possibility of hiring a doula; make a referral to a childbirth education program and assist with the preparation of a birth plan; discuss childbirth options and prebirth preparations (see Childbirth and Perinatal Education section).
6. Woman in the second trimester—questions and concerns: see Follow-up Visits and Education for Self-Management sections.
   A. Purpose of fundal height measurement: indirect assessment of how her fetus is growing.
   B. Determining fetal health status: discuss fetal heart rate (FHR) and let her listen; discuss fetal movement assessments and tell her how they are done.
   C. Clothing choices during pregnancy: see Clothing section; consider safety and comfort in terms of low-heeled shoes and nonrestrictive clothing.
   D. Gas and constipation: see Table 14-2 (second trimester section); assess problem and lifestyle factors that may be contributing to the problem; determine what she has tried so far; discuss why it occurs and appropriate relief measures (fluids, roughage, activity).
   E. Itchiness: if the woman is experiencing noninflammatory pruritus, use Table 14-2 (second trimester section) for basis of discomfort and relief measures; be sure to rule out rashes related to infection or allergic reactions.
   F. Travel during pregnancy: see Travel section; tell her that she may travel if her pregnancy is progressing normally; emphasize importance of staying hydrated, wearing seat belt and shoulder harness, doing breathing and lower extremity exercises, ambulating every hour for 15 minutes, and voiding every 2 hours.
7. Woman experiencing supine hypotension syndrome: see Emergency—Supine Hypotension box.
   A. Explanation of assessment findings: supine hypotension.

B. Immediate action: turn her onto her side and maintain the position until vital signs stabilize and signs and symptoms diminish; place wedge to maintain a lateral tilt, then continue the assessment; when completed, help her to rise slowly to an upright position and observe for signs of postural hypotension.

8. Woman during third trimester—questions and concerns.
   A. Nipple condition for breastfeeding: see Preparation for Breastfeeding section and Figs. 14-9 and 14-10 for several measures she can use and what to avoid.
   B. Ankle edema: see Table 14-2 (third trimester section); discuss basis of the edema and encourage use of lower extremity exercises and elevation of legs periodically during the day (Fig. 14-15); emphasize importance of fluid intake and sleeping in a lateral position (Fig. 14-13) to enhance kidney function, increasing the amount of excess fluid mobilized and excreted in urine.
   C. Leg cramps: see Table 14-2 (third-trimester section) and Fig. 14-16; discuss basis of leg cramps, then demonstrate relief measures such as pressing weight onto foot when standing or dorsiflexing the foot while lying in bed; avoid pointing the toes; ensure adequate intake of calcium.

9. Choosing a doula: see Doulas section in Perinatal Care Choices and Box 14-7 to formulate your answer; include relevant Internet sites to recommend to the couple.
   A. Role of doula: describe what a doula does; cite research that illustrates the benefits of using a doula for labor support; emphasize that the doula's role is to provide physical, emotional, and informational care and that her role does not involve the performance of clinical tasks.
   B. Finding a doula: community contacts, other health care professionals especially those involved in childbirth care or education, organizations such as DONA, and persons who have used a doula; emphasize the importance of starting early so that there is time to make the right choice; discuss questions to ask during an interview with a prospective doula and put these questions in writing so that the woman can refer to them during the interview.

10. Sibling reactions to mother's pregnancy: see Sibling Adaptation section in Preparing for Childbirth and Box 14-2, which provides tips for sibling preparation; emphasize importance of considering each child's developmental level; prepare children for prenatal events, time during hospitalization, and homecoming of the new baby; refer to sibling classes and encourage sibling visitation after birth; suggest books, DVDs, and Internet sites that parents could use to prepare their children for birth.

11. Expectant father concerned about wife's mood swings.
    A. Nursing diagnoses: deficient knowledge regarding pregnant spouse's mood changes related to lack of experience with pregnancy; Tom will explain basis for wife's mood swings and strategies he can use to cope with these changes and support his spouse.
    B. Nurse's response: see Maternal Adaptation section and Table 14-2 (first trimester section); discuss the basis for the mood swings and experiences during the first trimester, including ambivalence; identify measures he can use to support her.

12. Woman experiencing introspection: see Reordering Personal Relationships section; explain that she is concentrating on having a baby and forming a relationship with the fetus; emphasize her partner's important role as a caregiver and nurturer.

13. Birth plan development and deciding on a birth setting: see Birth Plan section and Box 14-7.
    ■ Purpose of birth plan: means of open communication about the childbirth process between the woman and her partner and with the health care providers in an effort to have a childbirth experience that meets their expectations and wishes as closely as possible; it is a tool that couples can use to stay in control and in this case to experience a more satisfying childbirth.
    ■ Guidelines for formation of birth plan: begin discussion early in pregnancy so that full consideration can be given to each option; identify components that should be included in the plan; facilitate decision making concerning the options available; recognize risk status implications for care options.
    ■ Topics for discussion and decision making: partner's role during childbirth and who will be present; setting for the birth; labor management measures, including pain control, comfort measures, positions, events at the birth, and newborn and postpartum care (e.g., celebratory activities, breastfeeding, mother-baby care).
    ■ Birth setting choice is an essential component of a birth plan.
    ■ Descriptions of each option, along with the criteria for use and the advantages and disadvantages.
    ■ Onsite visits and interaction with health care providers responsible for care at each site should be encouraged.
    ■ Recommend speaking to couples who gave birth in these settings to get their impressions.
    ■ Emphasize that the decision is theirs and that they should choose what is comfortable for them; their decision should be based on a full understanding of each option.

14. Home birth: see Home Birth section.
    A. Discuss decision-making process.
       ■ Fully review advantages and disadvantages of home birth so that an informed decision can be made and appropriate arrangements can be devised to enhance the advantages and offset the disadvantages.

- Recommend speaking to couples who have experienced a home birth.
  B. Preparation measures.
    - Preparation of home, including obtaining supplies and equipment and arranging for medical backup and transportation in the event of an emergency; measures to increase safety should be emphasized.
    - Choosing and preparing the persons who will be attending, including children and grandparents.

CHAPTER 15: MATERNAL AND FETAL NUTRITION

I. Learning Key Terms

1. Low birth weight (LBW)
2. Healthful diet before conception
3. Folate (folic acid); neural tube defects; 0.4 mg (400 mcg)
4. Dietary Reference Intakes (DRIs)
5. BMI; underweight; normal weight; overweight (high); obese
6. Ketonuria; preterm labor
7. Physiologic anemia
8. Lactose intolerance
9. Pica; clay; soil; laundry starch; ice/freezer frost; baking powder; baking soda; cornstarch
10. Food cravings
11. Listeriosis
12. Anthropometric measurements
13. MyPlate
14. Morning sickness (nausea and vomiting of pregnancy)
15. Hyperemesis gravidarum
16. Constipation
17. Pyrosis (heartburn)

II. Reviewing Key Concepts

18. Indicate nutrient requirements during pregnancy and food or fluid sources for each: see separate sections for each nutrient in Nutrient Needs During Pregnancy section and Table 15-1 to complete the table.
19. Indicators of nutritional risk: see Box 15-3 to identify the five risk indicators; consider the woman's lifestyle, age, culture, and socioeconomic status when developing risk-reduction strategies.
20. Cite pregnancy-related risks associated with nutritional problems: see Weight Gain, Pattern of Weight Gain, Hazards of Restricting Adequate Weight Gain, and Excessive Weight Gain sections and Box 15-3 to complete this activity.
21. Guidelines for strict vegetarians during pregnancy: see Vegetarian Diets section.
    - Begin by determining exactly what the woman eats.
    - Keep in mind that these diets tend to be low in vitamin B$_{12}$, protein, iron, calcium, zinc, and perhaps calories; supplements may be needed.

- Food needs to be combined to ensure that all essential amino acids are provided.
22. Signs of good and inadequate nutrition: see Table 15-6 for several signs of good and inadequate nutrition.
23. Determining recommended pregnancy weight gain pattern: see Weight Gain and Pattern of Weight Gain sections and Table 15-2 to determine weight gain patterns based on each woman's BMI; keep in mind that each woman should gain 1 to 2 kg in the first trimester; weight gain per week is recommended for the second and third trimesters.
    a. June: BMI 21 (normal weight); total 11.3 to 15.9 kg; 0.4 kg/week
    b. Alice: BMI 30 (obese); total 5 to 9.1 kg; 0.23 kg/week
    c. Ann: BMI 17 (underweight); total 12.7 to 18.1 kg; 0.5 kg/week
24. Choices A, D, and E are correct; oranges and tomatoes contain vitamin C, which enhances iron absorption.
25. Choice C is correct; BMI indicates that this woman is obese; she should not consider a weight loss regimen until healing is complete in the postpartum period; she should gain 5.0 to 9.1 kg; increase in calories should reflect energy expenditure of the pregnancy during the third trimester, which would be approximately 462 kcal.
26. Choice B is correct; BMI indicates that this woman is at a normal weight; total gain should be 11.3 to 15.9 kg, representing a gain of 0.4 kg/week and 1.6 kg/month during the second and third trimesters.
27. Choice C is correct; small, frequent meals are better tolerated than large meals that distend the stomach; hunger can worsen nausea; therefore meals should not be skipped; dry, starchy foods should be eaten in the morning and at other times during the day when nausea occurs; fried, fatty, and spicy foods should be avoided; a bedtime snack is recommended to avoid morning hunger.
28. Choices B, D, and E are correct; legumes are a good source of folic acid along with whole grains and fortified cereals, oranges, papaya, asparagus, liver, and green leafy vegetables; choices A, C, and F are not good sources of folic acid, though they do supply other important nutrients for pregnancy (see Box 15-1).
29. Choice A is correct; iron should not be taken at the same time as tea because tea decreases the absorption of iron, as do bran, coffee, milk, egg yolks, and oxalates in spinach and Swiss chard; vitamin C–containing foods such as citrus fruit and tomatoes enhance absorption of iron.
30. Choice A is correct; up to 5.5 to 6.5 oz. total are suggested from the protein foods group during pregnancy; choices B, C, and D are all appropriate for pregnancy (see Table 15-4).

304

Answer Key

Copyright © 2016 by Elsevier Inc. All rights reserved.
Copyright © 2012, 2007, 2004, 2000 by Mosby, an affiliate of Elsevier Inc. All rights reserved.

III. Thinking Critically

1. Nutrition and weight gain concerns during pregnancy.
   A. Concern regarding amount of recommended weight gain during pregnancy.
      - Identify the tissues and structures in the body (e.g., fetus, placenta, fluids, etc.) responsible for maternal weight gain (see Table 15-2); use Table 15-2 and Fig. 15-2 to illustrate how the weight gain is distributed over weeks of gestation.
      - Discuss effect of maternal weight gain on fetal growth and development; association between inadequate maternal weight gain and low birth weight and infant morbidity and mortality.
      - Discuss weight gain total and pattern recommended for a woman with a BMI of 24 (normal weight); discuss appropriate measures for weight loss after birth.
   B. Eating for two during pregnancy.
      - Place emphasis on quality of food that meets nutritional requirements, not on quantity of food.
      - Discuss expected weight gain total and pattern for a woman with an overweight BMI of 27.
      - Excessive weight gain during pregnancy may be difficult to lose after pregnancy and could lead to chronic obesity; excessive fetal size and childbirth problems could also result.
   C. Vitamin supplementation during pregnancy: determine what and how much she takes; compare to recommendations for pregnancy; discuss potential problems with toxicity, especially with overuse of fat-soluble vitamins.
   D. Factors that increase nutritional needs during pregnancy: growth and development of uterine-placental-fetal unit, expansion of maternal blood volume and RBCs, mammary changes, increased basal metabolic rate (BMR); discuss how she can reduce her fast-food intake during the week.
   E. Weight reduction diets during pregnancy.
      - BMI indicates overweight status; a gain of 6.8 to 11.3 kg during pregnancy is recommended.
      - Discuss hazards of inadequate caloric intake during pregnancy in terms of growth and development of fetus and pregnancy-related structures; effect of ketoacidosis and ketonuria.
      - Discuss quality foods and development of good nutritional habits to be used during the postpartum period as part of a sensible weight loss program.
      - Discuss importance of exercise and activity during pregnancy.
   F. Reduction of water intake: discuss importance of fluid to meet demands of pregnancy-related changes, regulate temperature, and prevent constipation and UTIs; consider possible association between dehydration and preterm labor and oligohydramnios.
   G. Lactose intolerance: discuss basis for problem; reduce lactose intake by using lactose-free products, nondairy sources of calcium, and calcium supplements; take lactase supplements; see Calcium section and Box 15-4.
   H. Weight loss lactation: discuss weight loss patterns with lactation; emphasize that pregnancy fat stores are used during lactation with a resultant weight loss; inform her of increased need for nutrients, calories, and fluids, which are used up with lactogenesis.
   I. Nutrition guidelines for lactation: see Nutritional Needs During Lactation section and Table 15-1 for details regarding nutritional requirements for the breastfeeding woman.
2. Taking iron supplements effectively: see Iron section in Nutrient Needs, Teaching for Self-Management—Iron Supplementation box and Table 15-1 for iron sources.
   - Discuss importance of iron.
   - Emphasize importance of vitamin C for iron absorption; discuss food sources high in iron and vitamin C.
   - Discuss ways to take iron supplements to enhance absorption and minimize side effects including gastrointestinal (GI) upset and constipation.
3. Nursing measures appropriate for each nursing diagnosis: see appropriate section for each nutrition-related discomfort in Coping with Nutritional-Related Discomforts of Pregnancy section.
   A. Imbalanced nutrition: less than body requirements related to inadequate intake associated with nausea and vomiting: see Nausea and Vomiting section and Box 15-6 for several relief measures.
   B. Constipation related to decreased intestinal motility associated with effects of increased progesterone and enlarging uterus: see Constipation section; begin with a discussion of woman's usual prepregnant bowel elimination patterns and practices; in your teaching include adequate fluid, roughage, and fiber intake, exercise and activity, and regular time for elimination.
   C. Acute pain related to reflux of gastric contents into esophagus associated with progesterone effect on gastric motility: see Pyrosis section; identify foods that help her to avoid pyrosis and those that cause her to experience it; discuss effectiveness of small frequent meals, drinking fluids between and not with meals, avoiding spicy foods, and remaining upright after eating.
4. Native-American woman—nutritional needs.
   A. Counseling approach.
      - Assess her current nutritional status and habits; obtain a diet history (see Box 15-5).
      - Analyze current patterns as a basis for menu planning.
      - Discuss weight gain pattern for an underweight woman.

- Use a variety of teaching methods; keep woman actively involved.
- Emphasize importance of good nutrition for herself and her newborn.

B. Menu plan: use Table 15-7 for Native-American foods and Table 15-4 for servings of required nutrients for a 1-day menu; distribute throughout day—meals and snacks.

ANSWER KEY UNIT IV

CHAPTER 16: LABOR AND BIRTH PROCESSES

I. Learning Key Terms

1. Passenger (fetus and placenta); passageway; powers; position of the mother; psychologic response
2. Fontanels
3. Molding
4. Presentation; cephalic; breech; shoulder
5. Presenting part; occiput; chin (mentum); sacrum; scapula
6. Vertex presentation
7. Fetal lie; longitudinal (vertical) lie; transverse (oblique, horizontal) lie
8. Attitude; general flexion
9. Biparietal diameter
10. Suboccipitobregmatic diameter
11. Fetal position
12. Engagement
13. Station; centimeters; descent
14. Effacement
15. Dilation
16. Lightening ("dropping")
17. Involuntary uterine contractions; effacement; dilation; descent
18. Frequency; duration; intensity
19. Voluntary bearing-down efforts (abdominal muscle contraction)
20. Bloody show
21. Cardinal movements of labor (mechanism of labor); engagement; descent; flexion; internal rotation; extension; external rotation (restitution); expulsion
22. Ferguson reflex
23. Regular uterine contractions; effacement and dilation of cervix; latent; active; transition
24. Cervix is fully dilated; birth of the fetus
25. Birth of the fetus; placenta is delivered
26. Recovery following birth
27. Maternal position; maternal blood pressure; uterine contractions; umbilical cord blood flow

II. Reviewing Key Concepts

28. Label illustrations.
    Fetal skull: A. mentum (chin); B. occipitofrontal diameter; C. frontal bone (sinciput); D. suboccipito-bregmatic diameter; E. parietal bone (vertex); F. occipitomental diameter; G. occiput; H. sagittal suture; I. lambdoid suture; J. posterior fontanel; K. biparietal diameter; L. coronal suture; M. frontal suture; N. anterior fontanel (bregma)
    Maternal pelvis: A. symphysis pubis; B. anteroposterior diameter of inlet; C. transverse diameter of the inlet; D. sacral promontory; E. sacrum; F. sacroiliac joint; G. ischial spine; H. pubic bone; I. sacrotuberous ligament; J. pubic arch; K. ischial tuberosity; L. coccyx; M. sacroiliac joint

29. Indicate presentation, presenting part, position, lie, and attitude represented by each illustration.
    A. Cephalic (vertex), occiput, LOA, longitudinal, flexion
    B. Cephalic (vertex), occiput, LOT, longitudinal, flexion
    C. Cephalic (vertex), occiput, LOP, longitudinal, flexion
    D. Cephalic (vertex), occiput, ROA, longitudinal, flexion
    E. Cephalic (vertex), occiput, ROT, longitudinal, flexion
    F. Cephalic (vertex), occiput, ROP, longitudinal, flexion
    G. Cephalic (face), mentum, LMA, longitudinal, extension
    H. Cephalic (face), mentum, RMP, longitudinal, extension
    I. Cephalic (face), mentum, RMA, longitudinal, extension
    J. Breech, sacrum, LSA, longitudinal, flexion
    K. Breech, sacrum, LSP, longitudinal, flexion
    L. Shoulder, scapula, ScA, transverse, flexion

30. Choices A, C, D, and E are correct; the presenting part is 1 cm above the ischial spines as indicated by the "−1"; attitude is flexion of head and neck, as indicated by the occiput ("O") as the presenting part; the lie is longitudinal, as indicated by the cephalic presentation; effacement is 75% complete and is 3 cm dilated, requiring 7 cm more for full dilation to 10 cm.

31. Choices A, C, and D are correct; white blood cell count increases; a decrease in blood glucose and proteinuria of 1+ can be expected; see Box 16-2.

32. Choice D is correct; quickening refers to the woman's first perception of fetal movement at 16 to 20 weeks of gestation; lightening accompanied by urinary frequency and weight loss of 0.5 to 1 kg occur to signal that the onset of labor is near; backache, stronger Braxton Hicks, and bloody show are also noted; see Box 16-1.

III. Thinking Critically

1. Teaching a class on the process of labor.
   A. Describe the five Ps and how they affect the process of childbirth: see Factors of Labor section and Chapter 19; consider the factors of passenger, passage, powers, position of mother, and psychologic response of mother; be sure to identify the visual aids you would use to facilitate learning.

B. Explain how the cardinal movements of labor facilitate birth: see Mechanism of Labor section in Process of Labor; describe engagement and descent, flexion, internal rotation, extension, external rotation and restitution, and expulsion.

2. Analysis of vaginal examinations.
   - Exam I: ROP (right occiput posterior, cephalic [vertex] presentation, longitudinal lie, flexed attitude), –1 (station at 1 cm above the ischial spines), 50% effaced, 3 cm dilated.
   - Exam II: RMA (right mentum anterior, cephalic [face] presentation, longitudinal lie, extended attitude), 0 (station at the ischial spines, engaged), 25% effaced, 2 cm dilated.
   - Exam III: LST (left sacrum transverse, breech presentation, longitudinal lie, flexed attitude), +1 (station at 1 cm below the ischial spines), 75% effaced, 6 cm dilated.
   - Exam IV: OA (occiput anterior, cephalic [vertex] presentation, longitudinal lie, flexed attitude), +3 (station at 3 cm below the ischial spines near or on the perineum), 100% effaced, 10 cm (fully) dilated.

3. Woman with questions and concerns about process of labor.
   A. Onset of labor: see Onset of Labor section; explain in simple terms the interaction of maternal and fetal hormones, uterine distention, placental aging, increase in prostaglandin level, increase in estrogen level, and decrease in progesterone.
   B. Signs of preceding labor: see Signs Preceding Labor section and Box 16-1 for a discussion of all of the signs that occur prior to the onset of labor; keep in mind that she is a primigravida.
   C. Position changes during labor; see Position of Laboring Woman section; answer should include each of the following:
      - Emphasize that the position of the woman is one of the 5 Ps of labor.
      - Discuss each position and describe its effect.
      - Demonstrate each position and have her practice each of them with her partner.
      - Emphasize the beneficial effects of ambulation and changing positions on fetus, circulation, comfort, and progress; tell her to express how she feels in each position to ensure that she is as comfortable as possible.

CHAPTER 17: PAIN MANAGEMENT

I. Learning Key Terms

1. B, 2. F, 3. H, 4. A, 5. G, 6. J, 7. M, 8. D, 9. I, 10. L, 11. C, 12. E, 13. K
14. Visceral pain
15. Somatic pain
16. Referred pain
17. Pain threshold
18. Pain tolerance
19. Gate control
20. Beta-endorphins
21. Slow-paced breathing
22. Modified-paced breathing
23. Deep cleansing breath
24. Patterned-paced (pant-blow) breathing
25. Hyperventilation; respiratory alkalosis
26. Effleurage
27. Counterpressure
28. Water therapy (hydrotherapy)
29. Transcutaneous electrical nerve stimulation (TENS)
30. Acupressure
31. Acupuncture
32. Therapeutic touch
33. Hypnosis
34. Biofeedback
35. Aromatherapy
36. Intradermal water block

II. Reviewing Key Concepts

37. Theoretic basis for effectiveness of massage, stroking, music, and imagery in reducing sensation of pain: discuss the gate-control theory of pain; see Childbirth Preparation and Nonpharmacologic Management of Pain and Gate-Control Theory of Pain sections; each of the methods listed is an example of the gate-control technique.

38. Complete table related to nerve block analgesic and anesthetic methods: see appropriate sections in Pharmacologic Management of Pain for each method cited in the table.

39. Choice C is correct; beginning in active labor reduces the risk that labor will slow down; there is no limit to the time a woman can stay in the tub; woman can and should change her position while in the bath, using lateral and hand-and-knees positions when indicated; there is no evidence indicating an increased risk for infection when membranes are ruptured; however, tubs must be carefully cleansed; contractions may slow if bath is begun in the latent phase.

40. Choice B is correct; naloxone hydrochloride (Narcan) is an opioid antagonist; promethazine (Phenergan) is a phenothiazine that can decrease anxiety and nausea but it has been found to diminish the effectiveness of opioids in terms of pain relief; fentanyl citrate (Sublimaze) is an opioid agonist analgesic.

41. Choice D is correct; nalbuphine hydrochloride (Nubain) is an opioid agonist-antagonist analgesic; a 10-mg dose is appropriate for IV administration; the antagonist component of this medication could precipitate withdrawal symptoms if the woman is opioid dependent.

42. Choice C is correct; as an opioid antagonist it will reverse the effects of the opioid agonist analgesic administered for pain; maternal adverse reactions include hypotension or hypertension, tachycardia, hyperventilation, nausea, and vomiting; Narcan is administered intravenously at a dose of 0.4 to 2.0 mg depending on the amount of opioid agonist analgesic

given and the degree of CNS depression; it may be repeated at 2- to 3-minute intervals if needed for adequate reversal; Narcan is only given parenterally.

43. Choices A, B, D, and F are correct; position with a curved back separates the vertebrae and facilitates administration of the anesthetic; alternating lateral positions after administration will prevent supine hypotension; she should be encouraged to empty her bladder every 2 hours; because the dura is not punctured, there is no leakage of cerebrospinal fluid, making spinal headache rare; the dosage can be adjusted to allow her to push during the second stage of labor.

44. Choices A, C, and D are correct; sneezing, rhinorrhea, sweating, lacrimation, and mydriasis also occur; see Signs of Potential Complications—Maternal Opioid Abstinence Syndrome box.

45. Choice B is correct; changing the woman to a lateral position will enhance cardiac output and raise her BP; because compression of the abdominal aorta and vena cava is removed, the other actions will follow; see Emergency—Maternal Hypotension with Decreased Placental Perfusion box.

III. Thinking Critically

1. Factors influencing nursing diagnosis of acute pain: see Factors Influencing Pain Response section for a discussion of many factors, such as endorphin level, anxiety and fear, culture, previous experience, knowledge and expectations, childbirth preparation, available support and comfort, physical condition of the woman at the onset of labor, history of substance abuse or sexual abuse, and environmental factors.

2. Systemic analgesic administration to a woman in labor: see Systemic Analgesia section of Pharmacologic Pain Management and Medication Guide box.
   A. Approach nurse should follow in pain relief: consider importance of a full assessment of this woman regarding her pain and what this assessment should include.
   B. Administering meperidine.
      1. Maternal reactions: discuss effect on pain and relaxation as well as on her vital signs, including breathing and blood pressure.
      2. Factors influencing effect of systemic analgesics on fetus/newborn: maternal dosage, characteristics of the specific drug, route, time administered during labor.
      3. Fetal/newborn effects: describe CNS depression as a result of the direct effect of the drug when it crosses the placenta and/or the indirect effect of the mother, resulting in respiratory depression, decreased alertness, and delayed sucking after birth.

3. IV administration of systemic analgesics as the preferred route: see Care Management—Pharmacologic Interventions section.
   A. Explanation of the rationale: include in answer that IV administration results in a faster, more predictable onset of action; a higher level of analgesia occurs at a lower dosage.
   B. Guidelines for administration: answer should include port used, timing of administration in terms of labor progress and occurrence of contractions, and assessment measures to complete before and after administration

4. Explaining basis of childbirth pain to expectant fathers: see Neurologic Origins of Pain section and Box 17-1; describe why pain occurs and its very real basis; discuss visceral, somatic, and referred pain, how women experience the pain, and factors that influence the experience; identify measures they can use to help their partners reduce and cope with the pain.

5. Nurse sensitivity to client's pain experience.
   A. Experience and expression of pain in labor: see Perception of Pain, Expression of Pain, and Factors Influencing the Pain Response sections; discuss physiologic effects, sensory responses, emotional responses, and affective expressions.
   B. Measures to alter perception of pain: see Perception of Pain and Nonpharmacologic Management of Pain sections; consider the specific factors influencing each woman's response when determining measures to use.

6. Working with couple with unrealistic, inaccurate views regarding pain and pain relief during labor.
   ■ Inform couple regarding the basis of pain and, as a stressor, its potentially adverse effects on the maternal-fetal unit and the progress of labor.
   ■ Discuss a variety of nonpharmacologic and pharmacologic measures that are safe and effective to use during labor and that can have beneficial effects on the maternal-fetal unit and can enhance the progress of labor.
   ■ Emphasize that the mother and fetus will be thoroughly assessed before, during, and after use of any measure to ensure safety.

7. Benefits of water therapy: see Water Therapy (Hydrotherapy) section.
   ■ Describe the beneficial effects of water therapy and how it can facilitate the labor process and create a more positive experience with less use of pharmacologic measures and fewer complications; use research findings to substantiate these claims.
   ■ Describe the successful experiences of other agencies that have implemented water therapy; state how it has affected the number of births.
   ■ Use favorable reports of women who have used water therapy; consider how this could affect other women preparing for childbirth.
   ■ Prepare a cost-benefit analysis.

8. Occurrence of hypotension after administration of epidural block during labor: see Emergency—Maternal Hypotension with Decreased Placental Perfusion box.
   A. What is being experienced by this woman: maternal hypotension related to effect of epidural

anesthesia/analgesia (block); fully describe why this happens and its effect on the maternal-fetal unit.

B. Nursing diagnosis: ineffective tissue perfusion to placenta related to maternal hypotension associated with epidural block anesthesia.

C. Immediate nursing actions: in answer, take a data, action, response approach; discuss measures used to enhance perfusion and ensure oxygenation, then determine response to actions taken; consider when to notify primary health care provider.

9. Woman receiving an epidural block: see Epidural Analgesia/Anesthesia [Block] and Care Management—Pharmacologic Interventions sections and Boxes 17-5 and 17-6.

A. Assessment prior to induction of block: describe how you would determine status of maternal-fetal unit and progress of labor in terms of phase and contraindications to use.

B. Preparation measures: answer should reflect actions related to explanation of procedures used, informed consent, hydration, and bladder condition.

C. Positions for induction: lateral (modified Sims with back curved forward) or sitting with back curved forward to separate vertebrae; assist her with assuming and maintaining the position without movement during the induction; it is important to avoid severe spinal flexion.

D. Nursing management during the epidural block: include in the outline assessment of the response, maintenance of fluid balance, assistance with elimination and positioning, and prevention of complications.

CHAPTER 18: FETAL ASSESSMENT DURING LABOR

I. Learning Key Terms

1. I, 2. H, 3. G, 4. J, 5. F, 6. C, 7. B, 8. D, 9. E, 10. A, 11. K
12. Hypoxemia
13. Hypoxia
14. Intermittent auscultation
15. Ultrasound transducer; maximal intensity of FHR
16. Tocotransducer (tocodynamometer); fundus above the umbilicus
17. Spiral electrode
18. Intrauterine pressure catheter (IUPC)
19. Fetal scalp stimulation; vibroacoustic stimulation
20. Amnioinfusion
21. Oligohydramnios
22. Anhydramnios
23. Tocolysis; terbutaline (Brethine)
24. Umbilical cord acid-base determination
25. Intrauterine resuscitation; supplemental oxygen; maternal position change; increasing IV infusion rate

II. Reviewing Key Concepts

26. Factors that affect fetal oxygen supply and characteristics of FHR and uterine activity.

A. Factors that can reduce fetal oxygen supply: see Fetal Response section for a discussion of these factors.

B. Characteristics of Category I FHR patterns: see Fetal Response section, Table 18-1, and Box 18-1.

C. Characteristics of Category II FHR patterns: see Fetal Response section, Table 18-1, and Box 18-1.

D. Characteristics of Category III FHR patterns: see Fetal Response section, Table 18-1, and Box 18-1.

E. Characteristics of normal and abnormal uterine activity: see Table 18-1.

27. 30 minutes; 15 minutes
28. 15 minutes; 5 minutes
29. Baseline rate; baseline variability; accelerations; decelerations; changes or trends over time

30. Legal responsibilities related to fetal monitoring during childbirth: see Nurse Alert in Intermittent Auscultation section and Legal Tip—Fetal Monitoring Standards; evaluate FHR pattern at frequency that reflects professional standards, agency policy, and condition of maternal-fetal unit; consider the correct interpretation of FHR patterns in terms of Categories; take appropriate action; evaluate response to actions taken; notify primary health care provider in a timely fashion; know the chain of command if a dispute about interpretation occurs; document assessment findings, actions, and responses.

31. Choice D is correct; the average resting tone during labor should be 10 mm Hg; choices A, B, and C are all findings within the expected ranges.

32. Choices C and F are correct; Leopold maneuvers are used to locate the PMI for correct placement of the ultrasound transducer; the tocotransducer is always placed over the fundus; the ultrasound transducer's position needs to change with fetal movement; the tocotransducer cannot assess intensity of contractions; therefore periodic palpation is an essential assessment measure; effleurage can be used around the transducers or on other parts of the woman's body.

33. Choices B, D, and E are correct; the baseline rate should be 110 to 160 beats/minute; accelerations should occur with fetal movement; no late deceleration pattern of any magnitude is normal (reassuring), especially if it is repetitive or uncorrectable; early deceleration patterns are expected findings when fetal head compression by the cervix occurs.

34. Choice C is correct; the FHR increases as the maternal core body temperature elevates; therefore tachycardia is the pattern exhibited; it is often a clue of intrauterine infection because maternal fever is often the first sign; diminished variability reflects hypoxia, variable decelerations are characteristic of cord compression, and early decelerations are characteristic of head compression by the cervix.

309

35. Choice B is correct; the pattern described is an early deceleration pattern, which is considered to be benign, requiring no action other than documentation of the finding; changing a woman's position and notifying the physician would be appropriate if abnormal (nonreassuring) signs such as late or variable decelerations were occurring; prolapse of cord is associated with variable decelerations as a result of cord compression.

36. Choice B is correct; see Box 18-5 for the rationale.

III. Thinking Critically

1. Intermittent auscultation to assess fetal status during labor: see Intermittent Auscultation section and Figs. 18-1 and 18-2.
   A. State advantages and disadvantages.
      - Advantages: high-touch/low-tech approach, natural method facilitating activity, comfortable, noninvasive.
      - Disadvantages: inconvenient and time consuming, increased anxiety if nurse has difficulty locating PMI, less information about FHR pattern is obtained, less accurate.
   B. Protocol to follow: cite the specific guidelines that should be used; see Box 18-2.

2. Nonreassuring pattern noted on evaluation of a monitor tracing: see Nursing Management of Abnormal Patterns section and Box 18-8; evaluate the tracing according to the five essential components and implement intrauterine resuscitation measures as appropriate; actions most often involve repositioning the mother, administering oxygen, altering rate of IV, discontinuing oxytocin (Pitocin), assessing for possible causes, notifying primary health care provider, and preparing for emergency treatment.

3. Woman concerned about use of external monitoring to assess her fetus and labor.
   A. Client and family teaching when EFM is used: see Box 18-9 and Client and Family Teaching section.
      - Discuss how fetus responds to labor and how the monitor will assess these responses.
      - Explain the advantages of monitoring.
      - Show her a monitor strip and explain what it reveals; tell her how to use the strip to help her with breathing techniques.
   B. Nursing care measures for woman being monitored externally: see Care Management section, including Client and Family Teaching and Documentation and Boxes 18-7 and 18-9 for a detailed outline related to assessing tracings and maternal responses, palpation of contractions, and caring for woman in terms of comfort, changing position, transducer placement and site care, and keeping her and her family informed about fetal and maternal status and progress of labor.

4. Woman whose labor is being induced and monitored externally.
   A. Pattern described and causative factors: late deceleration patterns as a result of uteroplacental insufficiency associated with intense uterine contractions, supine position (supine hypotension), and placental aging related to postterm gestation of 43 weeks (see Figs. 18-8, 18-15, and 18-16).
   B. Nursing interventions: see Nursing Management of Abnormal Patterns, Table 18-3, and Boxes 18-5 and 18-8; discontinue oxytocin to stop stimulation of contractions but continue primary infusion; change to lateral position and elevate legs to enhance uteroplacental perfusion; administer oxygen via mask to increase oxygen availability to fetus; assess response to actions and notify primary health care provider; see Documentation section for guidelines related to recording findings organized around data, action, and response.

5. Evaluation of monitor tracing following rupture of membranes.
   A. Nurse should be alert for variable deceleration pattern; see Variable Deceleration section and Figs. 18-17 and 18-18.
   B. Actions to take if variable decelerations occur: see Nursing Management of Abnormal Patterns section and Boxes 18-6 and 18-8.

CHAPTER 19: NURSING CARE OF THE FAMILY DURING LABOR AND BIRTH

I. Learning Key Terms

1. Regular uterine contractions; effacement; dilation; mucous plug
2. 3; 6; 8; 4; 7; 3; 6; 20; 40; 8; 10
3. Infant is born; dilation; effacement; baby's birth; latent; active pushing (descent); cervix
4. Birth of the baby; placenta is expelled; fundus; discoid; globular ovoid; gush of dark blood; lengthening of umbilical cord; vaginal fullness; fetal membranes
5. 1 to 2 hours
6. Emergency Medical Treatment and Active Labor Act (EMTALA)
7. Partogram
8. Doula
9. Lithotomy
10. P, 11. F, 12. G, 13. J, 14. H, 15. B, 16. M, 17. A, 18. Q, 19. E, 20. K, 21. N, 22. D, 23. O, 24. C, 25. I, 26. R, 27. L
28. Uterine contractions
29. Increment
30. Acme
31. Decrement
32. Frequency
33. Intensity
34. Duration
35. Resting tone
36. Interval
37. Bearing-down effort

II. Reviewing Key Concepts

38. Assessing uterine contractions using palpation: see Assessment of Uterine Contractions section; place hand on fundus to time several contractions to establish a pattern of frequency and duration; palpate entire uterus periodically to note differences in tone; use comparisons of tip of nose, chin, and forehead to gauge intensity and tone during the peak of a contraction and during the period of rest.

39. Admission of woman in labor: see Assessment section of Care Management, First Stage of Labor section and Tables 19-1 and 19-2.
    A. Information from prenatal record: see Prenatal Data section; include such information as age, weight gain, health status and medical problems during pregnancy, past and present obstetric history (gravida, para), including outcomes and problems encountered, laboratory and diagnostic test results, EDB, and baseline data from pregnancy, including vital signs and FHR.
    B. Information regarding status of labor: see Teaching for Self-Management—How to Distinguish True Labor from False Labor box; factors distinguishing false from true labor, uterine contractions (onset, characteristics), show, status of membranes, fetal movement, discomfort (location, characteristics), and any other signs of the onset of labor experienced.
    C. Information regarding current health status: health problems, respiratory status, allergies, character and time of last oral intake, and emotional status.

40. Signs of potential complications during labor: see Signs of Complications box.

41. Labor positions and their advantages: see Box 19-8 and Ambulation and Positioning section in Nursing Care—First Stage of Labor.

42. Critical maternal-fetal factors to assess during first stage of labor: see appropriate sections that discuss general systems assessment, vital signs, Leopold maneuvers, assessment of FHR and pattern, assessment of uterine contractions, vaginal examination, and tests for ruptured membranes; see Table 19-1, Boxes 19-1, 19-3, 19-5, and 19-6, and Physical Examination section.
    ■ Maternal factors: vital signs, uterine activity, cervical changes, show/bleeding/amniotic fluid, behavior, appearance, mood, energy level, and use of childbirth preparation methods.
    ■ Fetal factors: FHR pattern, activity level, progress in cardinal movements of labor, and passage of meconium.

43. Laboratory and diagnostic tests during labor: see Laboratory and Diagnostic Tests section in Assessment, First Stage of Labor; complete blood count (CBC), blood type and Rh factor, analysis of urine, dipstick for protein, glucose, acetone, Nitrazine and ferning tests for amniotic fluid; additional tests such as human immunodeficiency virus (HIV) or drug screening and vaginal cultures may be done depending on state laws and maternal condition.

44. Factors influencing duration of second stage of labor: use of regional anesthesia such as epidural block; quality of bearing-down efforts and positions used; parity; size, presentation, and position of fetus; maternal pelvic adequacy; maternal physical status, including energy level; and support measures provided.

45. Second stage positions: see Maternal Position section and Figs. 19-14, 19-15, and 19-16; describe squatting, side-lying, semirecumbent, standing, and hands-and-knees positions.

46. Encouraging breastfeeding during the fourth stage of labor: stimulates the production of oxytocin to contract the uterus and decrease blood loss; takes advantage of newborn's alert state to interact with the newborn, facilitates the process of attachment, and enhances the success of breastfeeding because the newborn is ready to feed and success is likely; colostrum stimulates peristalsis, thereby facilitating excretion of bilirubin in meconium; be sure to provide support, privacy, and positive reinforcement; keep breastfeeding period short related to maternal fatigue; see Fourth Stage of Labor—Care of Family section.

47. Choice A is correct; although choices B, C, and D are all important questions, the first question should gather information regarding whether or not the woman is in labor.

48. Choice C is correct; pH of amniotic fluid is alkaline at 6.5 or higher, ferning is noted when examining fluid with a microscope, and the fluid is relatively odorless; a strong odor is strongly suggestive of infection; white flecks indicate vernix caseosa.

49. Choices A, B, D, and E are correct; pain of true labor is usually felt in the lower back radiating to the lower portion of the abdomen.

50. Choice C is correct; O, or occiput, indicates a vertex presentation with the neck fully flexed and the occiput in the right anterior pelvic segment (R, A) of the woman's pelvis; the station is 2 cm below the ischial spines (+2); the woman is in the active phase of labor, as indicated by 4 cm of dilation, and effacement is 75%; the lie is longitudinal because the head (cephalic/vertex) is presenting.

51. Choice B is correct; research has indicated that enemas are not needed during labor; according to research findings, choices A, C, and D have all been found to be beneficial and safe during pregnancy.

III. Thinking Critically

1. Woman thinking she is in labor calls nurse: see Teaching for Self-Management—How to Distinguish True Labor from False Labor box.
    A. Nursing approach: determine the status of her labor, asking her to describe what she is experiencing and comparing her description to the characteristics of true and false labor.

B. Write questions: questions should be clear, concise, open-ended, and directed toward distinguishing her labor status and determining the basis for action.

C. Instructions for home care of woman in latent labor: discuss comfort measures, distracting activities, measures to reduce anxiety, and measures to enhance the labor process; inform regarding assessment measures to determine progress and identify signs of problems, when and whom to call, and when to come to the hospital; the nurse should notify the woman's primary health care provider to confirm plan for woman to stay home until labor progresses; follow-up calls should be made to check on progress.

2. Women in first stage of labor at various phases.

A. Identify phase of labor: see Table 19-1 to determine phase; Denise (active); Teresa (transition); Danielle (latent).

B. Describe behavior and appearance: see Table 19-1 for descriptions; consider the phase of the woman's labor when formulating your answer.

C. Specify physical care and emotional support required: see First Stage of Labor—Nursing Care section and Table 19-3 for information regarding care measures required by each woman according to her phase of labor.

D. Support of husband who is fatigued and "stressed": see Nursing Care section—Supportive Care During Labor and Birth, Box 19-9, and Support of the Father or Partner section in Second Stage of Labor for several measures the nurse can use to help the support person of the laboring woman.

3. Procedure for locating point of maximum intensity (PMI) before auscultation of FHR or application of ultrasound transducer: realize that presentation and position affect location of PMI (see Box 19-5) and that Leopold maneuvers will facilitate location of this point; the PMI will change as the fetus progresses through the birth canal.

4. Woman experiencing difficulty with vaginal examinations during labor: see Vaginal Examination section in Physical Examination First Stage of Labor and Box 19-6.

A. Nurse's response to concern: explain purpose of the examination and the information that will be obtained during each examination in terms of the progress of labor and the status of the fetus; compare findings obtained from a vaginal examination with information on the monitor tracing.

B. Measures to enhance comfort and safety: deep breathing and gentleness during the examination; limit frequency and explain why each examination is needed, what you are doing, and the results you are obtaining; acknowledge her feelings and ensure her privacy; use infection control measures such as perineal care before and sterile gloves and lubricant to perform; never perform when active bleeding is present.

5. Actions and rationale when membranes rupture: immediate assessment of the FHR and pattern (prolapse of the cord could have occurred, compressing the cord and leading to hypoxia and variable deceleration patterns); vaginal examination (status of cervix, check for cord prolapse); assess fluid, document findings, and notify primary health care provider; cleanse perineum as soon as possible once status of fetus, mother, and labor is determined; strict infection control measures are critical after rupture because risk for infection increases.

6. Sara, a 17-year-old primigravida in the latent phase of labor.
   ▪ Nursing diagnosis: anxiety related to lack of knowledge and experience regarding the process of childbirth.
   ▪ Expected outcome: couple will actively participate in measures to enhance progress of labor as their anxiety level decreases.
   ▪ Nursing measures: provide full, simple explanations about each aspect of labor and care measures required as they occur; demonstrate and assist with simple breathing and relaxation techniques; make use of phases of labor to tailor health teaching (doing more during latent phase and less as labor progresses); model coaching and comfort measures that the father can perform.

7. Cultural and religious beliefs and practices during labor.

A. Questions to determine cultural and religious preferences: see Cultural Factors and Culture and Father Participation sections; use questions to determine support persons, gender of caregivers, acceptable comfort measures, oral intake, and positions to use.

B. Importance of determining cultural preferences: see Cultural Considerations box; consider preferences so couple can act in ways that are comfortable to enhance the progress of labor and their view of health care providers; such an approach demonstrates respect, concern, and caring and provides the couple with positive memories of their childbirth experience that will be helpful should they experience childbirth again.

8. Couple surprised by changes in approaches to facilitate the labor process.
   ▪ Discuss advantages of new approaches: internal locus of control (listening to her own body); maternal positions that enhance circulation to the placenta and apply the principle of gravity to facilitate and even shorten labor; new bearing-down efforts are safer (better oxygenation for fetus) and more effective (less tiring while applying effective force to facilitate descent).
   ▪ Use illustrations, model, and DVD to help couple learn techniques since she is still in latent labor.
   ▪ Demonstrate positions; help them to try.

312

Answer Key

Copyright © 2016 by Elsevier Inc. All rights reserved.
Copyright © 2012, 2007, 2004, 2000 by Mosby, an affiliate of Elsevier Inc. All rights reserved.

9. Home birth: see Mechanism of Birth Vertex Presentation, Immediate Assessment and Care of Newborn, and Fourth Stage sections and Boxes 19-10, 19-11, 19-12, 19-13, and 19-14.

  A. Measures to reassure and comfort: use eye contact; assume a relaxed, calm, and confident manner; explain what is happening and what you are going to be doing to help her give birth; inform her and her husband about what they will need to do.

  B. Crowning (guideline 6): break membranes; tell her to pant or blow to reduce force; use Ritgen maneuver to control delivery of the head without trauma to fetus or to maternal soft tissues

  C. Actions after appearance of head (guideline 7): check for cord around neck, support head during external rotation and restitution, and ease shoulders out one at a time with anterior first, then posterior.

  D. Prevention of neonatal heat loss (guidelines 11 and 12): dry baby; wrap up with mother; cover head.

  E. Infection control (Box 19-4): use Standard Precautions during childbirth, adapting to the home setting; use handwashing and clean materials and wear gloves if available.

  F. Prevention of bleeding (guideline 17): breastfeed; assess fundus and massage as needed; expel clots if present once fundus is firm; assess bladder and encourage voiding; allow placenta to separate naturally.

  G. Documentation (guideline 20): include date, time, assessment of mother and newborn, family present, events, blood loss, and Apgar score.

10. Criteria of effective pushing: see Maternal Position and Bearing-Down Efforts sections in Second Stage of Labor and Box 19-10; cleansing breaths to begin and end each contraction; open-glottis pushing with no breath holds longer than 6 to 8 seconds; frequent catch breaths; strong expiratory grunt; upright or lateral position.

11. Is an episiotomy needed? See Perineal Trauma Related to Childbirth section; compare episiotomies with lacerations in terms of tissue affected, long-term sequelae, healing process, and discomfort; compare reasons given for performing an episiotomy with what research findings demonstrate to be true.

12. Siblings at childbirth: include research findings regarding effect of sibling participation on family and on the sibling; consider the developmental readiness of the sibling and use developmental principles to prepare him or her for the experience; offer family and sibling classes to prepare them for participation in the birth process; evaluate parental comfort with this option; arrange for a support person to remain with the sibling during the entire childbirth process.

13. Primipara during the fourth stage of labor: see Fourth Stage of Labor section and Box 19-14.

  A. Essential nursing assessment and care measures during the fourth stage of labor: see Box 19-14 and Fourth Stage of Labor—Assessment section.

  B. Factors accounting for disinterest in newborn: exhaustion, discomfort, cultural beliefs, disappointment, difficult labor and birth, taking-in stage of recovery.

  C. Nursing measures to encourage maternal-newborn interaction: continue to assess response to newborn; provide time for close contact with newborn when she is more comfortable and rested; help her to meet her needs during the taking-in stage in terms of comfort, rest, and desire to review what happened during the process of labor and birth.

14. Breastfeeding in the fourth stage of labor: recognize that the reluctance is related to lack of experience, knowledge, and fatigue; take these factors into consideration when formulating answer, which should include measures to ensure privacy and to support and encourage her attempt; take note of signs of fatigue and keep the session short, praise her attempt, and explain the benefits of breastfeeding at this time for both her and her baby.

ANSWER KEY UNIT V

CHAPTER 20: POSTPARTUM PHYSIOLOGIC CHANGES

I. Learning Key Terms

1. Postpartal diaphoresis
2. Afterpains
3. Prolactin; oxytocin
4. Episiotomy
5. Atony
6. Hemorrhoid
7. Involution
8. Autolysis
9. Puerperium; fourth trimester
10. Diastasis recti abdominis
11. Lochia
12. Lochia rubra
13. Lochia serosa
14. Lochia alba
15. Engorgement
16. Subinvolution; retained placental fragments; infection
17. Exogenous oxytocin (Pitocin)
18. Dyspareunia
19. Kegel exercises
20. Colostrum
21. Postpartal diuresis
22. Pelvic relaxation

II. Reviewing Key Concepts

23. Assessing the bladder for distention: see Urethra and Bladder section in Urinary System.

  A. Risk for bladder distention: birth-induced trauma to urethra and bladder; edematous urethra; increased bladder capacity and diuresis; diminished sensation of bladder fullness related to use

313

of conduction anesthesia; pelvic soreness, lacerations, and episiotomy

B. Implications of bladder distention.
- Bladder pushes uterus up and to side, inhibiting uterine contraction, which leads to excessive bleeding.
- Distention can lead to stasis of urine, increasing risk for UTI.

24. Factors interfering with bowel elimination: see Gastrointestinal System section; decreased muscle tone, effect of progesterone on peristalsis, prelabor diarrhea, limited oral intake and dehydration from labor, anticipated discomfort related to hemorrhoids and perineal trauma lead to resisting the urge to defecate.

25. Hypovolemic shock is less likely: see Blood Volume section; pregnancy-induced hypervolemia allows most women to tolerate a considerable blood loss; size of maternal vascular bed decreases with expulsion of placenta, there is loss of stimulus for vasodilation, and extravascular water stores of pregnancy are mobilized back into vascular system for excretion.

26. Risk for thrombophlebitis: see Coagulation Factors section; increase in clotting factors and fibrinogen levels during pregnancy continues into the postpartum period; hypercoagulable state combined with vessel damage during childbirth and decreased activity level of the postpartum period increase risk for thrombus formation.

27. Compare and contrast lochial and nonlochial bleeding: see Box 20-1 for the information needed to complete your answer.

28. Choice D is correct; fundus should be at or 1 cm above the umbilicus and at midline; deviation from midline (in this case to the right) could indicate a full bladder; bright to dark red uterine discharge refers to lochia rubra; edema and erythema are common shortly after repair of a wound; decreased abdominal muscle tone and enlarged uterus result in abdominal protrusion; separation of the abdominal muscle walls, diastasis recti abdominis, is common during pregnancy and the postpartum period.

29. Choice B is correct; the woman is describing the normal finding of postpartum diaphoresis, which is the body's attempt to excrete fluid retained during pregnancy; documentation is important but not the first nursing action; infection assessment and physician notification are not needed at this time.

30. Choice D is correct; afterpains are most likely to occur in the following circumstances: multiparity, overdistention of the uterus (macrosomia, multifetal pregnancy), breastfeeding (endogenous oxytocin secretion), and administration of an oxytocic.

III. Thinking Critically

1. Postpartum women express questions and concerns.
   A. Afterpains: breastfeeding with newborn sucking causes the posterior pituitary to secrete oxytocin, stimulating the let-down reflex; uterine contractions are also stimulated, leading to afterpains, which will occur for the first few days postpartum.
   B. Length of time fundus can be palpated: see Involution Process section in Uterus and Fig. 20-1; progress of uterine descent in the abdomen is described; within 2 weeks of childbirth the uterus is again located within the pelvis and is no longer palpable.
   C. Stages and duration of lochia: see Lochia section in Uterus; discuss characteristics of rubra, serosa, and alba lochia in terms of color, consistency, amount, odor, and duration; explain that the contents of the flow, including the amount of blood, change as progress is made from stage to stage.
   D. Protruding abdomen: see Abdomen section; enlarged uterus along with stretched abdominal muscles with diminished tone creates a still-pregnant appearance for the first few weeks after birth; by 6 weeks the abdominal wall will return to approximately its prepregnant state; skin will regain most of its elasticity and striae will fade but remain; discuss exercise and a sensible weight loss program to facilitate the return of tone and diminish protrusion.
   E. Diuresis: see Fluid Loss section in Urinary System; discuss normalcy of diuresis and diaphoresis designed to rid the body of fluid retained during pregnancy; be sure to ask questions related to characteristics of the urination, including amount, frequency, appearance of urine, and experience of pain such as burning to rule out urinary tract infection or urinary retention with voiding of overload in frequent, small amounts.
   F. Breastfeeding as a reliable contraceptive method: see Pituitary Hormones and Ovarian Function section; emphasize that breastfeeding is not a reliable method because return of ovulation is unpredictable and may precede menstruation; discuss appropriate contraceptive methods for a breastfeeding woman, taking care to avoid hormonal-based methods until lactation is well established.
   G. Lactation suppression in bottle-feeding woman: see Nonbreastfeeding Mothers section in Breast; congestion of veins and lymphatics along with some filling with milk begins to occur when estrogen and progesterone levels fall with expulsion of the placenta; because milk is not removed, the cycle shuts down and the milk is absorbed into the circulatory system; she will need to support her breasts with a snug bra or binder and avoid applying warmth on her breasts and expressing any of the milk or stimulating her nipples; ice pack application and analgesics can be used for discomfort.
   H. Sexuality during the postpartum period of breastfeeding women: see Vagina and Perineum section in Reproductive System and Associated

Structures; discuss role of prolactin in suppressing estrogen secretion, thereby inhibiting vaginal lubrication and resulting in vaginal dryness and dyspareunia, which will persist until ovulation resumes; use of water-soluble lubricant or a spermicide used with a condom for birth control can reduce discomfort.

CHAPTER 21: NURSING CARE OF THE FAMILY DURING THE POSTPARTUM PERIOD

I. Learning Key Terms

1. Fourth trimester
2. Couplet care; mother-baby care (single-room maternity care)
3. Early postpartum discharge; shortened hospital stay; 1-day maternity stay
4. Oxytocic
5. Uterine atony
6. Sitz bath
7. Afterpains (postbirth pains)
8. Splanchnic engorgement; orthostatic hypotension
9. Homans sign
10. Kegel
11. Engorgement
12. Rubella
13. RhoGAM (Rh immunoglobulin)
14. Warm line

II. Reviewing Key Concepts

15. Measures to assist with voiding: see Prevention of Bladder Distention section; help her to assume an upright position on bedpan or in bathroom, listen to running water, put hands in warm water, pour water over vulva with peribottle, stand in a shower, or sit in a sitz bath; provide analgesics.
16. Measures to prevent thrombophlebitis: see Ambulation section; exercise legs with active range of motion (ROM) of knees, ankles, feet, and toes; early ambulation; wear support hose (if varicosities are present); keep well hydrated.
17. Two interventions to prevent postpartum hemorrhage in early postpartum period: see Prevention of Excessive Bleeding section.
    - Maintain uterine tone: massage fundus if boggy, expel clots when fundus is firm, administer oxytocic medications, and breastfeed or stimulate nipples.
    - Prevent bladder distention.
18. Signs of potential psychosocial complications during postpartum period: see Signs of Potential Complications—Psychosocial Concerns box to formulate your answer.
19. Choice C is correct; follow principles for effective and accurate assessment of the abdomen; the woman should be assisted into a supine position with head and shoulders on a pillow, arms at sides, and knees flexed; this facilitates relaxation of abdominal muscles and allows deep palpation.

20. Choice A is correct; an oxytocic contracts the uterus, thereby preventing excessive blood loss; lochia will therefore reflect expected characteristics; this type of medication can cause uterine contractions that are severe enough to require an analgesic.
21. Choice B is correct; a direct and indirect Coombs test must be negative, indicating that antibodies have not been formed, before RhoGAM can be given; it must be given within 72 hours of birth; the newborn needs to be Rh positive; it is often given in the third trimester and then again after birth.
22. Choice D is correct; see Box 21-1; squeezing the buttocks together before sitting down will reduce pulling on any perineal repairs; this is a medical aseptic procedure; therefore clean, not sterile, equipment is used; the water should be warm at 38°C to 40.6°C; sitz bath is used at least twice a day for 20 minutes each time.
23. Choices C, E, and F are correct; squeeze bottle is always pointed backward and not upward into the vagina, which could carry debris through the cervix and into the uterus; topical medications should be used sparingly only three or four times per day; gloves are not needed but she should wash her hands before and after perineal care.
24. Choices B, D, and E are correct; temperature of 38°C during the first 24 hours may be related to deficient fluid and is therefore not a concern; fundus should be midline but firm, not boggy; saturation of the pad in 15 minutes or less would be a concern; a positive Homans sign could indicate DVT; usually women have a good appetite and eat well after birth; each voiding should be at least 100 to 150 mL.

III. Thinking Critically

1. Measures for bottle-feeding mother to suppress lactation and relieve discomfort of engorgement: see Lactation Suppression section; wear supportive bra continuously for at least the first 72 hours postpartum, avoid stimulating breasts (no warm water during shower, no infant sucking, no pumping or removal of milk), apply ice packs intermittently to relieve soreness, and use cabbage leaves and mild analgesics.
2. Pain relief for a postpartum breastfeeding mother: see Promotion of Comfort, Rest, Ambulation, and Exercise section; assess characteristics of pain (severity, location, relief measures already tried and effectiveness); use a combination of pharmacologic and nonpharmacologic measures as indicated by the nature of the pain being experienced; if breastfeeding, administer a systemic analgesic just after a feeding session; ensure that medication is not contraindicated for breastfeeding women.
3. Woman exhibiting signs of hemorrhage and early shock: see Prevention of Excessive Bleeding section and Emergency—Hypovolemic Shock box.
    A. Criteria to determine if flow is excessive: note length of time pad was worn and the degree to

which it was saturated with blood; check the bed to determine if lochia has pooled under buttocks; pad saturation in 15 minutes or less indicates a profuse flow.

B. Priority action: assess fundus and massage if boggy; once firm, express clots, check bladder for distention and assist to empty, and administer oxytocics if ordered; take note of vital sign findings and changes in behavior; notify the primary health care provider to discuss assessment findings, actions taken, and responses.

C. Additional interventions: see list of measures identified in Emergency—Hypovolemic Shock box.

4. Administering rubella vaccine to a postpartum woman: see Health Promotion for Planning Future Pregnancies and Children section; recheck titer results and order; determine if woman or any household members are immunocompromised; check allergies; inform her of side effects and emphasize that she must not become pregnant for at least 28 days after the immunization.

5. Administering RhoGAM to a postpartum woman: see Health Promotion for Planning Future Pregnancies and Children section and Medication Guide; check woman's and newborn's Rh status and Coombs test results; obtain RhoGAM and check all identification data; administer intramuscularly; woman must be Rh negative and indirect Coombs negative; newborn must be Rh positive and direct Coombs negative; ensure that it is administered within 72 hours after birth; provide woman with documentation that she received RhoGAM.

6. Sexual changes after pregnancy and childbirth: see Sexual Activity and Contraception section and Teaching for Self-Management—Resuming Sexual Activity after Birth box; identify changes that may occur; discuss physical and emotional readiness of the woman and potential for infection if healing is not complete; stress importance of open communication; discuss how to prevent discomfort in terms of position and lubrication; emphasize the importance of birth control because return of ovulation cannot be predicted with accuracy.

7. Postpartum women—nursing diagnoses, expected outcomes, and nursing management.

A. Nursing diagnosis: risk for infection of episiotomy related to ineffective perineal hygiene measures.
Expected outcome: episiotomy will heal without infection.
Nursing management: see Prevention of Infection section and Box 21-1 for full identification of measures to enhance healing and prevent infection.

B. Nursing diagnosis: constipation related to inactivity and lack of knowledge regarding bowel elimination patterns after childbirth.
Expected outcome: woman will have soft, formed bowel movement.

Nursing management: see Promotion of Normal Bladder and Bowel Patterns section; determine usual elimination patterns and measures used to enhance elimination; encourage activity, roughage, and fluids; obtain order for mild combination stool softener–laxative.

C. Nursing diagnosis: acute pain related to episiotomy and hemorrhoids.
Expected outcome: woman will experience a reduction in pain following implementation of suggested relief measures.
Nursing management: see Promotion of Comfort, Rest, Ambulation, and Exercise section, Nursing Care Plan, and Box 21-1; emphasize nonpharmacologic relief measures such as perineal care, sitz bath, topicals, side-lying position, Kegel exercises, and measures to enhance bowel and bladder elimination; use pharmacologic measures if local measures are ineffective or pain is severe.

8. Fundus above umbilicus and to the right of midline.

A. Most likely basis for finding: bladder distention; confirm by palpating the bladder and asking the woman to describe her voiding patterns.

B. Nursing action: assist woman to empty bladder; measure amount voided and assess characteristics of the urine; palpate bladder and fundus again to determine response; catheterization may be required if she is unable to empty her bladder fully because a distended bladder can lead to uterine atony with excessive bleeding and UTIs.

9. Resumption of physical activity after giving birth: see Promotion of Comfort, Rest, Ambulation, and Exercise section.

- Assess postanesthesia recovery and physical stability, including return of strength, mobility, and sensation in lower extremities.

- Assist and supervise first few times out of bed because orthostatic hypotension can cause her to be dizzy and fall.

- Show her where the call light is and what to do if she is alone and begins to feel dizzy or light-headed.

10. Early discharge option.

A. Decision making regarding early discharge: discuss the advantages and disadvantages of early discharge; the nurse should discuss these with the couple in terms of their own situation; explore the reasons why they are contemplating early discharge and determine the quality of support they will have after discharge.

B. Nurse's legal responsibility: assess woman, newborn, and family to confirm that criteria for discharge are fully met; notify primary health care provider if criteria are not met; document all assessment findings, actions, and responses.

C. Criteria for discharge—maternal, newborn: see Criteria for Discharge section.

D. Outline essential content that must be taught before discharge: see Discharge Teaching section; include information regarding self-care and newborn care, signs of complications, and prescribed medications; arrange for first postpartum checkup and for a follow-up telephone call or home visit, usually within 1 to 2 days after discharge.

11. Cultural beliefs and practices: see Impact of Cultural Diversity section and Cultural Considerations box.
    A. Importance of using a culturally sensitive approach: recognition of cultural beliefs and practices is essential to meet a woman's individual needs; such an approach demonstrates respect, caring, and concern and helps to foster trust and cooperation when creating a plan of care.
    B. Korean-American woman—heat and cold balance: ask woman about the substances and practices that she identifies as hot and cold, then intervene appropriately; realize that self-management may not be a priority and that she may seek guidance from older women in her family or community; see Cultural Considerations—Postpartum Period and Family Planning box.
    C. Muslim woman in postpartum period: emphasize diet modification and modesty.

12. Performing a postpartum assessment 8 hours after vaginal birth (see content of this chapter related to assessment, the content of Chapter 20, and the content related to the fourth stage of labor in Chapter 19).
    A. Position for fundal palpation: supine, head and shoulder on pillow, arms at sides, knees slightly flexed.
    B. Fundal characteristics to assess: consistency (firm or boggy), height (above, at, or below umbilicus), location (midline or deviated to the right or left).
    C. Position for assessment of perineum: lateral or modified Sims position with upper leg flexed on hip; wear gloves for this portion of the assessment, which will involve contact with body fluids, including blood (Standard Precautions).
    D. Episiotomy characteristics to assess: REEDA (redness, edema, ecchymosis, drainage, approximation); presence of hematoma; adequacy of hygiene, including cleanliness, presence of odor, method used to cleanse perineum and to apply topical preparations.
    E. Characteristics of lochia to assess: stage, amount, odor, clots.

13. Recovery room nurse report: see Transfer from Recovery Area section and Table 21-1 for a discussion of essential information that should be reported regarding the woman, the baby, and the significant events and findings from her prenatal and childbirth periods.

14. Using infection control measures: see Prevention of Infection section.
    A. Measures to prevent transmission of infection from person to person: clean environment, handwashing,

use of Standard Precautions, proper care and use of equipment.
    B. Infection prevention measures to teach the woman: avoid walking barefoot; handwashing; hygiene measures (general, breast, and perineal); prevention of bladder infection; measures to enhance resistance to infection, including nutrition and rest; correct breastfeeding techniques.

CHAPTER 22: TRANSITION TO PARENTHOOD

I. Learning Key Terms

1. Attachment; bonding
2. Acquaintance
3. Mutuality
4. Signaling behaviors
5. Executive behaviors
6. Claiming
7. En face (face to face)
8. Entrainment
9. Biorhythmicity
10. Reciprocity
11. Synchrony
12. Transition to parenthood
13. Dependent (taking-in)
14. Dependent-independent (taking-hold)
15. Interdependent (letting-go)
16. Becoming a mother
17. Maternal sensitivity
18. "Pink" period; "blue" period
19. Engrossment

II. Reviewing Key Concepts

20. Attachment of newborn to parents and parents to newborn: see Parental Attachment, Bonding, and Acquaintance section.
    A. Conditions that facilitate attachment: emotionally and physically healthy parents, competent in communication and caregiving; parent and newborn fit in terms of state, temperament, and gender; parental proximity to infant and time for interaction; adequate social support system; positive feedback and mutually satisfying interaction with newborn; health status of newborn.
    B. Assessment of process of attachment: see Assessment of Attachment Behaviors section and Box 22-1 for specific behaviors indicating the quality of the attachment that is developing; it is critical that nurses provide opportunities for parent-infant contact and be present during these contacts to observe the interaction.
    C. Facilitation of attachment process: see Tables 22-1, 22-2, and 22-3 for several measures nurses can use to help parents and newborns interact with each other and become attached; consider the conditions for attachment that you identified in A above to develop creative nursing approaches.

317

21. Parental tasks: see Parental Tasks and Responsibilities section for a description of each of the tasks of reconciling actual child with fantasy child, becoming adept in infant care, and establishing a place for the newborn within the family group.

22. Parent-infant contact: see specific sections for each form of contact in Parent-Infant Contact.
    A. Early contact: important to provide time for parents to see, touch, and hold their newborn as soon as possible after birth; stress that attachment is an ongoing process; interference with this early contact because of maternal and/or newborn problems should not have a long-term effect as long as it is balanced by opportunities for close contact as soon as possible after birth as appropriate for maternal and/or newborn condition.
    B. Extended contact: family-centered care, mother-baby care, rooming-in, and use of labor, delivery, recovery, and postpartum (LDRP) or labor, delivery, and recovery (LDR) rooms to facilitate this type of contact

23. Progress of a mother's touch as she becomes acquainted with her newborn: see Touch section for a description of touch as it progresses from an exploration with fingertips, gentle stroking, patting, and rubbing; indicate how touching the infant can vary among cultures.

24. Factors influencing parental responses to the birth of their child: see section for each factor in the Diversity in Transition to Parenthood and Parental Sensory Impairment sections and Boxes 22-2 and 22-3.

25. Compare and contrast two theories of maternal adjustment after birth: Mercer's theory (see Becoming a Mother section) and Rubin's theory (see Table 22-4); in your comparison, you should include a description of the stages proposed by Rubin and Mercer along with the behaviors of women and the tasks they must accomplish.

26. Choice D is correct; choice A reflects the first phase of identifying likenesses; choice B reflects the second phase of identifying differences; choice C reflects a negative reaction of claiming the infant in terms of pain and discomfort; choice D reflects the third or final stage of identifying uniqueness.

27. Choice B is correct; early close contact is recommended to initiate and enhance the attachment process.

28. Choice A is correct; engrossment refers to a father's absorption, preoccupation, and interest in his infant; choice B represents the claiming process phase I, identifying likeness; choice C represents reciprocity; choice D represents en face or face-to-face position with mutual gazing.

29. Choice B is correct; taking-in occurs in the first 1 to 2 days of recovery following birth; other behaviors exhibited include reliance on others to help her meet needs and being excited and talkative.

30. Choice C is correct; approximately 50% to 80% of women experience postpartum blues; new parents should be reassured that their skills as parents develop gradually and they should seek help to develop these skills; postpartum blues that are self-limiting and short lived do not require psychotropic medications; support and care of the postpartum woman and her newborn by her partner and family are the most effective prevention and coping strategies; feelings of fatigue from childbirth and meeting the demands of the newborn can accentuate feelings of depression.

III. Thinking Critically

1. Teaching parents communication skills with their newborns: see Communication between Parent and Infant section.
    A. Communication techniques: discuss touch, eye contact, voice, and odor; demonstrate techniques, have parents try them, and point out newborn response in terms of quieting, alerting, making eye contact, and gazing; help parents to interpret cues.
    B. Newborn's communication: point out infant responses; discuss processes of entrainment, biorhythmicity, reciprocity, synchrony, and repertoire of behaviors.

2. Woman following emergency cesarean birth: disappointment with lack of immediate bonding time with newborn.
    ■ Discuss concepts of early and extended contact.
    ■ Emphasize that the parent-infant attachment process is ongoing; her emotional bond with her baby will not be weaker.
    ■ Help her to meet her own physical and emotional needs so that she develops readiness to meet her newborn's needs.
    ■ Help her get to know her baby and interact with and care for her; point out newborn characteristics, including how the baby is responding to her efforts.
    ■ Show her how to communicate with her newborn and how her newborn communicates with her.
    ■ Arrange for follow-up after discharge to assess how attachment is progressing.

3. Sibling adjustment to newborn: see Sibling Adaptation section and Box 22-4, which identify strategies parents can use to help their other children accept a new baby; caution her that adjustment takes time and is strongly related to the developmental level and experiences of the sibling(s); give mother suggestions regarding what she can do now and what she did previously.

4. Parents unsure and anxious about caring for their newborn: see Nursing Care Plan, Home Care Follow-up, Communication between Parent and Infant, Transition to Parenthood, and Parental Role after Birth sections.
    A. Nursing diagnosis: risk for impaired parent-infant attachment related to lack of knowledge and feeling of incompetence regarding infant care.

B. Nursing measures to facilitate attachment can include the following:
- Perform newborn assessment with parents present, pointing out newborn characteristics and encouraging parents to participate and ask questions.
- Demonstrate newborn care measures and provide time for parents to practice and obtain feedback.
- Provide extended contact time with newborn, such as longer visiting hours and rooming-in, until discharge.
- Make referral for follow-up with telephone contacts and home visits; refer to parenting classes, support groups, lactation consultant, and La Leche League.
- Recommend books, magazines, DVDs, and interactive Internet sites that discuss newborns and their care.

5. Parental disappointment with newborn's gender and appearance: see Parental Tasks and Responsibilities section; foster attachment, acquaintance, and claiming; help parents to get acquainted with the infant and to reconcile the real child with the fantasy child; discuss the basis of molding, caput succedaneum, and forceps marks and how they will be resolved; be alert for problems with attachment and care so that follow-up can be arranged.

6. Grandparent adjustment: see Grandparent Adaptation section; observe interaction between grandparents and parents, taking note of signs of effective interaction and conflict; involve grandparents in teaching sessions as appropriate for this family; spend time with grandparents to help them be supportive without "taking over" or being critical; help the new parents to recognize the unique role grandparents can play as parenting role models, nurturers, and providers of respite care.

7. Woman experiencing postpartum blues.
- Nursing diagnosis: ineffective maternal coping related to hormonal changes and increased responsibilities following birth.
- Expected outcome: woman will report feeling more contented with her role as mother following the use of recommended coping strategies.
- Care management: see Postpartum Blues section and Teaching for Self-Management—Coping with Postpartum Blues box to identify behaviors that should be assessed to determine the level of blues she is experiencing; involve both Jane and her husband in the teaching session and in the development of a plan for coping with the blues; this must occur early to prevent development of postpartum depression.

8. Discussion of paternal adjustment: see Paternal Adjustment section and Table 22-5 to discuss the transition process to fatherhood and nursing measures that provide the father with support, teaching, demonstrations, and practice and interaction time with the newborn

ANSWER KEY UNIT VI

CHAPTER 23: PHYSIOLOGIC AND BEHAVIORAL ADAPTATIONS OF THE NEWBORN

I. Learning Key Terms

1. Surfactant
2. Thermoregulation
3. Thermogenesis
4. Nonshivering thermogenesis
5. Neutral thermal environment
6. Convection
7. Radiation
8. Evaporation
9. Conduction
10. Hyperthermia
11. Telangiectatic nevi (nevus simplex)
12. Molding
13. Caput succedaneum
14. Cephalhematoma
15. Mongolian spots
16. Acrocyanosis
17. Vernix caseosa
18. Milia
19. Jaundice
20. Physiologic jaundice
21. Acute bilirubin encephalopathy
22. Kernicterus
23. Breast milk jaundice
24. Meconium
25. Erythema toxicum (erythema neonatorum; flea bite dermatitis)
26. Hypospadias; epispadias
27. Hydrocele
28. Epstein pearls
29. Fontanel
30. Lanugo
31. Ecchymosis
32. Desquamation
33. Port-wine stain (nevus flammeus)
34. Strawberry hemangioma (nevus vascularis)
35. Pseudomenstruation
36. Prepuce
37. Developmental dysplasia of the hips (DDH)
38. Epithelial pearls
39. Oligodactyly
40. Polydactyly
41. Syndactyly
42. Sleep-wake states
43. Deep; light; 16 to 19; increasing
44. Drowsy; quiet-alert; active-alert; crying
45. Quiet-alert
46. State modulation
47. Habituation
48. Orientation
49. Temperament
50. K, 51. F, 52. B, 53. J, 54. D, 55. I, 56. H, 57. L, 58. A, 59. E, 60. G, 61. C, 62. M

319

II. Reviewing Key Concepts

63. Factors initiating breathing after birth: see Respiratory System section for a description of how a newborn begins to breathe, including effect of pressure changes, chilling, noise, light, and other sensations associated with birth and chemoreceptor activation of respiratory center.

64. Describe phases of newborn transition period to extrauterine life: see Transition to Extrauterine Life section for identification of each phase and descriptions of timing, duration, and typical newborn behaviors for each phase.

65. Factors affecting newborn behavior: see Behavioral Characteristics sections related to each factor to formulate your answer.

66. Choices A, B, and C are correct; the newborn at 5 hours old is in the second period of reactivity, during which tachycardia, tachypnea, increased muscle tone, skin color changes, increased mucus production, and passage of meconium are normal findings; respiratory rate should range between 30 and 60 breaths/minute; expiratory grunting and nasal flaring are signs of respiratory distress; crackles, which are commonly present in the first period of reactivity immediately following birth, should be absent during the second period, representing the absorption of lung fluid into the circulatory system.

67. Choice A is correct; the rash described is erythema toxicum; it is an inflammatory response that has no clinical significance and requires no treatment because it will disappear spontaneously.

68. Choices B and E are correct; physiologic jaundice does not appear until 24 hours after birth; further investigation would be needed if it appeared during the first 24 hours, because this is consistent with pathologic jaundice; glucose levels should range between 50 to 60 mg/dL and should not be lower than 40 mg/dL; acrocyanosis is normal for 7 to 10 days after birth.

69. Choice D is correct; choices B and C are common newborn reflexes used to assess integrity of neuromuscular system; syndactyly refers to webbing of the fingers.

70. Choice C is correct; telangiectatic nevi are also known as stork bite marks and can also appear on the eyelids; milia are plugged sebaceous glands and appear as white pimples; nevus vasculosus or a strawberry mark is a raised, sharply demarcated, bright or dark red swelling; nevus flammeus is a port-wine, flat red to purple lesion that does not blanch with pressure.

III. Thinking Critically

1. Newborn—risk for cold stress: see Thermogenic System section.
   A. Basis for cold stress: see Thermogenesis section to formulate answer, including newborn's ability to generate and conserve heat.
   B. Dangers of cold stress: see Fig. 23-2; metabolic and physiologic problems related to increased oxygen need and consumption; oxygen and energy diverted from brain cells and cardiac function and growth to thermogenesis; vasoconstriction results in respiratory distress, reopening of the ductus arteriosus, acidosis, and increasing the level of bilirubin; hypoglycemia can occur as a result of increased glucose use.
   C. Nursing diagnosis: risk for imbalanced body temperature— hypothermia related to immature thermoregulation associated with newborn status; expected outcome: newborn's temperature will stabilize between 36.5°C and 37.2°C within 8 to 10 hours of birth.
   D. Measures to stabilize newborn temperature and prevent cold stress: implement measures that reflect application of heat loss mechanisms of convection, radiation, evaporation, and conduction.
      - Dry infant and cover with warmed blankets or wrap with mother.
      - Cover head and feet; double-wrap.
      - Use radiant warmer to stabilize temperature, assess newborn, and perform procedures.
      - Adjust environment in terms of temperature and drafts (nursery and mother's room).
      - Place bassinet away from drafts and outside windows.
      - Maintain adequate nutrition (caloric intake).

2. Parental concern regarding head variations: see Integumentary System and Skeletal System sections; discuss each finding in terms of cause, significance for the newborn's health status and adjustment, and how and when it will be resolved; refer to Figs. 23-9 and 23-10 to facilitate parental understanding; perform a thorough newborn assessment with parents present to reassure the parents.

3. Physiologic jaundice: see Conjugation of Bilirubin and Newborn Jaundice section.
   A. Criteria for diagnosis: see Physiologic section for a full explanation of clinical manifestations.
   B. Explanation to parents: discuss why the jaundice occurs and its common occurrence among healthy newborns; emphasize that frequent feeding with associated bowel movements will be helpful in treating the jaundice by increasing the loss of bilirubin in the stool.

4. Parental interest in newborn's sensory capabilities: see Sensory Behaviors section.
   A. What nurse should tell parents: discuss and demonstrate newborn's capability regarding vision, hearing, touch, taste, and smell.
   B. Stimuli parents can provide to facilitate newborn development: face-to-face and eye-to-eye contact, objects (bright or black-and-white changing, complex patterns), sound (talking to infant, music, heartbeat simulator), and touch (infant massage, cuddling).

C. Best time to interact with newborn: during the quiet-alert state; describe what this state is and how they will know their child is in it.

5. Parental concern regarding "bruises" on newborn's back and buttocks: discuss the characteristics and cause of Mongolian spots (see Mongolian Spots section of Integumentary System and Fig. 23-5).

CHAPTER 24: NURSING CARE OF THE NEWBORN AND FAMILY

I. Learning Key Terms

1. Apgar score; heart rate; respiratory effort; muscle tone; reflex irritability; color
2. Bulb syringe
3. Thermistor probe
4. Eye prophylaxis
5. Ophthalmia neonatorum/neonatal conjunctivitis; 0.5% erythromycin; 1% tetracycline
6. Vitamin K
7. New Ballard Score
8. Appropriate for gestational age (AGA)
9. Large for gestational age (LGA)
10. Small for gestational age (SGA)
11. Preterm (premature)
12. Late preterm; early term
13. Full term; late term
14. Postterm
15. Postmature
16. Petechiae
17. Bilirubin
18. Physiologic jaundice
19. Blanch test
20. Transcutaneous bilirubinometry (TcB)
21. Thrush
22. Hypoglycemia
23. Hypocalcemia
24. Bradypnea
25. Tachypnea
26. Handwashing (hand hygiene)
27. Phototherapy
28. Circumcision
29. CRIES; crying; requires oxygen for saturation of 95%; increased vital signs; expression; sleeplessness

II. Reviewing Key Concepts

30. P, 31. N, 32. N, 33. P, 34. N, 35. N, 36. N, 37. P, 38. N, 39. N, 40. N, 41. N, 42. N, 43. P, 44. N, 45. N, 46. N, 47. P, 48. N, 49. N, 50. N, 51. P, 52. N, 53. N
54. Creation of a protective environment in terms of infection control and safety: see Protective Environment section to formulate answer that includes discussion of each of the following:
    - Environmental modifications
    - Infection control measures
    - Safety in terms of security precautions, identification measures, and falls prevention

55. Birth trauma: see Birth Injuries section; your answer should include factors leading to injuries and the types of injuries that can occur.
56. Health teaching in preparation for discharge: see Teaching for Self-Management boxes and Discharge Planning and Parent Education sections; be sure to include methodologies that reflect cognitive, psychomotor, and affective learning.
57. Guidelines for weighing and measuring newborn: see Table 24-3 and Baseline Measurements of Physical Growth section for guidelines to follow and expected findings; wear gloves when performing immediately after birth before infant's first bath.
    A. Weight: balance scale, cover scale with clean scale paper, place undressed infant on scale, keep hand hovering over infant, never turn away; weigh at the same time of day when hospitalized.
    B. Head circumference: measure the widest part of head just above ears and eyebrows; repeat if molding is present at birth.
    C. Chest circumference: measure across nipple line.
    D. Abdominal circumference: measure just above the level of umbilicus.
    E. Length: measure from crown to rump, then rump to heels.
58. Specimen collection guidelines: see Collection of Specimens section and Figs. 24-11 and 24-12 for procedure to follow for heelstick, venipuncture, and urine collection bag; include a description of restraint methods that should be used (see Fig. 24-19).
59. Maintaining a patent airway and supporting respirations: see Airway Maintenance section.
    A. Four conditions essential for maintaining an adequate oxygen supply: clear, patent airway; adequate respiratory effort; functioning cardiopulmonary system; adequate thermoregulation.
    B. Signs of respiratory distress: see Signs of Potential Complications—Abnormal Newborn Breathing box for a list of the signs to observe for; consider how respiratory signs change from the first period of reactivity to the second period of reactivity.
    C. Relieving airway obstruction using a bulb syringe: see Airway Maintenance and Maintaining an Adequate Oxygen Supply sections, Teaching for Self-Management—Suctioning with Bulb Syringe box, and Fig. 24-4; reposition infant, use a bulb syringe, and take note of effectiveness.
60. Shaken baby syndrome—teaching new parents: see Box 24-5 regarding the Period of PURPLE Crying program.
61. Choices D, E, and F are correct; thinning of lanugo with bald spots, absence of scarf sign, and descended testes are assessed with the New Ballard Scale and are consistent with full-term status; pulse and weight are not part of the New Ballard Scale; the popliteal angle for a full-term newborn is 100 degrees or less.
62. Choices C and E are correct; glucose should be 45 to 65 mg/dL; serum calcium should be at least 7.8 to

8 mg/dL; choices A, B, and D all fall within the expected ranges.

63. Choice B is correct; signs of hypoglycemia include apnea, jitteriness or twitching, respiratory distress, high-pitched cry, difficulty feeding, hunger, lethargy, hypotonia, hypothermia, and seizures; laryngospasm and a high-pitched cry are signs of hypocalcemia.

64. Choice A is correct; the control panel should be set between 36°C and 37°C; the probe should be placed in one of the upper quadrants of the abdomen below the intercostal margin, never over a rib; axillary, not rectal temperatures should be taken.

65. Choice B is correct; use the CRIES scale to determine pain level of newborns; the New Ballard Score is used to determine gestational age; the site should be checked every 30 minutes for the first hour, then every hour for 4 to 6 hours; diaper wipes should not be used on the site because they contain alcohol, which delays healing and causes discomfort; the yellow exudate is a protective film that forms in 24 hours and should not be removed.

66. Choices B, C, and D are correct; mother does not have to be hepatitis B positive for the vaccine to be given to her newborn; use a 5/8-inch 25-gauge needle and insert it at a 90-degree angle.

67. Choices B, C, E, and F are correct; administer within 1 to 2 hours and squeeze a 1- to 2-cm ribbon of ointment into the lower conjunctival sac.

III. Thinking Critically

1. Apgar scoring: see Table 24-1 and Initial Physical Assessment and Apgar Scoring sections.
   A. Baby boy Smith: heart rate: 160 (2); respiratory effort: good, crying (2); muscle tone: flexion, active movement (2); reflex irritability: cry with stimulus (2); color: acrocyanosis (1); score is 9; interpretation: score of 7 to 10 indicates that the infant is having minimal to no difficulty adjusting to extrauterine life.
   B. Baby girl Doe: heart rate: 102 (2); respiratory effort: slow, irregular, weak cry (1); muscle tone: some flexion (1); reflex irritability: grimace with stimulus (1); color: pale (0); score is 5; interpretation: score of 4 to 6 indicates moderate difficulty adjusting to extrauterine life.

2. Assessment of newborn girl.
   A. Protocol for assessment during first 2 hours: see Tables 24-1 (Apgar Score) and 24-2 (Initial Physical Assessment of Newborn) and Initial Assessment and Apgar Scoring sections to prepare your outline.
   B. Nurse's responsibility for newborn identification at birth: see Immediate Care after Birth and Protective Environment sections; complete the identification process before mother and newborn are separated; attach matching identification (ID) bands to both (father also, in some cases) immediately after birth; take newborn's footprint and mother's fingerprint(s) and place on appropriate form.

C. Priority nursing diagnosis for the first 24 hours: consider nursing diagnoses related to breathing and thermoregulation.
   D. Priority nursing care measures: discuss each of the following areas:
      ■ Stabilization of respiration and airway patency; ongoing assessment
      ■ Maintenance of body temperature
      ■ Immediate interventions in terms of identification, prophylactic medications, and promotion of parent-infant interaction
   E. Benefits of early contact between mother and newborn: see Promoting Parent-Infant Interaction section.

3. Performing a physical examination of newborn before discharge: see Protective Environment section.
   A. Actions to ensure safety and accuracy: well-lighted, warm, and draft-free environment; undress as needed; place on firm surface with constant supervision; progress in a systematic manner from cleanest to dirtiest area.
   B. Major areas assessed: see Table 24-3 and Chapter 23, Assessment of Newborn Reflexes section; areas to include are general appearance and posture, vital signs and weight, integument, head and neck, abdomen and back, genitalia and anus, elimination patterns, extremities, neurologic system including reflexes, and behavioral characteristics.
   C. Rationale for presence of parents: chance to observe parent-infant interactions and to identify and meet learning needs; foster active involvement in assessment and care of their newborn; encourage discussion of concerns and asking of questions; chance to explain and demonstrate newborn characteristics and capabilities.

4. Newborn with mucus in airway: see Airway Maintenance and Maintaining an Adequate Oxygen Supply section, Teaching for Self-Management—Suctioning with a Bulb Syringe box, and Fig. 24-4.
   A. Nursing diagnosis: impaired gas exchange related to upper airway obstruction with mucus.
   B. Steps using bulb syringe: suction mouth first, then nose; compress bulb before insertion; insert tip along the side of mouth, not over tongue, which could stimulate the gag reflex and sucking; release compression slowly; continue until breathing sounds clear; teach parents how to use bulb syringe.

5. Care of circumcision and umbilical cord sites.
   A. Nursing diagnosis: risk for infection related to removal of foreskin and healing umbilical cord site.
   B. Expected outcome: cord and circumcision site will heal without infection.
   C. Teaching parents care: see Umbilical Cord Care and Circumcision sections, Nursing Care Plan, and Teaching for Self-Management boxes; emphasize importance of assessing sites for infection

and progress of healing; discuss measures to keep areas clean and dry and to enhance comfort; teach parents how to assess circumcision site for bleeding and what to do if it occurs; emphasize importance of assessing urination and what to do if the newborn has difficulty voiding; demonstrate skills and assist parents to redemonstrate.

6. Newborn with hyperbilirubinemia: see Common Newborn Problems section.

   A. Responding to parental concerns: tell parents in simple terms that their newborn is exhibiting physiologic jaundice, explaining why it occurs, what effect it will have on their newborn's health, and how it will be resolved; emphasize that their newborn's form of jaundice is a common and naturally occurring physiologic process as the newborn adjusts to extrauterine life.

   B. Blanch test: apply pressure with finger over a bony area (nose, forehead, sternum) for several seconds to empty capillaries at the spot; if jaundice is present, the blanched area will appear yellow before the capillaries fill.

   C. Expected findings of physiologic hyperbilirubinemia: jaundice (cephalocaudal, proximodistal progression), watery greenish stools, sleepiness, alteration in bilirubin levels that follows a specific pattern and degree of elevation (see Chapter 23).

   D. Precautions and care measures during phototherapy: see Phototherapy section; increase fluids and feed at least every 3 hours; cover eyes, removing periodically to assess condition and allow for interaction with parents; monitor temperature for increases or decreases; cleanse stools promptly; do not put lotions on skin; place undressed under lights and change position every 2 to 3 hours to expose as much skin to the lights as possible; remove from under lights for feeding, cuddling, and interaction with parents.

7. Newborn scheduled for a circumcision—pain concerns: see Neonatal and Circumcision—Procedural Pain Management sections, Table 24-5, Box 24-4, and Figs. 24-18 and 24-19.

   A. Common behavioral responses to pain: see Neonatal Responses to Pain section for several examples.

   B. Changes in vital signs and integument: see Assessment of Neonatal Pain section and Table 24-5 for several examples.

   C. CRIES tool: see Table 24-5.

   D. Nonpharmacologic and pharmacologic relief measures: see Management of Neonatal Pain section.

   - Nonpharmacologic: swaddle, nonnutritive sucking, take to parent, distract, apply Vaseline ointment, change diaper promptly, avoid pressure on site when holding or positioning.

   - Pharmacologic: local anesthesia, topical preparations, systemic analgesics.

8. Administration of medications to newborns after birth: see Medication Guide for each of the medications to develop the guidelines to ensure safe and effective administration of erythromycin ophthalmic ointment 0.5% and vitamin K 0.5 mg IM.

9. Parental concern about weight loss: see Baseline Measurements of Physical Growth section and Table 24-3; determine percentage of weight loss, ensuring that it does not exceed 10%; explain that their newborn's weight loss of 6% is within the expected range for weight loss after birth; discuss the cause of the loss and feeding measures and inform them that the birth weight should be regained within 2 weeks.

CHAPTER 25: NEWBORN NUTRITION AND FEEDING

I. Learning Key Terms

1. Lobes
2. Alveoli
3. Milk ducts
4. Myoepithelial cells
5. Areola
6. Lactation (lactogenesis)
7. Prolactin
8. Oxytocin
9. Nipple erection reflex
10. Everted; inverted
11. Breast shell
12. Colostrum
13. Nipple confusion
14. Feeding cues
15. Let-down; milk ejection reflex (MER)
16. Rooting reflex
17. Latch (latch-on)
18. Engorgement
19. Football (clutch) hold
20. Cradle (traditional) hold
21. Lactation consultant
22. Mastitis
23. Thrush
24. Ankyloglossia (tongue-tie)
25. Weaning
26. Foremilk
27. Hindmilk (cream)
28. Prolactin; oxytocin
29. Galactogogues

II. Reviewing Key Concepts

30. Teaching group of women about breastfeeding: see Benefits of Breastfeeding section and Table 25-1; emphasize the importance and benefits of breastfeeding for infants, mothers, family, and society.

31. Breastfeeding positions: see Positioning section and Fig. 25-5; describe the positions of football hold, cradle (traditional), modified cradle (across the lap), and side-lying; included in the demonstration should be an explanation of the rationale for alternating positions.

32. Feeding cues: see Care Management section.
    A. Cues: hand-to-mouth or hand-to-hand movements, sucking motions, strong rooting reflex, mouthing, tongue movements; crying is a late sign.
    B. Rationale for feeding according to these cues: if cues are missed, baby may cry vigorously, become distraught, shut down, or withdraw into a deep sleep; these behaviors will make feeding more difficult or impossible; feeding when the infant exhibits readiness enhances the chance of success.
33. Proper latch: see Latch section.
    A. Steps to ensure proper latch: apply colostrum/milk to areola/nipple (lubricate and entice), support the breast (see Fig. 25-6), hold baby close, and tickle baby's lower lip with the nipple to stimulate the rooting reflex—mouth opening and extrusion of tongue occurs; pull baby onto nipple and areola; bring infant to the breast.
    B. Signs of proper latch: see Fig. 25-6; nose, cheeks, and chin touch the breast; firm, tugging sensation on the nipple but no pinching or pain; baby's cheeks are rounded and jaw glides smoothly with sucking; swallow is audible.
    C. Removal of baby from breast: see Fig. 25-7; break suction by inserting finger in the side of baby's mouth between gums and leaving the finger in until nipple is completely out of the baby's mouth.
34. Choice B is correct; soft, yellow, seedy stools are very characteristic of the stools of breastfed babies; birth weight is regained in 10 to 14 days; six to eight wet diapers are expected at this time; baby should be fed every 2 to 3 hours for a total of 8 to 10 times per day.
35. Choice A is correct; swaddling is recommended; choices B, C, and D are all appropriate actions to calm a fussy baby.
36. Choice D is correct; no soap should be used because it could dry the areola and nipple and increase the risk for irritation; vitamin E should not be used, especially before a feeding, because it is a fat-soluble vitamin that the infant could ingest when breastfeeding; lanolin or colostrum/milk are the preferred substances to apply to the area; plastic liners can trap moisture and lead to sore nipples.
37. Choice B is correct; a combination oral contraceptive could decrease the milk supply if given before lactation is well established during the first 6 weeks after birth; after 6 weeks a progestin-only contraceptive could be used, because it is the hormonal contraceptive least likely to affect lactation; even complete breastfeeding is not considered to be a reliable method, because ovulation can occur unexpectedly even before the first menstrual period; diaphragm used before pregnancy would have to be checked after healing has occurred and lochia has ceased to see if it fits properly before the woman uses it again.

38. Choice C is correct; nipple should allow only the passage of a slow drip; tap water can be used unless the water supply is unsafe or if otherwise instructed; formula should never be heated in the microwave because it could be overheated or heated unevenly.
39. Choices A, C, and D are correct; bring baby to breast, not breast to baby; feeding should occur when baby begins to exhibit feeding readiness cues; breast should be supported with thumb on top and four fingers under back edge of areola and gently compressed.
40. Choice C is correct; limiting length of feeding does not protect the nipples and areola; choices B and D are correct actions but not the most important one.

III. Thinking Critically

1. Bottle-feeding mother wishes to give her newborn skim milk to prevent cardiac problems: see Fat section in Nutrient Needs; emphasize the importance of fat in the newborn's diet for energy and supplying essential fatty acids for growth, neurologic development, tissue maintenance, cell membranes, and hormone production; skim and low-fat milk lack essential fatty acids; whole milk should not be given until after the first year of life.
2. Infant feeding method decision making during prenatal period: see Benefits of Breastfeeding and Choosing an Infant Feeding Method sections.
    A. Nursing diagnosis: decisional conflict regarding feeding method for their newborn related to lack of knowledge and experience with newborn feeding methods; expected outcome: couple will choose the feeding method for their newborn that is most comfortable for them.
    B. Rationale for couple making the decision together: both should learn about the pros and cons of feeding methods, with an emphasis on the benefits of breastfeeding and how the partner can help with that method.
    C. Making decision prenatally: the prenatal period is a less stressful time, allowing for full consideration of options, how feeding methods would be incorporated into life activities (such as work outside the home), and learning about breastfeeding by attending a prenatal breastfeeding class and reading.
    D. How the nurse can facilitate decision-making process: provide information about feeding methods in a nonjudgmental manner while still emphasizing the importance of breastfeeding as the preferred method; dispel myths; address personal concerns of the couple; make needed referrals to WIC, lactation consultant, breastfeeding classes, and La Leche League.
3. Breastfeeding mother's questions and concerns.
    A. Breast size: discuss development of lactation structures during pregnancy; emphasize the importance of this development and not the breast size for successful lactation.

B. Let-down reflex: explain what it is and why it happens, including physical and emotional triggers; emphasize its importance in providing the infant with hindmilk.

C. Signs that breastfeeding is going well: see Effective Breastfeeding section and Box 25-2, which identify maternal and newborn indicators of effective breastfeeding; put the indicators in writing and go over each one; provide contact person if mother is concerned.

D. Nipple soreness: see Breast Care and Sore Nipples sections; discuss and demonstrate measures to prevent and treat sore nipples, including, most important, good breastfeeding techniques such as latch, removal, and alternating starting breast and positions; discuss breast care measures such as air-drying nipples, avoiding soap, and applying colostrum/milk or purified lanolin after feeding; using breast shells.

E. Engorgement: see Engorgement section; begin by describing engorgement, what it is, why it occurs, and when it occurs; prevention of excessive engorgement includes frequency of feeding every 2 to 3 hours on each breast (use pumping to soften second breast if needed); relief measures include warm shower and massage before feeding, ice between feedings, and a supportive bra; emphasize the temporary, self-limiting nature of engorgement and analgesics such as ibuprofen or acetaminophen.

F. Afterpains and increased flow: explain that oxytocin is released as a result of infant sucking; this triggers the let-down reflex and stimulates the uterus to contract, causing afterpains; oxytocin also reduces excessive bleeding, though the contractions can cause flow already in the uterus to be expelled, giving the impression of an increased flow.

G. Breastfeeding as a birth control method: see Breastfeeding and Contraception section; emphasize that breastfeeding is not a reliable contraceptive method; although ovulation may be delayed, its return cannot be predicted with accuracy and may occur before the first menstrual period; discuss contraceptive methods that are safe to use with breastfeeding and resuming sexual intercourse during the postpartum period.

H. Weaning: see Weaning section; emphasize that weaning needs to be a gradual process, eliminating one feeding at a time, beginning with the one the baby is most likely to sleep through; discuss the use of bottles and cups; use of formula, cow's milk, and/or solids depends on the age of infant at the time of weaning.

4. Infrequent feeding of sleeping baby: see Frequency and Duration of Feeding, Indicators of Effective Breastfeeding, and Sleepy Baby sections, Nursing Care Plan, and Box 25-2.

A. Nursing diagnosis: imbalanced nutrition: less than body requirements related to infrequent feeding of newborn; expected outcome: mother will awaken infant every 2 to 3 hours during the day and every 4 hours at night to feed the infant, achieving approximately 8 to 12 feedings per day.

B. Nursing approach: discuss feeding cues to facilitate proper timing of feedings; discuss techniques to wake sleeping baby and signs indicating adequate intake; discuss potential problems associated with feedings that are too infrequent.

5. Bottle-feeding mother: see Formula Feeding section and Teaching for Self-Management—Formula Preparation and Feeding box.

A. Nurse's response to mother's concern: discuss how the mother can facilitate close contact and socialization with the infant during feeding by sitting comfortably, touching, singing, and talking quietly to newborn to make feeding a pleasant time for both; reassure mother that properly prepared formulas will fully meet her newborn's need for nutrients and fluid.

B. Guidelines for bottle-feeding: discuss how to choose a formula type; amount and frequency of feedings; how to prepare formula (follow directions for dilution exactly), warming formula correctly, discarding leftover formula, and bottle and nipple cleansing; principles of the feeding process, including semi-upright position, not propping bottles, fluid filling the nipple to limit air consumption, cues of feeding readiness and satiety, and burping.

6. Assessment of breastfeeding mother and infant to ensure that mother and infant are ready for discharge.

A. Factors to assess: see Care Management and Box 25-2 to determine what to assess; it is essential to assess maternal feeding technique, level of knowledge, and confidence as well as newborn responses and physical status.

B. Assessment 1 week after discharge: formulate questions that address the factors that you identified in A above; in addition, ask questions about such areas as frequency and duration of feedings, breastfeeding techniques used, how she feels about breastfeeding and how well she feels she is doing, family support for breastfeeding, her ability to rest, and nutrient and fluid intake.

ANSWER KEY UNIT VII

CHAPTER 26: ASSESSMENT OF HIGH RISK PREGNANCY

I. Learning Key Terms

1. High-risk pregnancy
2. Daily fetal movement count (DFMC); fetal alarm signal
3. Ultrasonography; transvaginal; transabdominal
4. Oligohydramnios
5. Polyhydramnios (hydramnios)
6. Nuchal translucency
7. Doppler blood flow analysis

8. Biophysical profile (BPP); ultrasound; electronic fetal monitoring; fetal breathing movements; fetal body movements; fetal tone; nonstress test (fetal heart rate reactivity); amniotic fluid volume
9. Magnetic resonance imaging (MRI)
10. Amniocentesis
11. Percutaneous umbilical blood sampling (PUBS)/cordocentesis
12. Chorionic villus sampling (CVS)
13. Maternal serum alpha-fetoprotein (MSAFP); 16; 18
14. Triple-marker; 16; 18; MSAFP; unconjugated estriol; hCG; age; quad screen
15. Indirect Coombs test
16. Cell-free DNA screening
17. Nonstress test
18. Vibroacoustic stimulation test (fetal acoustic stimulation test)
19. Contraction stress test; nipple-stimulated contraction stress; oxytocin-stimulated contraction stress
20. Diagnosis of fetal anomalies
21. Determine if the intrauterine environment continues to be supportive of the fetus; determine the timing of childbirth for women at risk for uteroplacental insufficiency (UPI)

II. Reviewing Key Concepts

22. Factors placing a pregnant woman and her fetus or newborn at risk and identification of strategies to eliminate or reduce the risk: see Box 26-1, which describes several risk factors in each category listed.
23. Role of nurse when caring for high-risk pregnant women undergoing antepartal testing: see Nurse's Role in Assessment and Management of the High-Risk Pregnancy section; answer should emphasize education, support measures, assisting with or performing the test, and follow-up care.
24. Risk factors for pregnancy-related problems: see Box 26-2, which lists risk factors for each pregnancy-related problem identified.
25. Choice D is correct; an amniocentesis with analysis of amniotic fluid for the lecithin/sphingomyelin (L/S) ratio and presence of phosphatidylglycerol (Pg) is used to determine pulmonary maturity; choice B refers to a contraction stress test; choice C refers to serial measurements of fetal growth using ultrasound.
26. Choice C is correct; food and fluid are not restricted before the test; the test will evaluate the response of the FHR to fetal movement—acceleration is expected; external, not internal, monitoring is used.
27. Choice B is correct; the quad marker test is used to screen the older pregnant woman for the possibility that her fetus has Down syndrome; serum levels of AFP, unconjugated estriol, human chorionic gonadotropin (hCG), and inhibin A are measured; maternal serum AFP alone is the screening test for open neural tube defects such as spina bifida; a 1-hour, 50-g glucose test is used to screen for gestational diabetes; amniocentesis and Coombs testing are used to check for Rh antibodies and sensitization.

28. Choice C is correct; an equivocal suspicious result is recorded when late decelerations occur with fewer than 50% of the contractions; see Table 26-5 for a full explanation of the results.
29. Choice A is correct; a supine position with hips elevated enhances the view of the uterus; a lithotomy position may also be used; a full bladder is not required for the vaginal ultrasound but is needed for most abdominal ultrasounds; during the test the woman may experience some pressure but medication for pain relief before the test is not required; contact gel is used with the abdominal ultrasound; water-soluble lubricant may be used to ease insertion of the vaginal probe.
30. Choice A is correct; choices B and D are types of results for the contraction stress test; see Box 26-8 for a full explanation of results for the nonstress test and Table 26-5 for the contraction stress test.

III. Thinking Critically

1. Woman scheduled for transvaginal ultrasound: see Ultrasonography section.
   A. Cite reasons for test for this woman: to determine location of gestational sac because PID could have resulted in narrowing of fallopian tube, thereby increasing risk for ectopic pregnancy; in addition, a determination of gestational age and estimation of date of birth would be done related to irregular cycles and unknown date of LMP.
   B. Preparation for the test: explain purpose of test, how it will be performed, and how it will feel; assist her into a lithotomy position or supine position with hips elevated on a pillow; point out structures on monitor as test is performed.
2. Nurse's role in transabdominal ultrasound for monitoring fetal growth: see Ultrasonography section; instruct woman to come for test with full bladder if appropriate; explain purpose of test and method of examination; assist her into a supine position with head and shoulders elevated on pillow and hips slightly tipped to right or left side; observe for supine hypotension during test and orthostatic hypotension when rising to upright position after test; indicate how the fetus is being measured and point out fetus and its movements if the woman wishes to know.
3. Woman having biophysical profile: see Biophysical Profile section and Tables 26-2 and 26-3 for identification of variables tested and scoring.
   A. Nursing diagnosis: anxiety related to unexpected need to undergo a biophysical profile.
   B. Nurse's response to woman's concern about the test: describe how the test will be performed using real-time ultrasound and external electronic fetal monitoring; explain that the purpose of the test is to view the fetus within its environment, to determine the amount of amniotic fluid, and to assess the FHR response to fetal activity.
   C. Meaning of score obtained: a score of 8 to 10 is a normal result.

4. Amniocentesis: see Amniocentesis and Nurse's Role in the Assessment and Management of the High-Risk Pregnancy sections.
   A. Preparing woman: explain procedure; witness informed consent; assess maternal vital signs and health status and FHR before the test; ensure that ultrasound is performed to locate placenta and fetus before the test.
   B. Supporting woman during the procedure: explain what is happening and what she will be feeling; help her to relax; encourage her to ask questions and voice concerns and feelings; assess her reactions.
   C. Postprocedure care and instructions: monitor maternal vital signs and health status and FHR; tell her when test results should be available and whom to call; administer RhoGAM because she is Rh negative; teach her to assess herself for signs of infection, bleeding, rupture of membranes, and uterine contractions; make a follow-up phone call to check her status.
5. Nonstress test: see Nonstress Test section and Box 26-8.
   A. Tell woman about purpose of test: test measures response of FHR to fetal activity to determine adequacy of placental perfusion and fetal oxygenation.
   B. Preparation of woman for test: tell her that she can eat before and during the test; schedule test at a time of day that fetus is usually active; assist woman into a reclining chair or semi-Fowler position with a left or right tilt.
   C. Indicate how test is conducted: attach tocotransducer over the fundus and ultrasound transducer at site of PMI; instruct woman to indicate when fetus moves; assess change, if any, in FHR following the movement.
   D. Analyze the results: see Box 26-8 and Figs. 26-10 and 26-12 for the criteria to determine the test result and to document it as reactive: good variability and normal baseline with accelerations following fetal movement that meet criteria for a reactive result; or as nonreactive: no accelerations with movement or the accelerations that do occur do not meet the criteria and limited variability.
6. Contraction stress test: see Contraction Stress Test section and Table 26-5.
   A. Tell woman about purpose of test: the test is a way of determining how her fetus will react to the stress of uterine contractions as they would occur during labor; uterine contractions decrease perfusion through placenta, leading to fetal hypoxia; late decelerations during this test could be interpreted as an early warning of fetal compromise.
   B. Preparation: assess woman's vital signs, general health status, and contraindications for the test; attach external electronic fetal monitor and assess FHR and uterine activity; assist woman into a lateral, semi-Fowler, or seated position; determine if an informed consent is required since contractions will be stimulated.
   C. Indicate how the test is performed: see Nipple-Stimulation Contraction Stress Test section; stimulate nipple(s) according to protocol until three contractions of good quality occur in a 10-minute period; ensure that contractions subside after the test and assess maternal and fetal responses.
   D. Use of oxytocin to stimulate contractions: see Oxytocin-Stimulated Contraction Stress Test section; administer oxytocin (Pitocin) intravenously (similar to induction of labor but with lower dosages) according to protocol, increasing rate until uterine contractions meet criteria indicated for a nipple-stimulated CST; monitor woman, fetus, and contractions during the test and afterward until contractions subside.
   E. Analyze the results: see Table 26-5 and Fig. 26-14 for criteria used to interpret the test results and to document result as negative, positive, equivocal suspicious, equivocal hyperstimulatory, or unsatisfactory.

CHAPTER 27: HYPERTENSIVE DISORDERS

I. Learning Key Terms

1. E, 2. C, 3. B, 4. A, 5. F, 6. D
7. Gestational hypertension
8. Chronic hypertension
9. Preeclampsia
10. Hypertension; 2; 4 to 6; 1
11. Proteinuria
12. Dependent edema; ankles; sacrum
13. Eclampsia
14. HELLP syndrome; hemolysis; liver enzymes; platelets
15. Vasospasm

II. Reviewing Key Concepts

16. Assessment techniques to determine findings associated with preeclampsia: see Care Management—Physical Assessment section and use a physical assessment textbook to further explain each assessment technique.
    ■ Hyperreflexia and ankle clonus: see Table 27-4, which grades DTR responses, and Fig. 27-5 for illustrations depicting performance of DTRs and ankle clonus.
    ■ Proteinuria: describe dipstick and 24-hour urine collection methods to determine level of protein in urine.
    ■ Pitting edema: see Figs. 27-3 and 27-4, which illustrate assessment of pitting edema and classifications.
17. Choice A is correct; the woman should rest for at least 10 minutes after assuming her position and the cuff should cover 80% of the upper arm or be 1.5 times the length of the upper arm; either Korotkoff phase V alone or with phase IV should be used when recording the diastolic pressure.

327

18. Choice C is correct; with severe preeclampsia the DTRs should be ≥3+ with positive ankle clonus indicating increased cerebral involvement, the BP should be >160/110 mm Hg, with a platelet count of <100,000/mm^3, which reflects thrombocytopenia; serum creatinine would be greater than 1.1 mg/dL.

19. Choices C, D, and F are correct; a respiratory rate of less than 12 breaths/minute indicates central nervous system (CNS) depression caused by the magnesium sulfate; the solution should be 40 g in 1000 mL of Ringer lactate; assessment should occur every 15 to 30 minutes and the maintenance dose should be 1 to 3 g/hour; calcium gluconate is the antidote for magnesium sulfate toxicity.

20. Choice B is correct; magnesium sulfate acts as a CNS depressant and is given to prevent seizures.

21. Choices B, C, D, and E are correct; a clean catch midstream urine specimen should be used to assess urine for protein using a dipstick; fluid intake should be six to eight 8-ounce glasses a day along with roughage to prevent constipation; gentle exercise improves circulation and helps to preserve muscle tone and a sense of well-being; no sodium restriction is required except for limiting excessively salty foods; diversional activities, including contact with friends, will decrease boredom and stress.

22. Choice C is correct; nifedipine (Procardia) is a calcium channel blocker used to decrease blood pressure.

23. Choice B is correct; magnesium sulfate is a CNS depressant that potentiates the action of other CNS depressants such as opioid analgesics; it reduces the risk for seizures but is unlikely to cause hypotension; diuresis is a common expected finding in the postpartum period.

24. Choice C is correct; oxytocin (Pitocin) as an oxytocic medication is safe and effective to use to contract the uterus and reduce blood loss because it will not increase blood pressure as can methylergonovine (Methergine), another oxytocic medication; calcium gluconate is the antidote used for magnesium sulfate toxicity; labetalol (Normodyne) is an antihypertensive medication.

25. Choice B is correct; although choices A, C, and D are all appropriate actions, they are not the first priority; remember the ABCs—airway, breathing, circulation—when considering the priority action.

III. Thinking Critically

1. Protocol to ensure accurate blood pressure measurement: see Box 27-2; emphasize consistency in position of woman and her arm, the arm used, size of cuff, and provision of a rest period prior to the measurement; consider teaching these principles to the pregnant woman and her family.

2. Profile of two women at risk for preeclampsia: see Preeclampsia section and Box 27-1 for information on risk factors to use when creating the profiles; be sure to use different risk factors for each profile created.

3. Preeclampsia and eclampsia—effect on fetal well-being.
   A. Describe effect: see Significance and Incidence and Pathophysiology sections and Figs. 27-1 and 27-2; many major effects on fetal health are described.
   B. Fetal surveillance measures: see Mild Gestational Hypertension and Preeclampsia without Severe Features—Maternal and Fetal Assessment section for the surveillance measures commonly used; emphasize to woman the importance of ongoing prenatal care.

4. Woman with preeclampsia—home care.
   A. Clinical manifestations: see Tables 27-2, which differentiates between preeclampsia with and without severe features in terms of maternal and fetal effects, and 27-3, which lists the changes in laboratory values.
   B. Three priority nursing diagnoses: see Nursing Care Plan; nursing diagnoses should consider physiologic effects of preeclampsia such as ineffective tissue perfusion—placenta and risk for injury to mother or fetus; psychosocial effects: anxiety, ineffective individual and family coping, powerlessness, ineffective role performance, interrupted family processes; assessment findings should guide the choice and priority of nursing diagnoses, especially regarding those that apply to psychosocial effects.
   C. Organization of home care: see Mild Gestational Hypertension and Preeclampsia without Severe Features section and Teaching for Self-Management boxes; help couple to mobilize their support system, make referrals to home care if needed, and discuss frequency of prenatal visits and antepartum testing.
   D. Teaching regarding assessment of status and signs of a worsening condition: see Table 27-2, Box 27-2, and Teaching for Self- Management—Assessing and Reporting Clinical Signs of Preeclampsia box; discuss signs and put them in writing so couple can refer to them at home; have woman keep a daily diary of her findings, feelings, and concerns; teach woman and family to take BP, weigh accurately, assess urine, and take daily fetal movement counts and about whom to call if problems or concerns arise.
   E. Instructions about nutrition and fluid intake: see Diet section and Teaching for Self-Management—Diet for Preeclampsia box for several food and fluid recommendations.
   F. Coping with bed rest: see Activity Restriction section and Teaching for Self-Management—Coping with Activity Restriction box; explain rationale for bed rest and activity restrictions; clarify what this restriction means; discuss importance of lateral position when in bed, gentle range-of-motion (ROM) exercises, relaxation exercises, and non-stressful and calming diversional activities.

G. Risk for constipation: see Teaching for Self-Management—Diet for Preeclampsia and Coping with Activity Restriction boxes; discuss roughage, fluid, and activity.

5. Woman with severe preeclampsia—hospital care: see Severe Gestational Hypertension and Preeclampsia with Severe Features section.

A. Signs and symptoms: see Tables 27-2, which differentiates between preeclampsia with and without severe features in terms of maternal and fetal effects, and 27-3, which lists changes in laboratory values.

B. Three priority nursing diagnoses: see Nursing Care Plan; impaired tissue perfusion, risk for impaired gas exchange, and injury take priority as the physiologic nursing diagnoses because her condition is worsening and the safety of the maternal-fetal unit is jeopardized; anxiety or fear is the priority psychosocial nursing diagnosis.

C. Measures to protect mother and fetus: see Box 27-3, which lists precautionary measures in terms of environmental modifications, seizure precautions, and readiness of emergency medications and equipment.

D. Administration of magnesium sulfate: see Box 27-4 and Magnesium Sulfate section.

   1. Create a protocol: list the guidelines for preparing and administering the medication solution safely including dosage, IV solution, and infusion rate; identify essential assessment measures that must be completed and documented before and during the infusion.

   2. Nursing diagnosis: risk for ineffective breathing pattern related to the CNS depressant effects of magnesium sulfate infusion.

   3. Explain expected therapeutic effect: discuss that this medication is used for its CNS depressant effects to prevent convulsions; describe how it will be given, how she will feel, and what will be done while she is receiving the infusion.

   4. Maternal and fetal assessments: maternal vital signs, FHR pattern, intake and output, urine for protein, DTRs and ankle clonus, signs of improvement or worsening condition including signs of an imminent seizure.

   5. Signs of magnesium sulfate toxicity: hyporeflexia, respiratory depression, oliguria, diminished level of consciousness (LOC).

   6. Immediate actions: discontinue the magnesium sulfate infusion, administer calcium gluconate slowly, and IV push according to protocol.

E. Seizure occurs: see Eclampsia section and Emergency—Eclampsia box.

   1. Emergency measures at onset of convulsion and immediately following:
      - Emphasize importance of maintaining a patent airway, preventing injury, and calling for help.
      - Observe effect of seizure on mother and fetus.
      - Document the event and care measures implemented during and after seizure.
      - Provide comfort and reassurance after the convulsion; orient to what happened; never leave alone because another seizure could occur or signs of complications can begin; inform family.

   2. List problems that can occur: rupture of membranes, preterm labor and birth, altered LOC, abruptio placentae, fetal distress.

F. Postpartum period recovering from eclampsia: see Postpartum Care section; discuss each of the following components of care:
   - Comprehensive assessment with emphasis on signs of hemorrhage, impending seizures, and status of preeclampsia
   - Precautionary measures
   - Medications that may be given
   - Emotional and psychosocial support for woman and her family; parent-infant interaction
   - Information to give to woman and family

CHAPTER 28: HEMORRHAGIC DISORDERS

I. Learning Key Terms

1. Miscarriage (spontaneous abortion); reduced cervical competence (premature dilation of the cervix); ectopic pregnancy; hydatidiform mole (molar pregnancy)
2. Placenta previa; premature separation of the placenta (abruptio placentae or placental abruption)
3. Spontaneous miscarriage (abortion); threatened; inevitable; incomplete; complete; missed
4. Recurrent (habitual) miscarriage
5. Human chorionic gonadotropin (hCG)
6. Dilation and curettage (D&C)
7. Premature dilation of the cervix (reduced cervical competence)
8. Cerclage
9. Ectopic (tubal) pregnancy
10. Cullen sign
11. Hydatidiform mole (molar pregnancy)
12. Gestational trophoblastic disease (GTD)
13. Complete hydatidiform mole
14. Partial hydatidiform mole
15. Placenta previa
16. Accreta; increta; precreta
17. Premature separation of the placenta (abruptio placentae)
18. Couvelaire uterus
19. Velamentous insertion of the cord
20. Battledore placenta
21. Succenturiate placenta
22. Disseminated intravascular coagulation (DIC) or consumptive coagulopathy

329

II. Reviewing Key Concepts

23. DIC in pregnancy: see Clotting Disorders in Pregnancy section.
    A. Obstetric risk factors for DIC: abruptio placentae, retained dead fetus, anaphylactoid syndrome, severe preeclampsia, HELLP syndrome, and gram-negative sepsis.
    B. Pathophysiology of DIC: see Disseminated Intravascular Coagulation section for an explanation of what goes wrong with clotting and why.
    C. Clinical manifestations: see Box 28-3 for a list of manifestations.
    D. Priority nursing care measures: see Management section; discuss thorough assessment, treatment of underlying cause, positioning, administration of fluid and blood/blood products and oxygen as ordered, education and emotional support of woman and family; closely monitor renal function, including urinary output.
24. Effect of bleeding during pregnancy: see chapter introductory section for a discussion of the harmful effects of blood loss for the mother and fetus.
25. Choice A is correct; the woman is experiencing a threatened miscarriage; therefore expectant management is attempted first, although there are no research-proven therapies; choices B and C reflect management of an inevitable and complete or incomplete abortion; cerclage or suturing of the cervix is done for recurrent spontaneous miscarriage associated with premature dilation of the cervix (reduced cervical competence).
26. Choice C is correct; choices A, B, and D are appropriate nursing diagnoses but deficient fluid volume is the most immediate concern since it places the woman's well-being at greatest risk.
27. Choices B, C, and D are correct; methotrexate destroys rapidly dividing cells, in this case the fetus and placenta, to avoid rupture of tube and need for surgery; folic acid increases the risk for side effects with this medication; the woman should not put anything into her vagina; she needs to return to check her hCG level.
28. Choice C is correct; the clinical manifestations of placenta previa are described; bleeding and clots with abdominal pain and uterine tenderness are characteristic of abruptio placentae; massive bleeding from many sites is associated with DIC; bleeding is not an expected sign of preterm labor.
29. Choice A is correct; hemorrhage is a major potential postpartum complication because the implantation site of the placenta is in the lower uterine segment, which has a limited capacity to contract after birth; infection is another major complication but it is not the immediate focus of care; choices B and D are also important but not to the same degree as hemorrhage, which is life threatening.

III. Thinking Critically

1. Woman with ruptured ectopic pregnancy: see Ectopic Pregnancy section.
    A. Risk factors: see Incidence and Etiology section for several risk factors.
    B. Assessment of findings: see Clinical Manifestations section; discuss findings beginning with signs of an unruptured tubal pregnancy, which are subtle and often missed; signs of rupture are more acute and may be mistaken for other acute abdominal conditions.
    C. Differential diagnosis (other health problems): see Diagnosis section; miscarriage, appendicitis, salpingitis, ruptured ovarian cyst, torsion of ovary, UTI, etc.
    D. Major care management problem: hemorrhage; much of the blood accumulates in the abdominal cavity.
    E. Two priority nursing diagnoses: deficient fluid volume and acute pain as well as fear/anxiety and anticipatory grief
    F. Nursing measures in the preoperative and postoperative periods: see Surgical Management, Initial Care, and Follow-up Care sections; assessment, general preoperative and postoperative care measures, fluid replacement, major emphasis on emotional support to facilitate grieving, discussion of effect of rupture on future pregnancies, referral for counseling as appropriate, prepare for discharge with instructions for postoperative self-care including self-assessment for complications such as infection, measures to enhance healing, importance of follow-up appointment to assess progress of physical and emotional recovery.
2. Woman with signs of miscarriage: see Miscarriage (Spontaneous Abortion) section and Table 28-1.
    A. Basis for signs and symptoms: signs indicate the woman is experiencing a threatened miscarriage.
    B. Expected care management: bed rest, sedation, avoidance of stress and orgasm; follow progress with hCG levels and ultrasound to assess integrity of gestational sac; watch for signs of progress to inevitable abortion; caution her to save peripads and tissue passed.
3. Woman with signs of miscarriage: see Miscarriage (Spontaneous Abortion) section, Table 28-1, and Teaching for Self-Management—Discharge Teaching for the Woman after Early Miscarriage box.
    A. Questions to ask: determine what she means by "a lot of bleeding" and if she is experiencing any other signs and symptoms related to miscarriage such as pain and cramping; determine the gestational age of her pregnancy and if there is anyone to bring her to the hospital for evaluation.
    B. Assessment findings indicative of an incomplete miscarriage: heavy, profuse bleeding, severe cramping, passage of tissue, cervix dilated with tissue present.

C. Priority nursing diagnosis at this time: deficient fluid volume related to blood loss secondary to incomplete abortion.

D. Outline nursing measures: prepare woman for the prompt termination of her pregnancy—assess before and after procedure (e.g., dilation and curettage), explain what will occur, provide emotional support, refer for counseling if needed, prepare for discharge, and arrange for follow-up to assess physical and emotional status; include immediate and postprocedure care.

E. Discharge instructions: see Follow-up Care section and Teaching for Self-Management—Discharge Teaching for the Woman after Early Miscarriage box; advise regarding signs and symptoms of complications (bleeding, infection), what to expect regarding progress of healing (pain, discharge), and measures to prevent complications (hygiene, nutrition, rest); advise her to allow for physical and emotional healing before considering another pregnancy.

F. Nursing measures for anticipatory grieving: see Follow-up Care section and Teaching for Self-Management—Discharge Teaching for the Woman after Early Miscarriage box; acknowledge her loss and provide time for her to express her feelings; inform her about how she may feel (mood swings, depression); refer her to grief counseling, support groups, clergy; make follow-up phone calls (see Chapter 37).

4. Care of woman following cerclage: see Cervical Insufficiency section; answer should include the following care measures:
   - Assessment for uterine contractions, rupture of membranes, infection
   - Explanation of activity restrictions, warning signs including those that may require immediate transfer to the hospital
   - Discussion of her feelings regarding the pregnancy and her understanding of her health problem and its treatment
   - Identification and involvement of support system as appropriate

5. Woman with complete hydatidiform mole: see Hydatidiform Mole section.
   A. Typical signs and symptoms: see Clinical Manifestations section for a description of assessment findings.
   B. Posttreatment instructions: see Management and Follow-up Care sections; frequent physical and pelvic examinations and regular measurement of serum hCG levels following protocol for frequency; emphasize importance of follow-up assessments and strict birth control (avoid use of IUD) to prevent pregnancy until hCG levels have been normal for a specified period of time; provide time to discuss knowledge of disorder, treatment, and follow-up and to express feelings; referral to support group may be helpful.

6. Comparison of a woman with marginal placenta previa to a woman with abruptio placentae, grade II.
   A. Comparison of findings: see Placenta Previa and Abruptio Placentae sections and Table 28-2 to compare findings for each disorder in terms of characteristics of bleeding, uterine tone, pain and tenderness, and ultrasound findings regarding location of placenta and fetal presentation/position, hypertension associations, and fetal effects.
   B. Priority nursing diagnoses: consider diagnoses related to major physical problems such as deficient fluid volume related to blood loss, ineffective tissue perfusion (placenta), and risk for fetal injury; acute pain would be another major nursing diagnosis as the placenta continues to separate; major psychosocial nursing diagnoses could include fear/anxiety, interrupted family processes, and anticipatory grieving.
   C. Comparison of care management approaches: consider home care versus hospital care for woman with placenta previa; hospital care is the safest approach for woman experiencing abruptio placentae; discuss active versus expectant management for each disorder.
   D. Postpartum considerations: potential complications should be the basis for the special postpartum care requirements; describe each major complication and the basis for its occurrence: hemorrhage and infection are the major physiologic complications that need to be addressed; emotional and psychosocial support are important related to the high-risk nature of the pregnancy, especially if fetal loss, maternal loss, or both was the outcome.

CHAPTER 29: ENDOCRINE AND METABOLIC DISORDERS

I. Learning Key Terms

1. Interrelationship of the clinical manifestations of diabetes mellitus: see Pathogenesis section in Diabetes Mellitus for a full description of each of the clinical manifestations listed in terms of cause and interrelationship with one another.
2. Diabetes mellitus
3. Polyuria
4. Polydipsia
5. Polyphagia
6. Glycosuria
7. Type 1 diabetes mellitus
8. Type 2 diabetes mellitus
9. Pregestational diabetes
10. Gestational diabetes
11. Glycemic control
12. Hydramnios (polyhydramnios)
13. Hypoglycemia
14. Hyperglycemia
15. Diabetic ketoacidosis (DKA)
16. Euglycemia; 65 to 95 mg/dL; 130 to 140 mg/dL

17. Macrosomia
18. Glycosylated hemoglobin (hemoglobin A_{1c})
19. Fasting (preprandial) blood glucose; 60 mg/dL; 99 mg/dL
20. Postprandial (postmeal) blood glucose; 130 mg/dL; 140 mg/dL; $\leq$120 mg/dL
21. Phosphatidylglycerol
22. Maternal serum alpha-fetoprotein
23. Fetal nuchal translucency (NT)
24. Hyperemesis gravidarum

II. Reviewing Key Concepts

25. Maternal and fetal/neonatal risks and complications related to pregestational and gestational diabetes: see Pregestational Diabetes Mellitus—Maternal Risks/Complications and Fetal/Neonatal Risks and Gestational Diabetes sections for lists with explanations of the risks and complications; describe why these risks/complications are more likely to occur in women with diabetes; explain to the woman what she can do to reduce the risk by regular health care, maintaining euglycemia and a normal BMI, exercising, reducing stress etc.
26. Explain metabolic changes in pregnancy and effect on diabetes management: see Metabolic Changes Associated with Pregnancy section in Diabetes Mellitus for a description related to changes associated with pregnancy and the postpartum period; include how the need for insulin changes from trimester to trimester.
27. Types of insulin and how they work: see Insulin Therapy section and Table 29-4 for a discussion of each type of insulin with examples; you also may wish to use a nursing drug manual for further information on the types of insulin.
28. Recommendations for screening for and diagnosis of gestational diabetes: see Screening for Gestational Diabetes Mellitus section for current guidelines related to screening and criteria for diagnosis.
    A. Recommendations for screening: explain to woman the risk factors she presents for gestational diabetes mellitus; discuss what it is and why screening is important for her and her baby.
    B. Test result and further testing: result of 130 to 140 mg/dL is a positive screen and requires further testing by an oral glucose tolerance test (OGTT); explain to the woman what this means and how to prepare for the diagnostic test.
    C. Confirmation of diagnosis: diagnosis is made if two or more of the values are met or exceeded.
29. State effect of thyroid disorders on reproduction and pregnancy: see Thyroid Disorders section for a full description of hyperthyroidism and hypothyroidism; consider effects of these disorders on reproductive development, sexuality, and fertility in terms of ability to conceive and to sustain a pregnancy to viability; potential fetal/newborn complications related to maternal treatment of her thyroid disorder.

30. Choice D is correct; the woman is exhibiting signs of DKA; insulin is the required treatment, with the dosage dependent on blood glucose level; IV fluids may also be required; choice A is the treatment for hypoglycemia; although they may increase the woman's comfort, choices B and C are not the priority.
31. Choice C is correct; a 2-hour postprandial blood glucose should be 130 mg/dL or less; choices A, B, and D all fall within the expected normal ranges for premeal and postmeal levels (see Table 29-3).
32. Choices A, C, and D are correct; based on a normal BMI (19.8 to 26), calories should be 30 to 35 kcal/kg each day; the bedtime snack needs to be substantial to prevent starvation ketoacidosis; simple carbohydrates should be avoided.
33. Choices B, D, and F are correct; washing hands is important but gloves are not necessary for self-injection; vial should be rotated gently, not shaken; regular insulin should be drawn into the syringe first; because she is obese, a 90-degree angle with skin taut is recommended; vial tops should be cleansed with alcohol prior to each use.
34. Choice B is correct; oral hygiene is important when nothing by mouth (NPO) and after vomiting episodes to maintain the integrity of oral mucosa; taking fluids between (not with) meals reduces nausea, thereby increasing tolerance for oral nutrition; vitamin B_6 (pyridoxine) and/or doxylamine (Unisom) are often the first-line antiemetic drugs used.

III. Thinking Critically

1. Preconception counseling for a woman with diabetes mellitus: see Preconception Counseling section. In your answer:
   - Discuss purpose in terms of planning pregnancy for the optimum time when glucose control is established within normal ranges and why this is important.
   - Discuss how her diabetes management will need to be altered during pregnancy; include her husband, because his health is important, as is his support during pregnancy.
2. Pregnant woman with pregestational diabetes experiencing hypoglycemia: see Tables 29-2 and 29-4, Teaching for Self-Management—Treatment for Hypoglycemia box, and Metabolic Changes Associated with Pregnancy and Pregestational Diabetes Mellitus sections.
   A. Problem: signs and symptoms suggest hypoglycemia resulting from insufficient caloric intake with no adjustment in insulin dosage.
   B. Action: see Table 29-2 and Teaching for Self-Management box for a discussion of the action to take in sequence.
   C. Glucose boosters: see Teaching for Self-Management box for a list of substances that provide 15 g of simple carbohydrate.
   D. Follow-up actions: after ingesting the simple carbohydrate, the woman should rest for 15 minutes,

then check her blood glucose level again; based on the finding, further action may need to be taken; be sure to discuss with the woman how to reduce the risk that the problem will recur (see Teaching for Self-Management—Treatment for Hypoglycemia box).

3. Woman with pregestational diabetes: see Care Management section.
   A. Additional antepartal fetal assessments: see Fetal Surveillance section, which describes several tests.
   B. Stressors facing woman and family: alteration in daily living, including usual diabetes management; need for additional antepartal testing and prenatal visits; financial implications.
   C. Nursing diagnoses: see Nursing Care Plan; consider both physiologic and psychosocial concerns; consider areas of deficient knowledge, anxiety/fear, ineffective coping, risk for maternal or fetal injury, and imbalanced nutrition.
   D. Activity and exercise recommendations: see Exercise section; recommend exercises according to her diabetic status and usual exercise patterns; discuss when she should exercise and emphasize the importance of checking blood glucose level and adjusting caloric intake and insulin administration accordingly.
   E. Complete outline related to care management during antepartum, intrapartum, and postpartum periods: see specific sections for diet, blood glucose monitoring, and insulin therapy, the Teaching for Self-Management boxes, Tables 29-3 and 29-4, and Nursing Care Plan for information regarding interventions and health teaching.
   F. Birth control recommendations: see Postpartum section; discuss risks and benefits of a variety of methods, including their effect on glucose levels and infection; stress importance of delaying intercourse until healing is complete to prevent infection; discuss effect of another pregnancy and its timing.

4. Hispanic-American woman with gestational diabetes: see Gestational Diabetes section.
   A. Complication of pregnancy exhibited with validating findings: gestational diabetes; 50-g glucose test result is 152 mg/dL (130 to 140 mg/dL or greater); 3-hour glucose test reveals three values exceeding the normal range (fasting, 1-hour result, and 2-hour result—see Fig. 29-4).
   B. Risk factors exhibited: older than 25 years of age, Hispanic, BMI indicates obesity, woman's mother has type 2 diabetes, previous birth of baby >4500 g (9.9 lb).
   C. Pathophysiology of gestational diabetes: see Metabolic Changes Associated with Pregnancy and Gestational Diabetes sections for a description of the pathophysiology involved.
   D. Ongoing assessment: see Care Management—Antepartum section; emphasize importance of monitoring blood glucose levels at recommended times, antepartal fetal surveillance measures, and increased frequency of prenatal visits.
   E. Nursing diagnoses:
      - Anxiety related to diagnosis of ineffective glucose metabolism during pregnancy associated with gestational diabetes
      - Risk for fetal injury related to excessive intrauterine growth associated with uncontrolled gestational diabetes
   F. Dietary changes: see Diet section, which provides guidelines to follow in terms of nutrient proportion and meal distribution.
   G. Administration of insulin: see Pharmacologic Therapy section and Teaching for Self-Management—Self-Administration of Insulin box for the information required to respond to the woman's concern and what to teach her; commend her for her positive efforts to follow the prescribed diet and provide her with the emotional support she will need to perform the skill of administering insulin safely and effectively; enlist family support if needed; incorporate teaching methodologies that represent cognitive, psychomotor, and affective learning.
   H. Implications of gestational diabetes mellitus: see Postpartum section for a description of recovery of glucose control and implications for her future related to the development of diabetes for herself and her children; discuss what the woman can do to reduce her risk for future glucose metabolism problems, including diet modification, exercise, and weight loss.

5. Woman with hyperemesis gravidarum: see Hyperemesis Gravidarum section.
   A. Predisposing/etiologic factors: see Hyperemesis Gravidarum section, which identifies several physiologic and psychologic factors, including the factors present in this situation: nullipara, obesity, ambivalence about pregnancy, lifestyle alterations; additional factors include multifetal pregnancy, molar pregnancy, body change concerns, history of diabetes, gastrointestinal disorders, and thyroid dysfunction.
   B. Assessment of physiologic and psychosocial factors upon admission: see Care Management—Assessment section.
      - Physiologic: full description of nausea and vomiting; presence of other gastrointestinal (GI) symptoms; relief measures used; weight, including changes; vital signs; signs of fluid, electrolyte, and acid-base imbalances; urine check for ketones (ketonuria) and specific gravity; CBC; serum electrolytes; liver enzymes; bilirubin levels; thyroid testing.
      - Psychosocial: discuss concerns regarding self and pregnancy; assess support system.
   C. Priority nursing diagnoses: deficient fluid volume, risk for fetal and maternal injury, anxiety, powerlessness, ineffective individual or family

coping; woman's condition and circumstances will determine the priority, with physiologic diagnoses taking precedence in the acute phase

D. Care measures during hospitalization
- Restore fluid and electrolyte balance with IV administration of fluids, electrolytes, and nutrients.
- Restore ability to tolerate oral nutrition: gradual progression from NPO to full diet.
- Monitor progress to determine effectiveness of therapeutic regimen, readiness for discharge, and need for continuing treatment with home care.
- Provide psychosocial support for woman and her family; make referrals as appropriate; offer comfort measures, including oral care, and provide a calm, restful environment free of odors.
- Teach woman and family about the disorder, how it is treated, and its effect on pregnancy and fetus.

E. Home care:
- Discuss follow-up care requirements, types of foods to eat, and ways to eat (similar to recommendations for morning sickness); see Teaching for Self-Management—Diet for Hyperemesis box.
- Include family in plan of care, especially with regard to meal preparation and support and encouragement of the woman.
- Teach woman how to assess herself in terms of weight, urine for ketones, signs of developing problems that should be reported including weight loss, return of nausea and vomiting, pain, and dehydration.

CHAPTER 30: MEDICAL-SURGICAL DISORDERS

I. Learning Key Terms

1. Cardiac decompensation
2. Functional classification of organic heart disease; asymptomatic without limitation of physical activity; symptomatic with slight limitation of activity; symptomatic with marked limitation of activity; symptomatic with inability to carry on any physical activity without discomfort
3. Atrial septal defect (ASD)
4. Ventricular septal defect (VSD)
5. Patent ductus arteriosus (PDA)
6. Coarctation of the aorta
7. Tetralogy of fallot
8. Aortic stenosis
9. Myocardial infarction (MI)
10. Peripartum cardiomyopathy
11. Mitral valve stenosis
12. Infective endocarditis
13. Eisenmenger syndrome
14. Mitral valve prolapse
15. Marfan syndrome
16. Primary pulmonary hypertension
17. Anemia
18. Folic acid (folate) deficiency
19. Sickle cell hemoglobinopathy
20. Thalassemia
21. Asthma
22. Acute respiratory distress syndrome (ARDS)
23. Cystic fibrosis
24. Pruritus gravidarum
25. Pruritic urticarial papules and plaques of pregnancy (PUPPS)
26. Intrahepatic cholestasis of pregnancy (ICP)
27. Epilepsy
28. Multiple sclerosis (MS)
29. Systemic lupus erythematosus (SLE)
30. Myasthenia gravis (MG)
31. Cholelithiasis
32. Cholecystitis
33. Inflammatory bowel disease
34. Urinary tract infection (UTI); bacteruria; cystitis; pyelonephritis
35. Appendicitis
36. Bell palsy

II. Reviewing Key Concepts

37. Maternal and fetal complications related to maternal cardiovascular problems: see Cardiovascular Disorders section and Box 30-1; increased risk for miscarriage, preterm labor and birth, intrauterine growth restriction (IUGR), maternal mortality, and stillbirth; help the couple to recognize that MVS represents a low risk but that could change as pregnancy progresses; emphasize the importance of regular health care and lifestyle practices, including diet, rest and exercise balance, and stress reduction, including infection prevention.

38. Modifications in CPR and abdominal thrust maneuver when a woman is pregnant: see Cardiopulmonary Resuscitation of the Pregnant Woman section, Emergency—Cardiopulmonary Resuscitation for the Pregnant Woman box, and Fig. 30-2, which cover the recommended modifications, based on anatomic changes that occur during pregnancy, for safe and effective CPR and the abdominal thrust maneuver.

39. Choices B, D, and E are correct; other signs of cardiac decompensation include moist, frequent cough and crackles at bases of lungs; supine hypotension is a common finding during pregnancy related to compression of vena cava and aorta, not cardiac decompensation; wheezing is characteristic of narrowed air passages and not fluid in the lungs, as would occur with pulmonary edema associated with cardiac decompensation.

40. Choice A is correct; this woman is exhibiting signs of cardiac decompensation; further information regarding her cardiac status is required to determine what action would be needed.

41. Choice C is correct; furosemide (Lasix) is a diuretic; propranolol (Inderal) is used to manage hypertension and cardiac dysrhythmias; heparin is a large-molecule anticoagulant that does not cross the placenta or cause teratogenic effects, as does warfarin (Coumadin), which does cross the placenta and potentially causes teratogenic effects.

42. Choice B is correct; bed rest is not required for a woman with a class II designation; she will need to avoid heavy exertion and stop activities that cause fatigue and dyspnea; actions in choices A, C, and D are all appropriate and recommended for class II cardiac disorder.

43. Choice C is correct; fat should be reduced to 40 to 50 g; protein should be limited to 10% to 12% of total calories; fatty and fried foods should be avoided; spices, as long as tolerated, are permitted.

III. Thinking Critically

1. Pregnant women requiring abdominal surgery.
   A. Factors that complicate diagnosis and treatment for abdominal problems: see Surgery during Pregnancy section for several reasons why diagnosis is more difficult, including displacement of abdominal organs and changes in clinical manifestations; treatment is more complicated as a result of the cardiovascular and respiratory changes associated with pregnancy and presence of an enlarged uterus and fetus.
   B. Clinical manifestations: see Appendicitis section for a full discussion.
   C. Importance of treating appendicitis before rupture: see Appendicitis section for goal of early diagnosis and prompt treatment; consider maternal and fetal effects of late diagnosis, after rupture, including the need to use medications and the potential for preterm labor and fetal loss.
   D. Fears often expressed by women undergoing surgery and her family: fear of losing baby and effects of the procedure and medications on fetal well-being and the course of the pregnancy; women should be encouraged to express their fears, concerns, and questions.
   E. Outline preoperative and postoperative care requirements: see Management—Hospital Care section; outline should include assessment and care measures.
   F. Discharge planning: see Home Care section and Box 30-3; teach woman and family about what to watch for, care of incision site, activity and rest considerations, and nutrition guidelines for healing and recovery; include assessing for changes in fetal status (e.g., fetal movements) and for signs of preterm labor.

2. Pregnant woman with mitral valve stenosis class II: see Cardiovascular Disorders section.
   A. Two nursing diagnoses: see Nursing Care Plan, where several nursing diagnoses and expected outcomes of care are listed; evaluate assessment findings to determine the priority for a specific pregnant woman.
   - Fear/anxiety would be a top priority psychosocial nursing diagnosis for this woman because it is her first pregnancy and she does not really know what to expect; expected outcome: the woman and couple will openly express concerns and seek information as needed.
   - Physiologically, activity intolerance, risk for ineffective tissue perfusion, and decreased cardiac output would be priorities as pregnancy advances and the cardiac workload increases; expected outcome: woman will follow recommended therapeutic regimen to reduce stress on her heart.
   B. Recommended therapeutic plan for a pregnant woman designated as class II: see Care Management—Antepartum section and Nursing Care Plan focusing on specific guidelines for class II and descriptions of recommended care measures for each area; fully discuss measures for each area in your answer, including a rationale for use and effectiveness.
   - Rest, sleep, and activity pattern: activities to avoid and importance of rest (include rest recommendations).
   - Prevention of infection: infection is a major stressor that can increase risk for decompensation.
   - Nutrition: nutrients to include in a well-balanced diet; avoid weight that exceeds the recommended range for her BMI; discuss possible need to restrict sodium and fluid.
   - Bowel elimination: prevent constipation, which could lead to using the Valsalva maneuver and straining with passage of stool.
   C. Factors increasing stress.
   - Physiologic stress: anemia, infection, edema, constipation.
   - Psychosocial stress: depression, anxiety and fear, financial concerns, anger, impaired social interactions, feelings of inadequacy, cultural expectations, inadequate support system.
   D. Subjective symptoms of cardiac decompensation: see Signs of Complications—Cardiac Decompensation box.
   E. Objective signs of cardiac decompensation: see Signs of Complications—Cardiac Decompensation box.
   F. Care during labor: see Intrapartum section, which identifies specific measures related to:
   - Comprehensive assessment for decompensation along with routine assessments related to labor and birth.
   - Decreasing fear and anxiety with support measures and creating a calm environment.
   - Providing pain relief using pharmacologic and nonpharmacologic measures.

- Vaginal birth being the best approach; include recommendations for measures to enhance labor process, including positioning, breathing exercises, pushing techniques.
- Preventing postpartum bleeding; medications to use.
G. Risk for postpartum cardiac decompensation: see Postpartum Care—Safety Alert for a discussion of the basis of cardiac decompensation in first 24 to 48 hours after birth.
H. Nursing diagnoses for early postpartum period.
  - Risk for excess fluid volume related to extravascular fluid shifts following birth would be the top priority physiologic nursing diagnosis.
  - Ineffective breastfeeding, risk for impaired mother-infant attachment, *or* situational low self-esteem can be priority psychosocial nursing diagnoses related to the woman's need for activity reduction and limited ability to care for newborn on her own.
I. Stress reduction during postpartum period: see Postpartum section; encourage rest in a lateral position with head of bed elevated; assist with activities of daily living (ADL) and progressive ambulation; provide for pain relief and comfort; emphasize measures to prevent infection and constipation; assist with newborn care while keeping newborn nearby so she can see and touch her baby, facilitating attachment.
J. Breastfeeding: breastfeeding is allowed but the woman will need extra support and rest because of the increased energy demands associated with lactation; medications used for the mother must be evaluated for their effect on the newborn.
K. Discharge plan: emphasize the following:
  - Follow up with health care providers for assessment of postpartum recovery and cardiac status.
  - Contraception, future pregnancy, and sexuality issues.
  - Assistance with infant, self, and home care; make referrals as needed; enlist family support.
  - Importance of balancing rest and activity.
  - Instructions regarding the healing process and how to assess progress and prevent complications.
3. Pregnant woman with cardiac disorder needs to take heparin: see Antepartum section and Table 30-1.
A. Explain why heparin instead of warfarin (Coumadin) will be used: discuss importance of taking an anticoagulant to prevent thrombus formation; inform that warfarin will cross the placenta and could cause congenital anomalies and fetal hemorrhage; heparin does not cross the placenta.
B. Information to ensure safe use of heparin.
  - Safe administration; teach subcutaneous injection technique to Allison and family.
  - Stress importance of routine blood tests to assess clotting ability.

- Review side effects, including unusual bleeding and bruising, and measures to prevent injury (use soft toothbrush, no razors for shaving).
4. Pregnant woman with epilepsy: see Epilepsy section in Neurologic Disorders; inform her that effects of pregnancy on epilepsy are unpredictable; convulsions may injure her or her fetus and lead to miscarriage, preterm labor, or separation of the placenta; medications, which will be given in the lowest therapeutic dose, must be taken to prevent convulsions; folic acid supplementation is important because anticonvulsants deplete folic acid stores, increasing the risk for neural tube defects.

CHAPTER 31: MENTAL HEALTH DISORDERS AND SUBSTANCE ABUSE

I. Learning Key Terms

1. Mood disorders
2. Anxiety disorders
3. Phobia
4. Panic disorder
5. Generalized anxiety disorder (GAD)
6. Obsessive-compulsive disorder (OCD)
7. Posttraumatic stress disorder (PTSD)
8. Postpartum depression without psychotic features
9. Postpartum depression with psychotic features (postpartum psychosis)
10. Bipolar disorder
11. Panic attacks

II. Reviewing Key Concepts

12. Diagnostic criteria for major depression: see Perinatal Mood Disorders—Diagnosis section, which lists several criteria, at least five of which must be present nearly every day.
13. Difficulty of diagnosing depression during pregnancy: see Nurse Alert—Perinatal Mood Disorders, which explains the difficulty and provides several diagnostic cues.
14. Screening for substance abuse: see Perinatal Substance Abuse section and Box 31-4.
A. Purpose for using the 4 Ps Plus screen.
B. Questions to ask to determine if patient is using alcohol, tobacco, or drugs.
15. Maternal and fetal/newborn effects related to a variety of substances: see specific section for each substance to gather the information needed to complete your answer.
16. Choice C is correct; doxepin (Sinequan) is in the L5—high lactation risk category and should not be used because it can lead to neonatal respiratory depression; choices A, B, and D are antidepressants that are classified as L2, which is a low lactation risk category and therefore considered safe for breastfeeding women (see Table 31-1).
17. Choice C is correct; the woman needs to avoid being a superwoman and placing unrealistic expectations

on herself; sharing feelings, rest, and some time away from the baby are all adaptive coping mechanisms.

18. Choice A is correct; citalopram (Celexa), as a selective serotonin reuptake inhibitor (SSRI), if taken along with dextromethorphan increases the risk for serotonin syndrome.

19. Choice A is correct; although the other questions are all appropriate, the potential for harming herself or her baby represents the most serious and very real concern.

20. Choice B is correct; acute onset of labor with long hard uterine contractions and precipitous birth are characteristic of cocaine use; cocaine is a CNS stimulant; IV use increases the risk for bloodborne infections.

21. Choice D is correct; the nurse should follow a sequence that establishes trust by starting with questions about substances that are least problematic for the woman and her fetus and are therefore the easiest to answer and then progress to questions about substances that are more problematic and therefore more difficult to answer; questions about alcohol and tobacco and, lastly, illicit drugs such as cocaine should be asked.

III. Thinking Critically

1. Profiles of women at risk for postpartum depression: see Postpartum Depression section and Box 31-3 for the risk factors you will need to develop your profiles; be sure to use different risk factors for each profile.

2. Nursing diagnosis—impaired parent-infant attachment: see Psychiatric Hospitalization section, which discusses measures to facilitate maternal-infant attachment.

3. Discharge teaching plan related to postpartum depression: see Postpartum Depression section, Box 31-3, and Teaching for Self-Management—Activities to Prevent Postpartum Depression and Signs of Postpartum Blues, Depression, and Psychoses boxes; outline should cover such topics as what postpartum depression is, why it can occur, risks for its occurrence, and signs to look for; woman and her family should be part of the teaching; handout should include highlights of the teaching plan content along with who to contact, community agencies and supports, and Internet sites.

4. Woman suspected of drug use during pregnancy: see Perinatal Substance Abuse section.

   A. Warning signs: late entry into prenatal care, poor nutrition, history of depression, substance use within family or social relationships.

   B. Impact of use: discuss effect on woman, her fetus, and her childbirth experience.

   C. Legal implications and barriers: see Barriers to Treatment and Legal Considerations sections; answer should include the legal responsibilities of a nurse (e.g., reporting of positive test results), the barriers facing the woman, and—very

important—how you would try to break down these barriers so that this woman would be more receptive to entering a treatment program.

   D. Process of change and readiness for change: see Care Management—Perinatal Substance Abuse section and Box 31-5.
   - See pregnancy as a window of opportunity for motivation to change.
   - Identify the steps a nurse should follow to identify women who are ready for change and the degree of readiness and supportive nursing interventions to facilitate change.
   - Identify problem with abuse and readiness for change.
   - Use supportive interventions and motivational interviewing.

   E. Considerations when planning care:
   - Consider the characteristics of substance abusers, including depression related to negative life experiences (e.g., violence); substance abuse may serve as a means of relieving loneliness and emptiness; abusers may have grown up in an environment in which substance abuse is common and have had little opportunity to learn sober living skills.
   - These characteristics can make change and recovery very difficult and interfere with the ability to be caring and nurturing parents; follow-up care is critical for safety of mother and newborn.
   - Determine readiness for change and use measures that will facilitate change, including the window of opportunity for change that pregnancy presents.

   F. Nursing measures:
   - Assist with decreasing and then stopping substance abuse; educate about effects of substances on pregnancy and fetus; be clear and confront woman if necessary; make referrals for treatment and to help woman deal with negative life experiences that may be contributing to the abuse of substances as a coping mechanism; assess progress and perform toxicology screens as indicated.
   - Recognize that ability to cope with childbirth may be limited; plan for toxicology screens of newborn.
   - Assess progress of maternal-newborn attachment and mother's level of knowledge and skill regarding newborn care; plan for discharge with the safety of the newborn of utmost importance; make arrangements for home visit follow-up and referral to services that will help mother to care for her baby and continue treatment; notify child protective services if indicated.

5. Woman with postpartum depression: see Postpartum Depression section.

   A. Signs and symptoms indicative of postpartum depression: see Teaching for Self-Management—Signs of Postpartum Blues, Depression, and

Psychoses box; include in your answer fatigue, concern about being a good mother but low level of self-esteem and self-confidence regarding her effectiveness, expressed jealousy of her husband's seemingly greater enjoyment when spending time with baby than with her, and angry outbursts directed at husband.

B. Predisposing factors: see Box 31-3; prenatal anxiety, meager social support and stressful life events (recent relocation, husband busy with new job, no friends locally), bottle-feeding, mother unemployed and inexperienced with newborn care, 23 years of age.

C. Screening: see Screening for PPD section for several questions to ask; formulate questions related to risk factors for postpartum depression and also questions related to common manifestations; be sure to ask Mary directly about contemplating harm to self or baby; use open-ended questions that encourage full expression of feelings and thoughts.

D. Nursing diagnoses: several nursing diagnoses are listed in the Nursing Care Plan; at this point, fatigue, situational low self-esteem, ineffective individual coping, and risk for impaired parenting seem to be paramount but risk for violence toward self and infant is a critical ongoing nursing diagnosis, especially if postpartum depression is not identified and treated early.

E. Measures to cope with postpartum depression: see Care Management—Nursing Care in the Home and Community section and the Teaching for Self-Management—Preventing Postpartum Depression box; include husband in discussions and planning; consider relationship with partner and suggest changes and resources they could seek out from their church and child-rearing couples in their community; emphasize safety measures for mother or newborn; referral for psychiatric care with possible use of psychotropic/antidepressant medications if postpartum depression is determined to be moderate to severe; frequent follow-up to check progress is critical.

6. Principles to follow for providing care to women who abuse alcohol or drugs: see Perinatal Substance Abuse section for description of principles to follow; emphasize:
   - Family focus.
   - Empowerment building and breaking down barriers to seeking care among pregnant women.
   - A community-based multidisciplinary approach with multiplicity of services; comprehensive, co-ordinated, and holistic treatment.
   - Continuum of care with consistent caregiver that allows for development of a trusting, nonjudgmental relationship with health care provider and a mostly female staff.

CHAPTER 32: LABOR AND BIRTH COMPLICATIONS

I. Learning Key Terms

1. Preterm labor
2. Preterm birth
3. Late preterm birth
4. Very preterm birth
5. Low birth weight (LBW)
6. Intrauterine growth restriction (IUGR)
7. Fetal fibronectins
8. Premature rupture of membranes (PROM)
9. Preterm premature rupture of membranes (PPROM)
10. Chorioamnionitis
11. Dysfunctional labor (dystocia)
12. Hypertonic uterine dysfunction; primary dysfunctional labor
13. Hypotonic uterine dysfunction; secondary uterine inertia
14. Pelvic dystocia
15. Soft tissue dystocia
16. Fetal dystocia
17. Macrosomia
18. Cephalopelvic disproportion (CPD); fetopelvic disproportion (FPD)
19. Occipitoposterior
20. Breech
21. Multifetal pregnancy
22. Prolonged latent phase
23. Protracted active phase—dilation
24. Secondary arrest—no change
25. Protracted descent
26. Arrest of descent
27. Failure of descent
28. Precipitous labor
29. External cephalic version (ECV)
30. Trial of labor
31. Induction of labor
32. Bishop score; dilation (cm); effacement (%); station (cm); cervical consistency; cervical position
33. Amniotomy
34. Augmentation of labor; oxytocin; amniotomy
35. Uterine tachysystole
36. Forceps-assisted
37. Vacuum-assisted birth; vacuum extraction
38. Cesarean birth
39. Postterm; postdate; prolonged; dysmaturity syndrome
40. Shoulder dystocia; fetopelvic disproportion related to excessive fetal size (macrosomia); maternal pelvic abnormalities
41. Prolapse of umbilical cord
42. Rupture of the uterus; scarred uterus; trial of labor for attempted vaginal birth after cesarean (VBAC)
43. Amniotic fluid embolism (AFE); anaphylactoid syndrome of pregnancy

II. Reviewing Key Concepts

44. Identify factors associated with risk categories for preterm labor and birth: see Box 32-1 and Predicting

Spontaneous Preterm Labor and Birth section to complete this activity.

45. B, 46. C, 47. E, 48. A, 49. D, 50. F
51. E, 52. F, 53. C, 54. D, 55. A, 56. G, 57. H, 58. B
59. Five factors that cause dystocia: see Dysfunctional Labor (Dystocia) section and specific sections for each factor.
   - Powers: ineffective uterine contractions or bearing-down efforts.
   - Passage: altered pelvic diameters and shape, soft tissue abnormality.
   - Passenger: malpresentation or malposition, anomalies, size, number.
   - Psychologic response of mother: past experiences, preparation, culture, support system, stress and anxiety level.
   - Position of mother: ability and willingness to assume positions that facilitate uteroplacental perfusion and fetal descent.
60. Therapeutic rest: see Hypertonic Uterine Dysfunction section.
   - Purpose: help woman experiencing hypertonic uterine dysfunction to rest or sleep so active labor can begin, usually after a 4- to 6-hour rest period.
   - Actions: use of shower or warm bath for relaxation; comfort measures; administration of analgesics to inhibit contractions, reduce pain, and encourage rest or sleep and relaxation.
61. Compare and contrast hypertonic uterine dysfunction and hypotonic uterine dysfunction: see Dysfunctional Labor section and Table 32-1 for information related to each dysfunctional labor pattern in terms of causes and precipitating factors, maternal-fetal effects, changes in labor progress, and care management.
62. Indications and contraindications for oxytocin induction of labor: see Box 32-7, which lists several indicators and contraindications.
63. Choices B, C, D, and E are correct; women who are underweight or overweight/obese; have high-stress jobs; are members of the non-Hispanic African-American race; or have a history of preterm birth, multiple miscarriages, infections of the genitourinary tract (including UTIs) and reproductive tract (such as bacterial vaginosis), and bleeding in the second trimester are at increased risk for preterm labor and birth.
64. Choice A is correct; magnesium sulfate is a CNS depressant; woman should alternate lateral positions to decrease pressure on cervix, which could stimulate uterine contractions; calcium gluconate would be used if toxicity occurs; infusion should be discontinued if respiratory rate is less than 12 breaths/minute.
65. Choice C is correct; it is inserted in the posterior vaginal fornix; the woman should remain in bed for 2 hours; caution should be used if the woman has asthma; therefore ensure that physician is aware of asthma; the insert is removed for severe side effects

such as uterine tachysystole; dinoprostone (Cervidil) often stimulates contractions and may even induce the onset of labor, eliminating or reducing the need for oxytocin (Pitocin); it should be removed after 12 hours or with onset of active labor.
66. Choice D is correct; a Bishop score of 9 indicates that the cervix is already sufficiently ripe for successful induction; it is currently recommended that 30 units of oxytocin (Pitocin) be mixed in 500 mL of an electrolyte solution such as Ringers lactate; the oxytocin solution is piggybacked at the proximal port (port nearest the insertion site).
67. Choice A is correct; uterine contractions should not occur more frequently than five contractions in 10 minutes to allow for an adequate rest period between contractions; choices B, C, and D are all expected findings within the normal range.
68. Choice C is correct; the presentation of this fetus is breech; the soft buttocks are a less efficient dilating wedge than the fetal head; therefore labor may be slower; the ultrasound transducer should be placed to the left of the umbilicus at a level at or above it; passage of meconium is an expected finding as a result of pressure on the abdomen during descent; knee-chest position would be used for occipitoposterior positions.
69. Choice D is correct; the dosage is correct at 12 mg × 2 doses; this medication will stimulate her baby's lungs to produce surfactant and help the baby to breathe more easily should birth occur; dosages should be spaced 24 hours apart; therefore the second dose should be given at 11 am on the next day; this medication is administered intramuscularly.
70. Choice A is correct; the definitive sign of preterm labor is significant change in the cervix; while uterine contractions do occur, they must occur at a frequency of more than six contractions per hour and cause significant changes in the cervix; fetal fibronectin indicates that the risk for preterm labor exists but it does not mean that preterm labor is occurring.
71. Choices A, D, and E are correct; see Teaching for Self-Management—What to Do If Symptoms of Preterm Labor Occur box.
72. Choice C is correct; although choices A, B, and D are appropriate actions along with changes in her position, removing pressure from the cord to preserve perfusion is the priority; see Emergency—Prolapsed Umbilical Cord box.

III. Thinking Critically

1. Preterm labor and birth prevention program: see Predicting Spontaneous Preterm Labor and Birth and Prevention and Early Recognition and Diagnosis sections.
   - Preterm birth is a major factor contributing to perinatal morbidity and mortality; early detection is critical for successful tocolysis and antenatal glucocorticoid therapy.

- Many risk factors for preterm labor have been identified (see Boxes 32-1 and 32-2) but risk scoring systems miss many women who go into preterm labor.
- All women should be taught signs of preterm labor and measures to prevent based on risk factors identified that can be manipulated by changes in lifestyle behaviors (see Box 32-3).

2. Woman with a history of preterm labor and birth.
   A. Identify signs of preterm labor: see Box 32-3 as a guide for teaching Sara about preterm labor; see if Sara can retrospectively remember experiencing these vague signs with her first pregnancy.
   B. Implementation of plan to prevent preterm labor.
      - Evaluate Sara's lifestyle for risky behaviors and health history for risk factors for preterm labor.
      - Discuss how certain factors identified could be changed to reduce her risk, especially those related to lifestyle (see Lifestyle Modifications section).
      - Consider modification of sexual activity, stress level, activity (work, home), and hygiene (prevent genitourinary [GU] tract infections).
   C. Criteria for use of tocolysis: assess Sara to ensure that she is indeed in labor and that she does not exhibit contraindications to tocolysis (see Suppression of Uterine Activity section and Box 32-4).
   D. Nursing care measures during magnesium sulfate infusion to suppress preterm labor: see Box 32-5, Suppression of Uterine Activity section, and Medication Guide, Tocolytic Therapy for Preterm Labor.
      - Assess for labor progress and maternal-fetal responses to magnesium sulfate.
      - Monitor and regulate infusion following protocol for increments in dosage of magnesium sulfate.
      - Measure intake and output.
      - Provide support and encouragement.
      - Maintain bed rest in lateral position.
   E. Administration of betamethasone: see Promotion of Fetal Lung Maturity section.
      1. Purpose: stimulation of fetal surfactant production.
      2. Protocol: see Medication Guide, Antenatal Glucocorticoid Therapy; assess Sara for signs of infection and pulmonary edema; explain action and indications for use; administer IM deep into gluteal muscle, 12 mg, twice, 24 hours apart; observe for adverse effects.

3. Woman experiencing preterm labor discharged to home care: see Suppression of Uterine Activity and Home Care sections and Nursing Care Plan.
   A. Self-administration of nifedipine: teach her how to take the medication, how the medication works, the side effects of nifedipine (Procardia) to watch for, and who to call if they should appear; teach her how to assess her vital signs, especially her blood pressure.
   B. Side effects of nifedipine: see Medication Guide, Tocolytic Therapy for Preterm Labor, which lists signs that should be taught to the client.
   C. Instructions regarding palpating uterine activity: discuss how often to monitor (once or twice a day while lying on side); teach her how to palpate abdomen for uterine contractions: palpate over fundus where contractions are most intense to determine characteristics and then palpate over entire uterus to determine generalized tone; tell her what activity could indicate preterm labor and who to call.
   D. Coping with bed rest and activity restriction: see Home Care section, Teaching for Self-Management—Suggested Activities for Children of Women on Activity Restriction box, and Fig. 32-2; identify the members of her support system and include them in discussions of how bed rest and activity limitations will be managed and how they can help; make referrals to home care agencies if needed.

4. Woman with occipitoposterior position and difficulty bearing down: see Dysfunctional Labor (Dystocia)—Fetal Causes—Malposition section and Box 19-8.
   A. Identifying factors that have a negative effect on bearing-down efforts: amount of analgesia and anesthesia used, exhaustion, maternal position, lack of knowledge about how to push effectively, lack of sleep, inadequate food and fluid intake.
   B. Measures to facilitate bearing-down efforts (BDE): coach her in BDE, help her into an appropriate position, apply counterpressure to sacrum, demonstrate open-glottis pushing and coach her efforts with every contraction, help her to begin pushing when Ferguson reflex is perceived; reduce epidural medication to a minimum effective dose.
   C. Recommended positions: hand-and-knees or lateral position on the same side as the fetal back when the fetus is in an occipitoposterior position can be very effective in facilitating internal rotation and reducing back pain; see Box 19-8 for many additional techniques.

5. Unplanned (emergency) cesarean birth: see Cesarean Birth section.
   A. Preoperative measures: see Preoperative Care section; implement typical preoperative care measures as for any major surgery in a calm and professional manner, explaining the purpose of each measure that must be performed; use a family-centered approach; discuss what will happen; witness an informed consent; assess fetal-maternal unit, insert Foley catheter, start or maintain IV infusion, and provide emotional support.
   B. Immediate postoperative measures: see Immediate Postoperative Care section; assess for signs of hemorrhage, pain level, respiratory effort, renal function, circulatory status to extremities, signs of postanesthesia recovery, emotional status, and attachment and reaction to newborn.

340

C. Ongoing postoperative care measures: see Postoperative Postpartum Care section and Teaching for Self-Management: Postpartum Pain Relief After Cesarean Birth and Signs of Postoperative Complications After Discharge Following Cesarean Birth boxes; measures include assessment of recovery, pain relief, coughing and deep breathing, leg exercises and assistance with ambulation, nutrition and fluid intake (oral, IV); provide opportunities for interaction and care of newborn, assisting her as needed; provide emotional support to help her deal with her disappointment and feelings of failure; help her and her family to prepare for discharge, making referrals as needed.

D. Nursing diagnosis: situational low self-esteem related to inability to reach goal of a vaginal birth secondary to occurrence of fetal distress.
- Discuss and review why Anne needed a cesarean birth, how she performed during labor, and that she had no control over the fetal distress.
- Discuss vaginal birth after cesarean (VBAC) and likelihood of its being an option because the reason for her primary cesarean (fetal distress) may not occur again; discuss trial of labor next time to determine her ability to proceed to vaginal birth.
- Use follow-up phone calls to assess progress in accepting cesarean birth.

6. Fetal position and presentation—RSA: see Malpresentation section and Figs. 32-3 and 32-4; right sacrum anterior (RSA) indicates a breech presentation; consider that descent may be slower, meconium is often expelled, there is increasing danger of meconium aspiration, and risk for cord prolapse is increased; depending on progress of labor and maternal characteristics, cesarean or vaginal birth may occur or external cephalic version (ECV) may be attempted.

7. Induction of labor: see Induction of Labor section and Box 32-7.
A. Bishop score: see Table 32-3 for factors assessed to determine degree of cervical ripening in preparation for labor process; it is used to determine if a cervical ripening method will need to be used to increase the chances of a successful labor induction.

B. Score of 5 for a nulliparous woman: her score should be greater than 9 to ensure a successful induction; a score of 5 indicates a cervix that is not fully ripe; therefore cervical ripening will be needed before induction to enhance its success.

C. Administration of dinoprostone (Cervidil): see Cervical Ripening Methods section and Medication Guide for guidelines for use and adverse reactions; consider how and where it is inserted, protocol to follow after the insertion, and adverse reactions and what to do if they occur.

D. Amniotomy: see Amniotomy section and Box 32-8, Assisting with Amniotomy; explain what will happen, how it will feel, and why it is being done; assess

maternal-fetal unit before and after the procedure; document findings; support woman during procedure, telling her what is happening; document procedure and outcomes and reactions appropriately.

E. Induction protocol: see Medication Guide—Oxytocin (Pitocin).
1. A   2. A   3. A   4. NA   5. A
6. NA   7. NA   8. A   9. NA   10. A
11. NA

F. Major side effects of oxytocin (Pitocin) induction: tachysystole, uterine rupture, nonreassuring FHR patterns, abruptio placentae, postpartum hemorrhage and infection, water intoxication.

G. Actions if uterine tachysystole occurs: see Emergency—Uterine Tachysystole with Oxytocin box, which lists signs related to uterine contractions and abnormal (nonreassuring) FHR patterns as well as immediate interventions such as discontinuing the induction, maintaining the primary infusion of fluid, turning the woman onto her side, administering oxygen via face mask, monitoring response of maternal-fetal unit to actions, notifying primary health care provider, and preparing for possible administration of terbutaline to suppress contractions.

8. Postterm pregnancy: see Postterm Pregnancy, Labor, and Birth section.
A. Maternal-fetal risks related to postterm pregnancy: see Maternal-Fetal Risks section; maternal risk relates to excessive size of fetus and hardness of fetal skull, which increases risk for dystocia; fetal risk relates to postmaturity syndrome as the placenta ages and a stressful, prolonged labor and birth process, including increased risk for birth injury and neonatal hypoglycemia; macrosomia can result in shoulder dystocia and maternal/fetal birth injury.

B. Clinical manifestations: maternal weight loss, decrease in uterine size, meconium in amniotic fluid, advanced fetal bone maturation, including of the skull.

C. Care measures to ensure safety of maternal-fetal unit: see Care Management section.
- Continue prenatal care with more frequent visits.
- Antepartal assessments, including daily fetal movement counts, nonstress test (NST), amniotic fluid volume assessments, biophysical profile (BPP), contraction stress test (CST), Doppler blood flow measurements, cervical checks for ripening.
- Emotional support.
- Prepare for cervical ripening, induction of labor, monitoring for late and variable deceleration patterns, amnioinfusion, forceps- or vacuum-assisted or cesarean birth.

D. Instructions for self-care at home: see Teaching for Self-Management—Postterm Pregnancy box.
- Make sure Lora knows how to assess fetal movements and signs of labor.

- Emphasize importance of keeping all appointments for prenatal care and antepartal assessments.
- Identify who to call with concerns, questions, and reports of changing status, such as onset of labor or change in fetal movement pattern.

9. Planning care for a laboring woman who is obese: see Obesity section and Fig. 32-5 to formulate your answer, which should include the increased risks that this woman and her fetus face.

CHAPTER 33: POSTPARTUM COMPLICATIONS

I. Learning Key Terms

1. Postpartum hemorrhage (PPH); early (acute, primary); late (secondary)
2. Uterine atony
3. Perineal lacerations
4. Hematoma; vulvar hematomas
5. Placenta accreta
6. Placenta increta
7. Placenta percreta
8. Inversion of the uterus
9. Subinvolution; retained placental fragments; pelvic infection
10. Hemorrhagic (hypovolemic) shock
11. Coagulopathy
12. Thrombocytopenia
13. Idiopathic (immune) thrombocytopenic purpura (ITP)
14. von Willebrand disease
15. Venous thromboembolism (VTE)
16. Thrombophlebitis
17. Superficial venous thrombosis
18. Deep venous thrombosis (DVT)
19. Pulmonary embolism
20. Postpartum (puerperal) infection
21. Endometritis
22. Mastitis

II. Reviewing Key Concepts

23. Twofold focus of management of hemorrhagic shock: see Hemorrhagic (Hypovolemic) Shock—Medical Management section; restore circulating blood volume and perfusion and treat the cause of the hemorrhage.
24. Standard of care for bleeding emergencies: see Hemorrhagic (Hypovolemic) Shock—Legal Tip section for a description of the standard of care that focuses on provisions made for the nurse to implement actions independently and establishment of policies, procedures, standing orders or protocols, and clinical guidelines; the nurse should never leave the client alone.
25. Choice B is correct; although BP should be taken before and after administration of methylergonovine (Methergine), the woman's hypertensive status would be a contraindicating factor for its use, especially

if administered parenterally; therefore the order should be questioned; a more appropriate choice would be oxytocin (Pitocin); Methergine should not be given if the BP is greater than 140/90 mm Hg.

26. Choice D is correct; 15-methylprostaglandin F_{2a} (Hemabate) is a powerful prostaglandin that is given to treat excessive uterine blood loss or hemorrhage related to uterine atony; it has no action related to pain, infection, or clotting.
27. Choice A is correct; puerperal infections are infections of the genital tract after birth; pulse will increase, not decrease, in response to fever; choices B and C will also occur but are not the first signs exhibited.
28. Choices C and F are correct; heparin and warfarin are safe for use by breastfeeding women; heparin, usually administered intravenously for the first 3 to 5 days, is the anticoagulant of choice during the acute stage of DVT; after acute phase, warfarin (Coumadin) is begun orally while the patient is still receiving heparin; woman should be fitted for elastic stockings after the acute stage has passed when edema subsides; the woman should be encouraged to change her position when on bed rest.

III. Thinking Critically

1. Postpartum woman at risk for postpartum hemorrhage: see PPH section.
   A. Risk factors for early postpartum hemorrhage: see Etiology and Risk Factors and Uterine Atony sections and Box 33-1; discuss increased likelihood for uterine atony as a result of parity (6-5-1-0-7), vaginal full-term twin birth 1 hour ago, hypotonic uterine dysfunction treated with oxytocin (Pitocin), use of forceps for birth, increased manipulation with birth of twins; increased size and stretch of uterus with a multiple gestation.
   B. Nursing diagnosis: see Nursing Care Plan for Postpartum Hemorrhage; risk for deficient fluid volume related to moderate to heavy blood loss associated with vaginal birth of twins.
   C. Nurse's response to excessive blood loss in 15 minutes: see Medical Management and Nursing Interventions sections; most common cause of excessive blood loss 1 hour after birth would be uterine atony, especially because woman exhibits several risk factors; discuss each of the following with rationale for action:
   - Assess fundus; massage as the priority action.
   - Express clots if necessary once fundus is firm.
   - Check bladder and perineum for swelling and ask woman about experiencing perineal pressure.
   D. Guidelines for administering oxytocin (Pitocin) IV: see Medication Guide—Drugs Used to Manage Postpartum Hemorrhage to explain guidelines for administration in terms of dose and route, side effects, and nursing management, including assessment and maternal support.

E. Signs of developing hemorrhagic (hypovolemic) shock: see Hemorrhagic (Hypovolemic) Shock section, Box 33-2, and Emergency—Hemorrhagic Shock box, which identifies the priority assessment a nurse should perform and the findings that would indicate progress from hemorrhage to shock; assessment includes vital signs, skin, urinary output, level of consciousness, and mental status; assessment should be frequent and findings compared to one another to note change; ongoing documentation of data, action, and response is critical.

F. Nursing measures to support the woman and family: see Nursing Interventions section and Nursing Care Plan for Postpartum Hemorrhage.
- Explain progress.
- Discuss physiologic care; consider approach to take and organization of care.
- Comfort and support measures.
- Opportunities for interaction with newborn.

2. Puerperal infection: see Postpartum Infection section.
A. Risk factors: see Box 33-3; consider preconception, antepartal, and intrapartal factors.
B. Infection prevention measures: see Care Management section; emphasize measures to maintain resistance to infection (nutrition, rest, hygiene); use of standard precautions, including handwashing, proper use of gloves, and care of equipment; teach woman about prevention measures, including genital hygiene and safer sex practices.
C. Typical signs of endometritis: see Endometritis section for a description of typical clinical manifestations to guide assessment.
D. Nursing diagnoses: acute pain related to effects of infection in uterine tissue; interrupted family process or anxiety or ineffective individual or family coping related to unexpected postpartum complication; use assessment findings to determine priority psychosocial nursing diagnoses.
E. Nursing measures: see Care Management section and Chapters 20 and 21, which discuss many nursing interventions related to prevention and early detection of postpartum infection.

3. Woman with mastitis: see Postpartum Infection section and Chapter 25, Breastfeeding section.
A. Assessment findings associated with mastitis: fever; malaise; flulike symptoms; sore, warm, erythematous area on the breast (see Fig. 33-6).
B. Nursing diagnoses: acute pain related to inflammation of right breast associated with mastitis; ineffective breastfeeding or anxiety related to interruption of breastfeeding while taking antibiotics or related to concerns regarding transmission of infection to newborn.
C. Treatment measures: discuss several measures, including medications used including antibiotic therapy, local applications to enhance comfort, breast support, adequate hydration and nutrition, and pumping of breast to maintain lactation if breastfeeding is prohibited because of medications being used for treatment.

D. Measures to prevent recurrence of mastitis: focus on good breastfeeding techniques, breast care to maintain integrity of areolae and nipples, early detection and treatment of cracks, and cleanliness including strict hand hygiene measures.

4. Woman with deep vein thrombosis: see Thromboembolic Venous Disorders section.
A. Risk factors: see Incidence and Etiology section; in addition to venous stasis and hypercoagulability of pregnancy continuing into the postpartum period, other risk factors for this woman would be cesarean birth, obesity, age over 35 years, multiparity, and smoking.
B. Signs and symptoms indicative of DVT: see Clinical Manifestations section for a description of typical clinical manifestations.
C. Nursing diagnosis: anxiety related to unexpected development of a postpartum complication.
D. Expected care management: see Medical Management and Nursing Interventions sections; discuss what should be included in each of the following sections of your outline: assessment, anticoagulant therapy, activity level, pain management, leg support, reassurance that breastfeeding is safe, emotional support, and assistance with care of self and newborn.
E. Discharge instructions:
- How to assess leg and for signs of unusual bleeding; proper use of elastic/support stockings.
- How to take anticoagulant safely and importance of follow-up to assess progress; use a medication information resource to learn about safe and effective anticoagulant use.
- Practices to prevent bleeding while taking an anticoagulant and importance of avoiding pregnancy because warfarin is teratogenic.

ANSWER KEY UNIT VIII

CHAPTER 34: NURSING CARE OF THE HIGH RISK NEWBORN AND FAMILY

I. Learning Key Terms

1. Low-birth-weight (LBW)
2. Very low-birth-weight (VLBW)
3. Extremely low-birth-weight (ELBW)
4. Premature; preterm
5. Late preterm
6. Full term
7. Postmature; postterm
8. Large for gestational age (LGA)
9. Appropriate for gestational age (AGA)
10. Small for date (SFD) or small for gestational age (SGA)
11. Intrauterine growth restriction (IUGR)
12. Symmetric IUGR
13. Asymmetric IUGR
14. Live birth
15. Fetal death

16. Neonatal death
17. Perinatal mortality
18. Periodic breathing
19. Apnea
20. Oscillometry (Dinamap)
21. Neutral thermal environment
22. Surfactant
23. Insensible water loss (IWL)
24. Gavage feeding
25. Minimal enteral nutrition (MEN)
26. Gastrostomy tube feeding
27. Total parenteral nutrition (TPN)
28. Nonnutritive sucking
29. Kangaroo care
30. Anticipatory grief

II. Reviewing Key Concepts

31. Identify physiologic problems of the preterm newborn: physiologic functions and potential problems are discussed in specific sections in the Preterm Infant—Physiologic Function section.
32. B, 33. F, 34. C, 35. A, 36. G, 37. D, 38. E
39. Comparing needs of late preterm and full-term newborns: see Late Preterm Infants section and Table 34-3 to complete your comparison.
40. Choices B, D, and E are correct; retractions, nasal flaring, and expiratory grunting reflect increased effort and work to breathe; choices A, C, and F are all expected findings consistent with efficient respiratory effort in the preterm newborn.
41. Choice B is correct; although choices A, C, and D are appropriate and important, respiration with adequate gas exchange takes precedence, especially because adequate surfactant is not produced before 32 weeks of gestation.
42. Choices A, B, E, and F are correct; air, not sterile water, is used to check placement before feeding; because newborns are nose-breathers, the mouth is the preferred route for insertion unless the infant is unable to tolerate; see Box 34-5—Inserting a Gavage Feeding Tube and Fig. 34-6.
43. Choices A, B, and F are correct; see Table 34-2 for normal arterial gas values for neonates.
44. Choice D is correct; monitoring vital signs is an assessment measure; cleansing the skin and teaching parents are important but not the single most important action; hand hygiene practiced by everyone who has contact with the preterm newborn is critical.
45. Choices B, C, E, and F are correct; acrocyanosis and periodic breathing patterns are expected findings but central cyanosis and apnea reflect hypothermia (see Box 34-2).

III. Thinking Critically

1. Oxygen therapy for the newborn experiencing respiratory distress: see Respiratory Function and Oxygen Therapy sections.
   A. Criteria to determine need for oxygen: increased effort to breathe, respiratory distress with apnea, tachycardia or bradycardia, central cyanosis, Pao_2 less than 60 mm Hg, oxygen saturation less than 92%.
   B. Guidelines for safe and effective administration of oxygen: observe respiratory status every hour with continuous pulse oximetry and arterial blood gas measurement as warranted, vital signs, controlled oxygen concentration, volume, temperature and humidity; oxygen should be warm and humidified.
   C. Signs of readiness: see Weaning from Respiratory Assistance section to formulate your answer; include signs of respiratory distress that are no longer exhibited, arterial blood gases (ABGs) and oxygen saturation maintained within normal limits, newborn displays spontaneous adequate respiratory effort without difficulty and exhibits good color and improved muscle tone during increased activity.
   D. Guidelines: approach carefully, proceeding in a stepwise manner from one method to another with close observation for signs of good or poor tolerance of the change; reassure and keep parents informed throughout the process of weaning, pointing out signs that their newborn is breathing effectively and is well oxygenated.
2. Meeting nutritional needs of a preterm infant: see Nutritional Care and Gavage Feeding sections.
   A. Assessment to determine effectiveness of feeding method: observe for ability to suck and swallow and the coordination of each; signs of respiratory distress during the feeding; length of time for the feeding and the amount ingested; presence of regurgitation, vomiting, or abdominal distention after feeding; daily weight gains and losses and elimination patterns.
   B. Guidelines to follow when inserting a gavage tube: see Gavage Feeding section, Box 34-5—Inserting a Gavage Feeding Tube, and Fig. 34-6; emphasize tubing choice and measurement of length, insertion without trauma and securing to maintain placement, and checking placement.
   C. Nursing diagnosis: imbalanced nutrition: less than body requirements related to weak suck associated with premature status.
   D. Principles to follow before, during, and after a gavage feeding: discuss each of the following:
      ■ Assess nutritional status (e.g., weight, elimination patterns, abdominal circumference) and tolerance of feedings (volume of residual gastric aspirate); check skin at site where tubing is secured.
      ■ Initiate measures to prevent aspiration with proper tube insertion, removal, and position check techniques.
      ■ Instill breast milk or formula at rate prescribed; assist mother to pump breasts.
      ■ Cuddle and swaddle infant during feedings; involve parents; use nonnutritive sucking: see Fig. 34-7.

344

- Document assessment findings and specifics of the procedure.
  E. Advancing to oral feeding: see Advancing Infant Feedings section; proceed cautiously, checking for gastrointestinal (GI), nutritional, fluid, and electrolyte signs of tolerance or intolerance for advancement; decrease gavage feedings as ability to suck improves; keep parents involved in the process.
3. NICU environment: see Environmental Concerns section, Nursing Care Plan—High-Risk Preterm Infant, and Fig. 34-8.
   A. Common stressors.
      - Infant stressors: continuous exposure to light and noise; administration of sedatives and pain medications; invasive procedures and medications required for treatment.
      - Family stressors: size and compromised and often fluctuating health status of their newborn; difficulty interacting with newborn and making eye contact; increased learning needs regarding status of newborn and care needs; concern regarding potential disabilities.
   B. Identify approach and avoidance newborn behaviors: see Developmental Care section for a description of these behaviors.
   C. Measures to provide a balance of stimuli for the newborn: see Developmental Care section for many ideas, including waterbeds, kangaroo care, bundling, positioning, coordinated plan of care to provide for period of interrupted rest and sleep, using pain medications and sedatives as needed, providing diurnal light patterns, decreasing noise level; use stroking, talking, mobiles, decals, music, and windup toys for stimulation; kangaroo care.
   D. Guidelines for infant positioning: see Positioning section and Fig. 34-9; change position frequently, observing effect of position change on breathing and oxygenation and preventing aspiration; consider boundaries, body alignment, sense of security and comfort when positioning; teach parents; use facilitated tucking and blanket swaddling.
4. Postterm pregnancy: see Postmature Infants section.
   A. Rationale for increased mortality: increased oxygen demands are not met, especially during labor and birth when contractions combine with an aging placenta to diminish perfusion and increase the likelihood for impaired gas exchange, leading to hypoxia and passage of meconium into amniotic fluid; risk for aspiration of meconium into lungs.
   B. Typical assessment findings: thin, emaciated appearance (dysmature) due to loss of subcutaneous fat and muscle mass; peeling of skin; meconium staining on fingernails; long hair and nails; absence of vernix.
   C. Two major complications: meconium aspiration syndrome and persistent pulmonary hypertension

of the newborn (PPHN); see separate sections that describe each complication.
5. Birth of a small for gestational age newborn: see Small for Gestational Age and Intrauterine Growth Restriction sections.
   A. Major complications: perinatal asphyxia with possible passage of meconium and aspiration, hypoglycemia, polycythemia, heat loss (cold stress).
   B. Physiologic basis for each identified complication: see separate section for each complication.
6. Transport to a tertiary center: see Transport to and from a Regional Center section, Box 34-8, and Fig. 34-15.
   A. Advantages of transport before birth:
      - Associated neonatal morbidity and mortality are decreased.
      - Infant-parent attachment is supported because separation is avoided.
   B. Stabilization of needs before transport: vital signs, oxygenation and ventilation, thermoregulation, acid-base balance, fluid and electrolyte status, glucose levels, and developmental interventions.
   C. Support measures for family: provide information about center (location, visiting hours, phone number, caregivers' names, rules), one parent accompany infant, see infant before transport, get status updates.
7. Parents of a preterm newborn: see Parental Adaptation to a Preterm Infant, Figs. 34-11 and 34-12, and Nursing Care Plan—High Risk Preterm Newborn.
   A. Identify parental tasks and nursing measures to help parents: measures should include ideas regarding helping parents get to know their newborn, informing them of newborn's status, educating regarding care needs, providing emotional support and help with the grieving process, making referrals to parents groups and home care agencies, mobilizing family support system
   B. Assessment of attachment progress and coping ability of parents: see Parental Responses and Parental Maladaptation sections and attachment content in Chapter 22 to formulate your answer; include progress of touch, eagerness to help with care, asking questions and demonstrating interest in status, visiting practices, and bringing items from home to identify the newborn as their own and part of a family.
8. Surfactant administration to preterm infant born at 26 weeks of gestation: see Oxygen Therapy—Surfactant section and Medication Guide—Surfactant.
   A. Purpose of exogenous surfactant administration: preterm infant born at 26 weeks of gestation will be unable to produce enough surfactant to survive extrauterine life; exogenous surfactant will facilitate alveoli expansion and stability, easing respirations, and enhancing gas exchange until the newborn can produce sufficient quantities on its own; it is administered via an endotracheal tube directly into the lungs.

345

B. Informing and reassuring parents: show parents how their baby is having difficulty breathing; discuss surfactant—what it does, how it can help their baby by preventing complications and increasing their baby's chances of survival, and why their baby does not have enough, thereby causing difficulty breathing; show them how it will be administered, including how their baby's comfort needs will be met and then, after administration, point out how it is helping their baby to breathe.

9. Kangaroo care: see Kangaroo Care section and Fig. 34-10; explain what it is and why it is used; show pictures and film; report testimony of effectiveness from parents and nurses who have used kangaroo care; involve nurses and parents who had or have children in the NICU in creating the protocol that will be used to implement this form of care.

10. Pain of a newborn in NICU: see Infant Pain Responses section and Chapter 24.

A. Explain how the newborn expresses pain: see Pain Assessment section and Table 34-7 for a list of behavioral responses in several categories; describe behaviors such as crying, body movements, and facial expressions and how they differ when infant is in pain compared to common newborn responses.

B. Evidence of infant pain memory: see Memory of Pain section for defensive-type behaviors that an infant might exhibit when painful procedures are repeated.

C. Consequences of unrelieved pain: see Consequences of Untreated Pain in Infants section, which discusses physiologic and behavioral responses when pain is not relieved and how these responses can interfere with growth and development and positive adaptations to extrauterine life.

D. Management strategies: see Pain Management section and Chapter 24; several measures are discussed for each type of relief measure; consider involvement of family in pain relief and tell them what you are doing to keep baby comfortable; show them how their baby is indicating that relief measures are working.

CHAPTER 35: ACQUIRED PROBLEMS OF THE NEWBORN

I. Learning Key Terms

1. Birth trauma (birth injury)
2. Subconjunctival (scleral and retinal) hemorrhages
3. Ecchymoses
4. Petechiae
5. Clavicle
6. Erb-Duchenne palsy; brachial plexus injury
7. Renal agenesis
8. Caudal regression syndrome
9. Macrosomia
10. Hypoglycemia

11. Cardiomyopathy
12. Polycythemia; hyperbilirubinemia
13. Sepsis
14. Septicemia
15. Septic shock
16. Eye prophylaxis
17. Condylomata
18. Snuffles
19. Rhagades
20. Highly active antiretroviral therapy (HAART)
21. Opportunistic infection
22. Parvovirus B19
23. Group B streptococci
24. Listeriosis
25. Thrush
26. Fetal alcohol syndrome (FAS)
27. Neonatal abstinence syndrome

II. Reviewing Key Concepts

28. Common congenital anomalies experienced by infants of women with diabetes: see Infants of Diabetic Mothers—Congenital Anomalies section for the identification of anomalies in each category.

29. Infections represented by TORCH: see Transplacental Infections section and Box 35-1 for infections represented by each letter.

30. Sepsis: see Neonatal Infections section.

A. Modes of transmission of infection: see Sepsis section for a review of prenatal, perinatal, and postnatal transmission modes.

B. Risk factors: see Table 35-2, which lists risk factors according to maternal, intrapartum, and neonatal sources.

C. Signs of sepsis exhibited by neonate: see Table 35-3 for a list of signs according to body systems.

D. Effective nursing measures: see appropriate sections for Preventive Measures and Curative Measures in the Care Management section.

31. Choice B is correct; findings are consistent with a bone fracture, in this case the clavicle.

32. Choices B, C, and F are correct; macrosomic infants are at increased risk for hypoglycemia (e.g., a blood glucose level of 38 mg/dL would be considered hypoglycemia); hypocalcemia is also common; fracture and trauma are more common in the upper body, such as the humerus and clavicle; the newborn of a pregestational diabetic mother is more likely to experience congenital anomalies such as heart defects; there is no increased risk over the general population with gestational diabetes; the complexion is characteristically plethoric or flushed.

33. Choice A is correct; the second dose is given at 1 month and the third dose is given at 6 months.

34. Choice B is correct; isolation is not required and breastfeeding is contraindicated because of the potential for viral transmission; the nurse should be using standard precautions as would be used with all clients; HAART is used to prevent transmission of

HIV—the chance of this newborn becoming HIV positive is very low because the mother was treated during pregnancy.

35. Choices B, E, and F are correct; signs of abstinence syndrome also include little sleep, jitteriness, hyperactivity, shrill cry, vomiting, tachypnea, and fever; see Table 35-5.

III. Thinking Critically

1. Birth trauma: see Birth Trauma section.
   A. Risk factors for trauma: see Birth Trauma section for a discussion of maternal and fetal factors and intrapartum techniques that predispose a newborn to birth injury.
   B. Approach to reduce birth injuries; consider an approach that facilitates labor progress, including maternal movement, comfort measures, and support; use risk factors for injury to guide nursing measures.
   C. Signs of fractured clavicle: see Fig. 35-3 and Skeletal Injuries section; signs include limited motion of arm and absence of Moro reflex on affected side, crepitus over the bone.
   D. Treatment: there is no accepted standard treatment; care is limited to gently handling and supporting shoulder when changing clothes and moving and proper alignment; alert caregivers and parents regarding need for special handling; support and reassure parents.

2. Macrosomic infant: see Neonatal Complications—Macrosomia section.
   A. Pathophysiologic basis for macrosomia: discuss the effect of fetal insulin secretion in response to maternal blood glucose levels during pregnancy; discuss the rationale for frequent monitoring of the baby's blood glucose levels until stabilized after birth; it also is important to discuss the importance of good nutrition patterns, exercise habits, and maintaining a normal body mass index (BMI) for herself and the rest of her family, including her new baby; she is at risk for type 2 diabetes, as are her children.
   B. Characteristics: see Macrosomia section and Fig. 35-6, which describes several characteristics that can be noted with assessment of the newborn.
   C. After constant exposure to high circulating levels of glucose, hyperplasia of the fetal pancreas occurs, resulting in hyperinsulinemia. Disruption of the fetal glucose supply occurs with the clamping of the umbilical cord, and the neonate's blood glucose level decreases rapidly in the presence of fetal hyperinsulinism. It can take several days for the newborn to regulate the secretion of insulin in response to a lower postnatal supply of glucose. Hypoglycemia is most common in the macrosomic infant, but the nurse should monitor blood glucose levels in all infants of mothers with known or suspected diabetes.
   D. Signs of hypoglycemia include jitteriness, apnea, tachypnea, and cya Many infants with hypoglycemia remain asymptomatic. Significant hypoglycemia can result in seizures. Hypoglycemia is worsened by the presence of hypothermia or respiratory distress.

3. Newborn whose mother is hepatitis B positive: see Hepatitis B Virus section.
   A. Protocol for newborn care: discuss use of hepatitis B immunoglobulin and hepatitis B vaccine, including when and how to administer.
   B. Safety of breastfeeding: it is safe to breastfeed after the infant has been cleansed and the vaccine and immunoglobulin have been administered.

4. Newborn whose mother has active herpes at the time of birth: see Herpes Simplex Virus section.
   A. Four modes of transmission: transplacental, ascending by way of birth canal, direct contamination during passage through birth canal (mode for this baby), and direct transmission to the newborn by an infected person.
   B. Clinical signs of active infection in the newborn: see Herpes Simplex Virus section for signs of infection in each category.
   C. Recommended nursing measures related to:
      - Management after birth, prior to discharge: discuss assessment measures, including inspection of eyes, oral cavity, and skin for lesions; infection control measures, including use of glove when appropriate; specimen collection for culture with evaluation of results as criteria for discharge; and appropriateness of breastfeeding.
      - Pharmacologic therapy: discuss how and why each medication is used and for how long.

5. Newborn whose mother is HIV positive: see HIV/AIDS section.
   A. Potential for newborn infection: there is a 12% to 40% risk for transmission if the mother was not treated during pregnancy; the risk is reduced to less than 1% if she was treated.
   B. Strategies to prevent transmission: universal HIV testing, HAART treatment during pregnancy, labor, and to the newborn, elective cesarean section, and avoiding breastfeeding.
   C. Testing protocol: discuss tests used and time performed as well as factors that can influence test accuracy.
   D. Opportunistic infections: common infections can include *Pneumocystis jiroveci* pneumonia, candidiasis, cytomegalovirus (CMV) infection, cryptosporidiosis, herpes simplex or herpes zoster, and disseminated varicella.
   E. Care measures: discuss use of standard precautions, cleansing of skin, and antimicrobial and immunization administration; also discuss counseling, referrals, and follow-up care.
   F. Breastfeeding safety: because breast milk can contain the virus, the newborn should not be breastfed; teach mother how to bottle-feed and demonstrate how she can have close contact with

her newborn during feeding; discuss risk that breastfeeding poses, citing statistics; inform the mother about the safe use of immunizations for her newborn.

6. Infant with thrush: see Fungal Infections—Candidiasis section.
   A. Signs: white adherent patches and plaques on oral mucosa, gums, and tongue that bleed when touched.
   B. Modes of transmission: maternal vaginal infection during birth; person-to-person contact; contaminated hands, bottles, nipples, or other articles.
   C. Management: discuss assessment of mother for signs of fungal infection, use of Standard Precautions/infection control measures, cleanliness, measures to improve resistance to infection, and procedure for administration of an antifungal preparation; discuss treatment of infant (mouth) and mother (e.g., breasts) together.

7. Newborn with fetal alcohol syndrome (FAS): see Substance Abuse—Alcohol section, Fig. 35-12, and Table 35-4.
   A. Typical characteristics: fully describe appearance of the infant with FAS; consider that this infant may also exhibit signs related to alcohol withdrawal.
   B. Long-term effects: several are described in the Alcohol section, including those related to learning behaviors, socialization and judgment problems, and fine motor dysfunction; also increased incidence of congenital anomalies.
   C. Nursing measures: see Care Management section for several ideas; involve parents in care of newborn, encouraging attachment; teach parents what to expect about their child's behavior; help the parents to create a warm and caring home environment that enhances development; make appropriate referrals to community services for the newborn as well as treatment program for the mother to help her with her alcohol abuse problem (father may also need assistance).

8. Effect of maternal abuse of cocaine on the newborn: see Substance Abuse section.
   A. Effect of cocaine exposure: see Box 32-4 and Table 35-4 for list of neonatal effects in terms of physical and behavioral assessment findings.
   B. Care of newborn and mother: see Cocaine and Care Management section for a discussion of supportive care for the newborn and counseling for the mother; ensure that she is able to care for her newborn independently, making referrals as needed.

9. Newborn of mother suspected of abusing drugs during pregnancy: see Heroin and Care Management sections, Table 35-4, Fig. 35-13, and Nursing Care Plan for Infant Experiencing Withdrawal.
   A. Signs of neonatal abstinence syndrome: see Table 35-5 for a list of signs in terms of gastrointestinal, CNS, metabolic, vasomotor, and respiratory function.

   B. Nursing diagnoses: deficient fluid volume related to inadequate fluid intake and increased fluid loss associated with heroin withdrawal; disorganized infant behavior *or* disturbed sleep pattern related to withdrawal from heroin; risk for infection related to risky maternal behaviors associated with drug abuse.
   C. Care management: see Box 35-3; encourage parent participation in care of newborn, providing education and social support as needed; maintain nutrition, fluid, and electrolyte balance with careful management of feeding; infection control and respiratory care; swaddling and holding; stimulus reduction; pharmacologic treatment as appropriate; discharge planning and referral.

CHAPTER 36: HEMOLYTIC DISORDERS AND CONGENITAL ANOMALIES

I. Learning Key Terms

1. Hyperbilirubinemia
2. Jaundice (icterus); physiologic; pathologic
3. Rh incompatibility (isoimmunization)
4. Maternal sensitization
5. Fetal hemolytic anemia
6. Erythroblastosis fetalis
7. Hydrops fetalis
8. Acute bilirubin encephalopathy
9. Kernicterus
10. Indirect Coombs test
11. Direct Coombs test
12. Congenital anomaly
13. Inborn errors of metabolism
14. Microcephaly
15. Hypospadias
16. Epispadias
17. Exstrophy of the bladder
18. Hydrocephalus
19. Congenital heart defects
20. Talipes equinovarus
21. Choanal atresia
22. Spina bifida (neural tube defect)
23. Spinal bifida occulta
24. Meningocele (spina bifida manifesta)
25. Omphalocele
26. Gastroschisis
27. Esophageal atresia
28. Tracheoesophageal fistula
29. Imperforate anus
30. Developmental dysplasia of the hip (DDH)
31. Encephalocele
32. Anencephaly
33. Congenital diaphragmatic hernia
34. Myelomeningocele (spina bifida manifesta)
35. Cleft lip or palate
36. Polydactyly
37. Ambiguous genitalia
38. Hydramnios (polyhydramnios)

39. Oligohydramnios
40. Cytogenic studies

II. Reviewing Key Concepts

41. Physiologic basis for ABO incompatibility: see Hemolytic Disease of the Newborn section for an explanation of the pathophysiology.
42. Congenital anomalies—assessment techniques and considerations guiding diagnosis: see Care Management—Diagnosis section for an overview of techniques that are commonly used for diagnosis of congenital anomalies.
43. Congenital heart defects: see Cardiovascular System Anomalies section and Box 36-3.
    A. Maternal factors associated with higher risk: several factors are discussed in this section, including rubella, alcohol intake, certain medications, tobacco use, and maternal age and health status.
    B. Four physiologic classifications and one example of each: see Table 36-1 for the list of classifications with examples of each.
    C. Signs that could indicate CHD: discuss characteristics of cry, color of skin (e.g., cyanosis and when it occurs), activity level (e.g., restless, lethargic, responsiveness), and effect of activity such as crying, feeding, and stooling on color and breathing, vital signs, respiratory status, and pulse oximetry.
44. Choice B is correct; at 16 mg/dL the serum bilirubin exceeds the 12.9 mg/dL limit on the second day of life; other signs of pathologic hyperbilirubinemia include serum bilirubin concentration in cord blood >5 mg/dL, increase of >5 mg/dL in 24 hours, and appearance of jaundice within the first 24 hours after birth.
45. Choice D is correct; RhoGAM should be administered intramuscularly to the mother within 72 hours of birth; pathologic jaundice is unlikely because Coombs test results indicate that antibodies have not been formed to destroy the newborn's red blood cells (RBCs); RhoGAM is given to prevent formation of antibodies; it would not be given if antibodies have already been formed as indicated by positive Coombs test results.
46. Choice B is correct; kneeling or prone position prevents pressure on the sac that could cause damage; sterile, moist nonadherent dressings are used to protect the sac; a drape should be placed over the buttocks below the lesion—diapers are not used; 80% of affected newborns will also develop hydrocephalus, so measures of head circumference should be done.

III. Thinking Critically

1. Pathologic jaundice: see Hyperbilirubinemia section.
   A. Contrast pathologic and physiologic jaundice: see Physiologic and Pathologic sections for information regarding onset, resolution, and serum bilirubin levels to complete the comparison.
   B. Physiologic process that leads to hyperbilirubinemia: see Hyperbilirubinemia section; discuss the effect of RBC destruction, including the number of RBCs and the speed at which they are destroyed.
   C. Potential causes for pathologic jaundice: see Pathologic Jaundice section and Box 36-1 for a list of maternal causes and fetal/newborn causes.
   D. Effective prevention measures: see Hyperbilirubinemia—Care Management section, where measures are described; fully discuss:
      - Identification of mother and newborn at risk and institute appropriate measures; determine maternal blood type and Rh factor early in pregnancy.
      - Prevention of and prompt therapy for asphyxia, acidosis, sepsis, cold stress, and hypoglycemia.
      - Administration of RhoGAM promptly; take note of any potential for sensitization during pregnancy if the woman is Rh negative (e.g., postamniocentesis).
      - Promotion of early feeding to stimulate stooling and thereby removal of bilirubin.
2. Pregnant woman who is Rh negative: see Hyperbilirubinemia section.
   A. Physiologic basis: see Rh Incompatibility section; if an Rh-negative mother's blood comes into contact with the blood of her Rh-positive fetus, she will form antibodies against Rh-positive blood that can then be transferred via the placenta to the fetus; if a fetus is Rh positive, the presence of these antibodies in its bloodstream will result in destruction of its RBCs (hemolysis).
   B. Meaning of a positive indirect Coombs test: indicates that the woman has formed antibodies, probably as a result of her miscarriage and not receiving RhoGAM to prevent antibody formation.
   C. Candidate to receive RhoGAM: woman is not a candidate because RhoGAM cannot be given once antibodies or sensitization has occurred.
   D. RhoGAM purpose and use: prevents sensitization by injecting passive antibodies against the Rh factor that will destroy any fetal RBCs that may have entered maternal circulation before the maternal immune system is activated; Rh-negative mothers who are indirect Coombs negative should receive RhoGAM after an abortion, after specific invasive tests such as chorionic villus sampling (CVS) and amniocentesis, during the third trimester, and within 72 hours after the birth of an Rh-positive, direct Coombs–negative newborn.
   E. Newborn complications: see Rh Incompatibility section, in which both erythroblastosis fetalis and hydrops fetalis are described.
   F. Prevention of perinatal mortality: regular pregnancy testing to check bilirubin levels, anemia, and antibody titers; intrauterine transfusions and

early birth if the Rh antibody titer rises to dangerous levels and bilirubin is increasing.

3. Care management of newborn born with myelomeningocele: see CNS Anomalies—Spina Bifida section.
   - Preoperative and postoperative measures, including how to position newborn to protect the site; assessment of neurologic function; preventing trauma, rupture, and infection of the site; and site care.
   - Parental support, including facilitating the attachment process, providing information and emotional care, preparing for surgical interventions, and making referrals for long-term care for parents and child to help them adjust to and cope with the effects of the congenital anomaly.

4. Newborn with a diaphragmatic hernia: see Respiratory System Anomalies—Congenital Diaphragmatic Hernia section and Fig. 36-5.
   A. Clinical manifestations exhibited are influenced by the degree of the defect: respiratory distress, which worsens as intestine fills with air; diminished breath sounds; cyanosis; heart sounds in the right chest; low blood pressure; barrel-shaped chest with flat/scaphoid abdomen; bowel in the chest.
   B. Nursing diagnosis: impaired gas exchange related to inability to fully expand lungs associated with diaphragmatic hernia.
   C. Care measures in immediate postbirth period:
      - Position: head and chest elevated, affected side down to allow normal lung to fully expand.
      - Aspirate gastric contents to decompress gastrointestinal tract.
      - Oxygen therapy, mechanical ventilation, and correction of acidosis.

5. Newborn with cleft lip and palate: see Gastrointestinal System Anomalies—Cleft Lip and Palate section and Fig. 36-6.
   A. Nursing diagnoses: imbalanced nutrition: less than body requirements, risk for ineffective airway clearance, risk for impaired parent-infant attachment; all of these are related to defective and incomplete development of the lip and palate.
   B. Nursing measures:
      - Maintain airway patency while ensuring adequate hydration and nutrition using devices that prevent passage of milk into airway.
      - Support and facilitate parental attachment to infant and skill with feeding; prepare parents for discharge.
      - Explain the condition, how it occurs, what it entails, and how and when it will be repaired.
      - Refer to support group.

CHAPTER 37: PERINATAL LOSS, BEREAVEMENT, AND GRIEF

I. Learning Key Terms

1. Losses
2. Bereavement; grief
3. Acute distress
4. Intense grief
5. Disorganization
6. Reorganization
7. Bittersweet grief
8. Caring theory; knowing; being with; doing for; enabling; maintaining belief
9. Complicated grief (complicated bereavement), prolonged grief, pathologic grief, or mourning
10. Perinatal palliative care (perinatal hospice)
11. Mourning
12. Ambiguous loss
13. Disenfranchised grief

II. Reviewing Key Concepts

14. Pregnant woman at 24 weeks of gestation with suspected fetal death: see separate sections for a description of each phase and Box 37-1.
    A. Acute distress.
    B. Intense grief.
    C. Disorganization.
    D. Reorganization.
15. Father's grief responses: see Acute Distress section; discuss each of the following:
    - Distressed by grief of partner.
    - May be less able to share deep, intense grief; feels need to be stoic; special efforts are required to give fathers the support they may need.
    - Experience a variable response depending on the degree to which he identified with the pregnancy.
16. Use of the five components of the caring theory developed by Swanson and Kauffman to support grieving parents: see Caring Theory section for a description of each component; explain how you would use each of the following to help parents:
    - Knowing
    - Being with
    - Doing for
    - Enabling
    - Maintaining belief
17. Actualizing the loss: see Care Management for several sections that provide many ideas, such as tangible memories of the baby can help parents to actualize (make a reality) the loss; help them to participate in the options that are most appealing and comfortable for them; use baby's name and words such as "dead" and "died"; help parents to tell their story.
18. Complicated bereavement: see Complicated Grief (Bereavement) section.
    A. Characteristic behaviors: several behaviors are described in Complicated Grief (Bereavement) section.
    B. Nursing approach: refer for counseling to a therapist or counselor who is experienced in grief counseling; be persistent in getting individual or family into counseling, especially to the first visit, enlisting other family members to help.
19. Choice A is correct; telling her to be happy that one twin survived may be interpreted as that she should

not grieve the loss of the daughter who died; the loss must be acknowledged and the tasks for mourners accomplished; choices B, C, and D are all appropriate responses by the nurse, with choices B and C helpful in actualizing the loss.

20. Choice D is correct; choices A and B represent the intense grief phase and choice C represents the reorganization phase.

21. Choice B is correct; see Box 37-2; note that choices A, C, and D are in the category of what not to say whereas choice B represents a response that acknowledges the difficulty of the loss and offers an opportunity for expression of feelings.

III. Thinking Critically

1. Family experiencing miscarriage at 13 weeks of gestation.
   A. Approach to individualize support measures: see Care Management section.
      ■ Begin with assessment to determine best approach to take for this couple.
      ■ Determine nature of the parental attachment to the pregnancy and the meaning of the pregnancy and birth to the parents.
      ■ Circumstances surrounding the loss—listen to their story.
      ■ The immediate response of each parent to the loss—do they match?
      ■ Persons comprising their social network and how they can support them; do the parents want their support?
   B. Cite questions and observations to gather information required to create an individualized plan of care: use each of the areas identified in A to formulate questions and organize observations.
   C. Therapeutic communication techniques to help couple express feelings and emotions: see Caring Theory and Helping the Bereaved to Acknowledge and Express Their Feelings sections and Box 37-2; examples of therapeutic communication techniques include encouraging expression of feelings by leaning forward, nodding, reflection, and saying "tell me more"; observe nonverbal cues; use touch as appropriate; listen patiently and use silence while couple tell their story; avoid giving advice or using clichés, reassure regarding normalcy of emotions.
   D. Analysis of nurse responses: 1. N, 2. T, 3. N, 4. N, 5. T, 6. T, 7. N, 8. N, 9. T, 10. T

2. Physical needs of postpartum woman following stillbirth: see Meet the Physical Needs of the Bereaved Mother in Postpartum Period section.
   ■ Provide option of staying on maternity unit or transferring to another; discuss the advantages and disadvantages of each option.
   ■ Provide option for room assignment (away from nursery).
   ■ Assist with breast care (milk coming in is a reminder of the loss).
   ■ Emphasize the importance of analgesics and comfort measures to help with rest and sleep.
   ■ Encourage adequate nutrition, fluids, and balance of activity and rest to enhance strength and healing.

3. Birth of baby who died with anencephaly.
   A. Making the decision to see the baby: see Preparing and Holding the Baby's Body section.
      ■ Tell them about the option to see the baby; consider that each parent may have different feelings.
      ■ Give them time to think about the option so they can choose what is best for them.
      ■ Come back and ask them their decision; if they are unsure or say no, ask again before discharge.
   B. Measures to help the couple when they see their baby.
      ■ Explain to parents how the baby will look so they know what to expect.
      ■ Prepare baby, making it look as normal as possible—bathe, use powder, comb hair, put on ID bracelet, dress, wrap in a pretty blanket (get help from a funeral director if needed); give parents the opportunity to provide care because they may want to help bathe and dress the baby and leave mementos.
      ■ Treat baby as one would a live baby when bringing baby to parents—use name, touch cheek; talk about baby's features, emphasizing those that are normal or resemble family members, including themselves.
      ■ Provide time alone with baby and adjust length of time with the baby to meet their needs; observe for cues that tell you that they need more time or are done.
      ■ Determine what else they would need to make a memory: footprint, photograph, lock of hair, etc.

4. Role of the nurse in supporting a pregnant woman at 16 weeks of gestation who is told that her baby has anencephaly: see Prenatal Diagnoses with Poor Prognosis and Address Cultural and Spiritual Needs of Parents sections.
   ■ Fully explain anencephaly and discuss her options.
   ■ Be a good listener, encouraging her to express how she feels about the experience, including cultural and religious beliefs and values that will guide the option that she will choose.
   ■ Respect her decision and provide her with follow-up support, including referral to a perinatal hospice program if she decides to continue the pregnancy or after elective abortion if that is her choice; if elective abortion is her choice, determine if she wishes to see the fetus.